TSRA Clinical Sc

MW00914879

Edited by

Tom C. Nguyen, MD
Columbia University
Cardiothoracic Surgery Fellow
Emory University
Advanced TAVR Fellow
President TSRA 2012-2013

Gabriel Loor, MD
Cleveland Clinic
Cardiothoracic Surgery Fellow
Chair TSRA Projects Committee

Section Editors

Ryan A. Macke, MD
University of Pittsburgh Thoracic Surgery Fellow
Thoracic Section Editor

Damien J. LaPar, MD
University of Virginia Cardiothoracic Surgery Fellow
Adult Cardiac Section Editor

Jennifer C. Nelson, MD
University of Michigan Congenital Cardiac Surgery Fellow
Congenital Section Editor

Copy Editor

Monica A. Isabella, BA
Cleveland Clinic Lerner College of Medicine

Thoracic Surgery Residents Association
www.tsranet.org

Copyright © 2013 by the Thoracic Surgery Residents Association, Tom C. Nguyen and Gabriel Loor

TSRA/TSDA
633 N. Saint Clair Street
Suite 2320
Chicago, IL 60611
www.tsranet.org

Disclaimer

The material presented herein is, to the best of our knowledge, accurate and factual to date. The information is provided as a basic guideline for the study of cardiothoracic surgery and should be used in conjunction with a variety of other educational references and resources. The *TSRA Clinical Scenarios in Cardiothoracic Surgery* should not be construed as a definitive study guide for either the TSDA In-Training Exam or the ABTS Certification Exam. TSRA makes no claims regarding the study book's value in preparing for, or its contribution toward performance on either the TSDA In-Training Exam or the ABTS Certification Exam.

To Elizabeth, family, mentors, and Starbucks...

~ TCN

*To Michele, Jake, Camryn, and Ellie
for the time we've given together
and all my mentors*

~ GL

Forward

It has been a pleasure over the last few years for the Joint Council on Thoracic Surgery Education (JCTSE) to work closely with the Thoracic Surgery Resident Association (TSRA) and the Thoracic Surgery Directors Association (TSDA) in improving the depth, breadth, and quality of educational content for residents learning the complex world of cardiothoracic surgery. Two major contributions from the TSRA to that educational pool of content in the last 3 years was first the *TSRA Review of Cardiothoracic Surgery*, and now the *TSRA Clinical Scenarios in Cardiothoracic Surgery*. Information is quite readily available for the digital learner in 2013 but more advanced learning skills necessary for decision-making and judgment are best learned through case-based cognitive opportunities. This is the strategy that the TSRA has decided to pursue with this in-depth, comprehensive, and well-organized clinical scenarios approach. By simply focusing on learner needs, the residents in cardiothoracic surgery have made a significant and unique contribution to surgical education, which will complement many of the other exciting initiatives being pursued by the TSDA and the JCTSE. Cardiothoracic surgery will be better for this important contribution.

Edward D. Verrier, MD
Surgical Director of Education
Joint Council on Thoracic Surgery Education
K Alvin Merendino Endowed Professor of Cardiovascular Surgery
University of Washington

May 2013

Preface

The Thoracic Surgery Residents Association (TSRA) was established in 1997 under the guidance of the Thoracic Surgery Directors Association (TSDA) with the goal of representing residents in cardiothoracic surgery training. One of our core missions involves resident education. In 2010, we released the *TSRA Review of Cardiothoracic Surgery*, which has been a phenomenal success. The free pdf has been downloaded more than 7,000 times at the time of this publication and has also been translated into Turkish.

This current book, *TSRA Clinical Scenarios in Cardiothoracic Surgery*, completes the logical continuum of resident education aimed at the application of decision-making, surgical technique, and practical knowledge towards different clinical case scenarios. The book's goal is to review common, high-yield, and important scenarios that may surface during the course of a cardiothoracic surgeon's practice in congenital, thoracic, or adult cardiac surgery. As with prior TSRA projects, the book was written by residents for residents. We strived to maintain a high level of accuracy and clinical relevance, and as such, the book had four layers of peer review. Each chapter was meticulously reviewed by an established faculty member, a section editor, and two main editors. The book contains 72 chapters authored by over 50 residents and faculty from across the country. Contents of the book are organized into three major sections: General Thoracic Surgery, Adult Cardiac, and Congenital Cardiac Surgery. Chapters are designed to emulate possible conversation during the workup and treatment of a given patient.

Despite the rigorous review process it may be evident to the reader that there are differences in institutional practice regarding specific management schemes and technical details. The scenarios and their responses are a reflection of the safest practice as determined by the author and reviewers. The reader should not forgo what works best for him or her as long as their approach is reliable, reproducible and supported by published literature and guidelines. Furthermore, the review book is intended to be dynamic. At the end of each chapter, there is a section for notes and we encourage the reader to actively think of other potential clinical scenarios. We welcome feedback and submission of additional scenarios to Tom C. Nguyen (tom.c.nguyen@gmail.com) and Gabriel Loor (gabeloor@gmail.com).

We would like to express our gratitude to all the residents and faculty who have contributed to this project. We would also like to thank the TSDA and the Joint Council for Thoracic Surgery Education (JCTSE) for their continued support. We hope you enjoy reading through this book as much as we enjoyed compiling it.

Tom C. Nguyen, MD
TSRA President
Committee

Gabe Loor, MD
Chair TSRA Projects

May 2013

Contributors

Travis Abicht, MD
Northwestern University
Combined aortic and mitral valve disease

Muhammad Aftab, MD
Baylor College of Medicine/Texas Heart Institute
Aortic root aneurysm, Transposition of the great arteries

Shair Ahmed, MD
Emory University Medical Center
Small cell lung cancer, Pulmonary carcinoid

Gorav Ailawadi, MD
University of Virginia
Redo coronary artery bypass surgery, Ischemic mitral regurgitation, Redo mitral valve replacement, Operative management of pulmonary embolism

George Alfieris, MD
University of Rochester
Aortic coarctation

Carlos J. Anciano, MD
University of Pittsburgh Medical Center
Esophageal diverticula

Mara B. Antonoff, MD
Washington University School of Medicine
COPD, emphysema, and spontaneous pneumothorax

Michael Argenziano, MD
NYP-Columbia University Medical Center
Cardioprotection pitfalls

Vinay Badhwar, MD
University of Pittsburgh Medical Center
Hypertrophic obstructive cardiomyopathy, Cardiac tumors

Stephen Bailey, MD
Allegheny General Hospital
Descending aortic aneurysm

Faisal G. Bakaeen, MD, FACS
Baylor College of Medicine/Texas Heart Institute
Aortic root aneurysm

Bryan Barrus, MD
University of Rochester
Aortic coarctation

James Beck, CCP
NYP-Columbia University Medical Center
Cardioprotection pitfalls

Harold M. Burkhart, MD
Mayo Clinic
Cardiopulmonary bypass pitfalls, Aortic regurgitation

Philip W. Carrott, MD
University of Virginia
Paraesophageal and diaphragmatic hernias

Joanna Chikwe, MD
Mount Sinai Medical Center
Post-infarction ventricular septal defect

Richard C. Cook, MD
University of British Columbia
Stable angina

Traves D. Crabtree, MD
Washington University School of Medicine
COPD, emphysema, and spontaneous pneumothorax

Sagar S. Damle, MD
University of Colorado Hospitals
Thoracic trauma

Marcelo C. DaSilva, MD
Brigham and Women's Hospital
Malignant pleural mesothelioma

James E. Davies, Jr., MD
University of Alabama at Birmingham
Acute myocardial infarction/unstable angina

Jonathan D'Cuhna, MD
University of Pittsburgh Medical Center
Mediastinal staging

Ismael de Armas, MD
Baylor College of Medicine/Texas Heart Institute
Aortic root aneurysm

Kristopher B. Deatrick, MD
University of Michigan
Patent ductus arteriosus

Pedro J. del Nido, MD
Children's Hospital of Boston
Ebstein's anomaly

Walter F. DeNino, MD
Medical University of South Carolina
Atrioventricular canal defects

George Dimeling, MD
Stanford University Medical Center
Ventricular septal defects

Emily Downs, MD
University of Virginia
Operative management of pulmonary embolism

Peter F. Ehrlich MD, MHS
C.S. Mott Children's Hospital and Von Voigtlander Women's Hospital
Congenital tracheoesophageal fistulae

Michelle C. Ellis, MD
University of Michigan
GERD and Barrett's esophagus

Michael P. Fischbein, MD, PhD
Stanford University Medical Center
Type B aortic dissection

Seth Force, MD
Emory University School of Medicine
Primary chest wall tumors, Esophageal motility disorders

Charles D. Fraser, Jr., MD
Baylor College of Medicine/Texas Heart Institute
Transposition of the great arteries

James Gangemi, MD
University of Virginia
Anomalous pulmonary venous return

Ravi Ghanta, MD
University of Virginia
Combined CABG/valve, Type A aortic dissection

David Griffin, MD
Allegheny General Hospital
Descending aortic aneurysm

Eric Griffiths, MD
University of Virginia
Redo coronary artery bypass surgery, Anomalous pulmonary venous return

Shawn S. Groth, MD
Brigham and Women's Hospital
Malignant pleural mesothelioma

Robert A. Guyton, MD
Emory University School of Medicine
Tricuspid regurgitation, Mitral stenosis

Katherine B. Harrington, MD
Stanford University Medical Center
Endocarditis, Type B aortic dissection

Jennifer C. Hirsch-Romano, MD
University of Michigan
Congenital cystic adenomatoid malformation

Monica A. Isabella, BA
Cleveland Clinic Lerner College of Medicine

Kaj H. Johansen, MD
University of Pittsburgh Medical Center
Thoracic outlet syndrome

Douglas R. Johnston, MD
Cleveland Clinic
Aortic stenosis, Combined coronary and carotid procedures

Mark Joseph, MD
University of North Carolina at Chapel Hill
Management of the porcelain aorta, Cardiac trauma

Andrew J. Kaufman, MD
Mount Sinai Medical Center
Esophageal perforation

Minoo N. Kavarana, MD
Medical University of South Carolina
Atrioventricular canal defects

Mark Kearns, MD
University of British Columbia
Stable angina

John A. Kern, MD
University of Virginia
Vascular injuries, Redo aortic valve replacement, Ascending aortic aneurysm

Armin Kiankhooy, MD
University of Virginia
Type A aortic dissection

Andy C. Kiser, MD
University of North Carolina at Chapel Hill
Management of the porcelain aorta, Cardiac trauma

Peter A. Knight, MD
University of Rochester
Iatrogenic aortic dissection, Aortic arch aneurysm, Pericardial disease/pericardiectomy

Brian Kogon, MD
Emory School of Medicine
Atrial septal defects

Igor E. Konstantinov, MD, PhD, FRACS
Cardiac Surgery Unit, Royal Children's Hospital, Melbourne
Pulmonary artery sling

Benjamin D. Kozower, MD, MPH, FACS
University of Virginia
Paraesophageal and diaphragmatic hernias

Fatuma Kromah, MD
Mayo Clinic
Pulmonary metastasectomy

Damien J. LaPar, MD, MSc
University of Virginia
Ebstein's anomaly

Christine L. Lau, MD, MBA
University of Virginia
Hemoptysis

John F. Lazar, MD
University of Rochester
Aortic arch aneurysm

Andrew J. Lodge, MD
Duke University Medical Center
Tetralogy of Fallot

Gabriel Loor, MD
Cleveland Clinic
Mediastinal masses, Aortic stenosis, Combined coronary and carotid procedures

Robroy MacIver, MD, MPH
Cardiac Surgery Unit, Royal Children's Hospital, Melbourne
Pulmonary artery sling

Ryan A. Macke, MD
University of Pittsburgh Medical Center
Chylothorax, Esophageal cancer

Katsuhide Maeda, MD, PhD
Stanford University Medical Center
Congenital aortic stenosis

Muhammad F. Masood, MD
University of Pittsburgh Medical Center
Hypertrophic obstructive cardiomyopathy, Cardiac tumors

David Mauchley, MD
University of Colorado
Infectious lung disease

Edwin McGee, MD
Northwestern University
Combined aortic and mitral valve disease

John Mitchell, MD
University of Colorado
Infectious lung disease

Michael C. Monge, MD
Ann & Robert H. Lurie Children's Hospital of Chicago
Anomalous origin of the left coronary artery from the pulmonary artery

Linda Mongero, CCP
NYP-Columbia University Medical Center
Cardioprotection pitfalls

Emmanuel Moss, MD
Emory University School of Medicine
Tricuspid regurgitation

Ashok Muralidaran, MD
Stanford University Medical Center
Congenital aortic stenosis

Alykhan S. Nagji, MD
University of Virginia
Vascular injuries

Basil S. Nasir, MBBCh
University of Alabama at Birmingham
Acute myocardial infarction/unstable angina

Robert C. Neely, MD
NYP-Columbia University Medical Center
Cardioprotection pitfalls

Jennifer Nelson, MD
University of Michigan
Congenital cystic adenomatoid malformation

Muhammad A.K. Nuri, MD
Pediatric Cardiac Surgery
Children's Healthcare of Atlanta
Congenital tracheoesophageal fistulae

David D. Odell, MD
University of Pittsburgh Medical Center
Early stage lung cancer (Ia-IIb), Mediastinal staging

William D. Ogden, MD
Stanford University Medical Center
Malignant lesions of the trachea

Richard G. Ohye, MD
University of Michigan
Patent ductus arteriosus

Juan G. Penaranda, MD
Mayo Clinic
Cardiopulmonary bypass pitfalls, Aortic regurgitation

Roman V. Petrov, MD
University of Pittsburgh Medical Center
Thoracic outlet syndrome, Esophageal cancer

Allan Pickens, MD
Emory University Medical Center
Small cell lung cancer, Pulmonary carcinoid

Timothy J. Pirolli, MD
Stanford University Medical Center
Malignant lesions of the trachea

Elizabeth Pocock, MD
Baylor College of Medicine/Texas Heart Institute
Transposition of the great arteries

Marek Polomsky, MD
Emory University School of Medicine
Esophageal motility disorders, Mitral stenosis

Daniel Raymond, MD
Cleveland Clinic
Pneumonectomy and sleeve resection, Pleural effusions and empyema, Tracheal strictures and fistulae, Mediastinal masses

Rishindra M. Reddy, MD
University of Michigan, Section of Thoracic Surgery
GERD and Barrett's esophagus

Olaf Reinhartz, MD
Stanford University Medical Center
Ventricular septal defects

Bruce A. Reitz, MD
Stanford University Medical Center
Endocarditis

Michael P. Robich, MD
Cleveland Clinic
Pneumonectomy and sleeve resection, Tracheal strictures and fistulae

Mark Roeser, MD
University of Virginia
Combined CABG/valve

Hyde M. Russell, MD
Ann & Robert H. Lurie Children's Hospital of Chicago
Anomalous origin of the left coronary artery from the pulmonary artery

Chittoor B. Sai-Sudhakar, MD
Ohio State University Medical Center
Non-ischemic mitral regurgitation

Matthew J. Schuchert, MD
University of Pittsburgh Medical Center
Early stage lung cancer (Ia-IIb)

Asad A. Shah, MD
Duke University Medical Center
Tetralogy of Fallot

Manisha Shende, MD
University of Pittsburgh Medical Center
Esophageal cancer, Esophageal diverticula

Christian C. Shults, MD
Emory University School of Medicine
Primary chest wall tumors

William Stein, MD
Emory School of Medicine
Atrial septal defects

David J. Sugarbaker, MD
Brigham and Women's Hospital
Malignant pleural mesothelioma

Matthew D. Taylor, MD
University of Virginia
Hemoptysis

Vakhtang Tchantchaleishvili, MD
Rochester University
Iatrogenic aortic dissection, Pericardial disease/pericardiectomy

Betty Tong, MD
Duke University Medical Center
Advanced non-small cell lung cancer

Yoshiya Toyoda, MD, PhD
Temple University
Arrhythmia surgery

Immanuel Turner, MD
University of Michigan
Congenital cystic adenomatoid malformation

Nakul Vakil, MD
Cleveland Clinic
Pleural effusions and empyema

Cynthia E. Wagner, MD
University of Virginia
Redo mitral valve replacement

Benjamin Wei, MD
Duke University Medical Center
Advanced non-small cell lung cancer

Aaron J. Weiss, MD
Mount Sinai Medical Center
Esophageal perforation, Post-infarction ventricular septal defect

Benny Weksler, MD
University of Pittsburgh Medical Center
Chylothorax

Michael J. Weyant, MD
University of Colorado Hospitals
Thoracic trauma

Dennis Wigle, MD
Mayo Clinic
Pulmonary metastasectomy

Jennifer M. Worth, MD
Ohio State University Medical Center
Non-ischemic mitral regurgitation

Leora Yarboro, MD
University of Virginia
Redo aortic valve replacement, Ascending aortic aneurysm

Kenan W. Yount, MD, MBA
University of Virginia
Ischemic mitral regurgitation

Muhammad Habib Zubair, MD
Temple University
Arrhythmia surgery

Abbreviations

AAA: Abdominal aortic aneurysm
ABG: Arterial blood gas
ABVD: Adriamycin, bleomycin, vinblastine, and dacarbazine
AC: Anticoagulation
ACC: American College of Cardiology
ACC: Adenoid cystic carcinoma
ACCF: American College of Cardiology Foundation
ACCP: American College of Chest Physicians
ACE: Angiotensin-converting enzyme
ACEI: Angiotensin converting enzyme inhibitor
ACOSOG: American College of Surgeons Oncology Group
ACS: Acute coronary syndrome
ACS: American College of Surgeons
ACT: Activated clotting time
ACTH: Adrenocorticotropic hormone
AF: Atrial fibrillation
AFP: Alpha fetoprotein
AHA: American Heart Association
AI: Aortic insufficiency
AJCC: American Joint Committee on Cancer
ALCAPA: Anomalous left coronary artery from the pulmonary artery
ALK: Anaplastic lymphoma kinase
AMI: Acute myocardial infarction
AML: Anterior mitral leaflet
AP: Anteroposterior
AR: Aortic regurgitation
ARB: Angiotensin receptor blocker
ARS: Anti-reflux surgery
ARVD: Arrhythmogenic right ventricular dysplasia
AS: Aortic stenosis
ASA: ACETYLSALICYLIC ACID
ASD: Atrial septal defect
ASM: Anterior scalene muscle
ASO: Arterial switch operation
ATLS: Advanced Trauma Life Support
AV: Atrioventricular
AVA: Aortic valve area
AVR: Aortic valve replacement
AVV: Atrioventricular valve
BE: Barrett's esophagus
B-HCG: Beta human chorionic gonadotropin
BID: *Bis in die* (twice a day)
BIS: Bispectral index

BMI: Body mass index
BMP: Basic metabolic panel
BNP: B-type natriuretic peptide
BP: Blood pressure
BPF: Bronchopleural fistula
bpm: Beats per minute
BRB: Bright red blood
BSA: Body surface area
BTS: Blalock-Taussig shunt
BUN: Blood urea nitrogen
CABG: Coronary artery bypass grafting
CAD: Coronary artery disease
CAVC: Complete atrioventricular canal
CBC: Complete blood count
CCAM: Congenital cystic adenomatoid malformation
CCS: Canadian Cardiovascular Society
CEA: Carotid endarterectomy
CHB: Complete heart block
CHF: Congestive heart failure
CI: Cardiac index
CKD: Chronic kidney disease
CMP: Complete metabolic panel
COAPT: Clinical Outcomes Assessment of the MitraClip Percutaneous
    Therapy
COL3a1: Collagen, type III, alpha I
COPD: Chronic obstructive pulmonary disease
CPB: Cardiopulmonary bypass
CPR: Cardiopulmonary resuscitation
Cx: Circumflex
CRP: C-reactive protein
CRT: Chemoradiation therapy
CSF: Cerebrospinal fluid
CT: Computed tomography
CTA: Computed tomographic angiography
CTEPH: Chronic thromboembolic pulmonary hypertension
CTPA: Computed tomography pulmonary angiogram
CV: Central venous
CVG: Composite valve graft
CVICU: Cardiovascular Intensive Care Unit
CVP: Central venous pressure
CVR: CCAM volume ratio
CWT: Chest wall tumor
CXR: Chest x-ray
DAA: Descending aortic aneurysm
DES: Diffuse esophageal spasm

DES: Drug-eluting stent
DHCA: Deep hypothermic circulatory arrest
DKA: Diabetic ketoacidosis
DLCO: Diffusing lung capacity for carbon monoxide
DM: Diabetes mellitus
DORV: Double outlet right ventricle
DVT: Deep venous thrombosis
EBUS: Endobronchial ultrasound
ECMO: Extracorporeal membrane oxygenation
ECV: Electrical cardioversion
ED: Emergency department
EDVI: End-diastolic volume index
EEA: End-to-end anastomosis
EEG: Electroencephalogram
EF: Ejection fraction
EFE: Endocardial fibroelastosis
EGD: Esophagogastroduodenoscopy
EGFR: Epidermal growth factor receptor
EKG: Electrocardiogram
EMG: Electromyography
EMR: Endomucosal resection
ENT: Ear, nose, and throat
EOA: Effective orifice area
EOAI: Effective orifice area index
EP: Electrophysiology
EPD: Extended pleurectomy/decortication
EPP: Extrapleural pneumonectomy
ERO: Effective regurgitant orifice
ESR: Erythrocyte sedimentation rate
ESRD: End stage renal disease
ESV: End systolic volume
ESVI: End systolic volume index
ETT: Endotracheal tube
EUS: Endoscopic ultrasound
FAST: Focused assessment with sonography in trauma
FDG: Fluorodeoxyglucose
FEV1: Forced expiratory volume in the first second
FFR: Fractional flow reserve
FiO2: Inspired fraction of oxygen
FMR: Functional mitral regurgitation
FNA: Fine needle aspiration
GCS: Glasgow Coma Scale
GCT: Germ cell tumor
GDMT: Guideline directed medical therapy
GEA: Gastroepiploic artery

GEJ: Gastroesophageal junction
GERD: Gastroesophageal reflux disease
GETA: General endotracheal anesthesia
GI: Gastrointestinal
GIA: Gastrointestinal anastomosis
GIST: Gastrointestinal Stromal Tumor
GOS: Great Ormond Street
GSV: Greater saphenous vein
GSW: Gunshot wound
GT: Genetic testing
H&P: History & physical examination
HACEK: Haemophilus, Actinobacillus, Cardiobacterium, Eikenella, and
    Kingella
HCT: Hematocrit
HGD: High grade dysplasia
H/H: Hemoglobin and hematocrit
HIAA: Hydroxyindoleacteic acid
HIV: Human immunodeficiency virus
HLD: Hyperlipidemia
HLHS: Hypoplastic left heart syndrome
HOCM: Hypertrophic obstructive cardiomyopathy
HR: Heart rate
HTK: Histidine, Tryptophan, and Ketoglutarate
HTN: Hypertension
IAA: Interrupted aortic arch
IABP: Intra-aortic balloon pump
ICA: Internal carotid artery
ICP: Intracranial pressure
ICS: Intercostal space
ICU: Intensive care unit
IE: Infective endocarditis
IEA: Inferior epigastric artery
IEM: Ineffective esophageal motility
IgG: Immunoglobulin G
IJ: Internal jugular
ILE: Ivor Lewis esophagectomy
IMA: Internal mammary artery
IMH: Intramural hematoma
IMR: Ischemic mitral regurgitation
iNO: Inhaled nitric oxide
INR: International Normalized Ratio
IV: Intravenous
IVC: Inferior vena cava
IVDU: Intravenous drug user
IVIG: Intravenous immunoglobulin

IVS: Intact ventricular septum
JET: Junctional ectopic tachycardia
JP: Jackson-Pratt
JVD: Jugular venous distention
KRAS: V-Ki-ras2
LA: Left atrium
LAA: Left atrial appendage
LAAL: Left atrial appendage ligation
LAD: Left anterior descending
LCA: Left coronary artery
LCCA: Left common carotid artery
LCSG: Lung Cancer Study Group
LDG: Low grade dysplasia
LDH: Lactate dehydrogenase
LES: Lower esophageal sphincter
LHB: Left heart bypass
LIMA: Left internal mammary artery
LLL: Left lower lobe
LM: Left main
LN: Lymph node
LPA: Left pulmonary artery
LSCA: Left subclavian artery
LSVC: Left sided superior vena cava
LUL: Left upper lobe
LV: Left ventricle
LVA: Left vertebral artery
LVAD: Left ventricular assist device
LVH: Left ventricular hypertrophy
LVEED: Left ventricular end diastolic diameter
LVESD: Left ventricular end-systolic diameter
LVOT: Left ventricular outflow tract
LVOTO: Left ventricular outflow tract obstruction
LVRS: Lung volume reduction surgery
MAC: Mitral annular calcification
MAP: Mean arterial pressure
MDR-TB: Multidrug-resistant tuberculosis
MFH: Malignant fibrous histiocytoma
MG: Myasthenia Gravis
MGH: Massachusetts General Hospital
MI: Myocardial infarction
MIBG: Metaiodobenzylguanidine
MICU: Medical Intensive Care Unit
MIDCAB: Minimally Invasive Direct Coronary Artery Bypass
MIE: Minimally invasive esophagectomy
MOPP: Mustargen, procarbazine, prednisone, vincristine

MPA: Main pulmonary artery
MPM: Malignant pleural mesothelioma
MR: Mitral regurgitation
MRA: Magnetic resonance angiography
MRI: Magnetic resonance imaging
MRSA: Methicillin sensitive *Staphylococcus aureus*
MS: Mitral stenosis
MSM: Middle scalene muscle
MV: Mitral valve
MVR: Mitral valve replacement
Nd:YAG: Neodymium:yttrium-aluminum garnet laser
NG: Nasogastric
NICU: Neonatal Intensive Care Unit
NIH: National Institutes of Health
NPO: *Nil per os* (nothing by mouth)
NPV: Negative predictive value
NS: Normal saline
NSAID: Nonsteroidal anti-inflammatory drug
NSCLC: Non-small cell lung cancer
NSE: Neuron-specific enolase
NSTEMI: Non-ST elevation myocardial infarction
NYHA: New York Heart Association
OK-432: Picibanil
OM: Obtuse marginal
OPCAB: Off-pump coronary artery bypass
OR: Operating room
OS: Overall survival
PA: Pulmonary artery
PA: Pulmonary atresia
PAB: Pulmonary artery band
PaCO2: Partial pressure of carbon dioxide in arterial blood
PAF: Paroxysmal atrial fibrillation
PAP: Pulmonary artery pressure
PAPVR: Partial anomalous pulmonary venous return
PASP: Pulmonary artery systolic pressure
PAU: Penetrating aortic ulcer
PAVC: Partial atrioventricular canal
PCA: Patient controlled analgesia
PCI: Percutaneous coronary intervention
PCP: Primary care physician
PCWP: Pulmonary capillary wedge pressure
PDA: Patent ductus arteriosus
PDT: Photodynamic therapy
PE: Pulmonary embolus
PEA: Pulseless electrical activity

PEEP: Positive end-expiratory pressure
PEG: Percutaneous endoscopic gastrostomy
PET: Positron emission tomography
PFO: Patent foramen ovale
PFT: Pulmonary function test
PGE: Prostaglandin E
PHTN: Pulmonary hypertension
PI: Pulmonary insufficiency
PIT: Primary intimal tear
PM: Pectoralis minor
PMBV: Percutaneous mitral balloon valvuloplasty
PML: Posterior mitral leaflet
PNET: Primitive neuroectodermal tumor
POD: Post-operative day
PPI: Proton pump inhibitor
PPM: Patient prosthesis mismatch
PPO: Postoperative predicted
Ppo: Postoperative pulmonary
PPV: Positive predictive value
PRBC: Packed red blood cells
PS: Pulmonary stenosis
PT: Physical therapy
PT: Prothrombin time
PTFE: Polytetrafluoroethylene
PTT: Partial thromboplastin time
PV: Pulmonary vein
PVC: Premature ventricular contraction
PVD: Peripheral vascular disease
PVE: Prosthetic valve endocarditis
PVI: Pulmonary vein isolation
PVOD: Pulmonary vascular obstructive disease
PVR: Pulmonary vascular resistance
Qp:Qs: Ratio of pulmonary blood flow to systemic blood flow
RA: Right atrium
RAA: Right atrial appendage
RB gene p53: Retinoblastoma gene
RBP: Retrograde brain perfusion
RCA: Right coronary artery
REV: Réparation à l'etage ventriculaire
RF: Radiofrequency
RF: Regurgitant fraction
RIMA: Right internal mammary artery
RIPV: Right inferior pulmonary vein
RLL: Right lower lobe
RLN: Recurrent laryngeal nerve

RML: Right middle lobe
RSPV: Right superior pulmonary vein
RUL: Right upper lobe
RV: Regurgitant volume
RV: Right ventricle
RVA: Right vertebral artery
RVH: Right ventricular hypertrophy
RVOT: Right ventricular outflow tract
SA: Sinoatrial
SAM: Systolic anterior motion
SBRT: Stereotatic body radiation therapy
SCA: Subclavian artery
SCC: Squamous cell carcinoma
SCD: Sudden cardiac death
SCLC: Small cell lung cancer
SCM: Sternocleidomastoid
SIADH: Syndrome of inappropriate antidiuretic hormone secretion
SLE: Systemic lupus erythematosus
SMA: Superior mesenteric artery
SOB: Shortness of breath
SRS: Stereotactic radiosurgery
STAT: *statim* (immediately)
STEMI: ST elevation myocardial infarction
STJ: Sinotubular junction
STS: Society of Thoracic Surgeons
SUV: Standardized uptake value
SVC: Superior vena cava
SVD: Structural valve deterioration
SVG: Saphenous vein graft
SVR: Systemic vascular resistance
TA: Truncus arteriosus
TAA: Thoracoabdominal aneurysm
TAPVR: Total anomalous pulmonary venous return
TAVC: Transitional atrioventricular canal
TAVR: Transcathether aortic valve replacement
TB: Tuberculosis
TBNA: Transbronchial needle aspiration
TEE: Transesophageal echocardiogram
TEF: Tracheoesophageal fistula
TGA: Transposition of great arteries
TGF-B: Transforming growth factor beta
THE: Transhiatal esophagectomy
TIA: Transient ischemic attack
TIF: Tracheoinnominate fistula
TNM: Tumor, nodes, metastasis

TOS: Thoracic outlet syndrome
TP: Transverse processes
TPN: Total parenteral nutrition
TR: Tricuspid regurgitation
TRAM: Transverse rectus abdominis muscle
TTE: Transthoracic echocardiogram
TTF1: Thyroid transcription factor 1
TV: Tricuspid valve
TVR: Tricuspid valve replacement
UA: Unstable angina
UNCV: Ulnar nerve conduction velocity
U/S: Ultrasound
UTI: Urinary tract infection
VACTERL: Vertebral defects, Anal atresia, Cardiac defects,
    Tracheoesophageal fistula, Renal anomalies, and Limb abnormalities
VO2: Volume of oxygen consumption
V/Q: Ventilation/ perfusion
VAD: Ventricular assist device
VATS: Video-assisted thoracic surgery
VSD: Ventricular septal defect
VT: Ventricular tachycardia
WBC: White blood cell
WPW: Wolff-Parkinson-White
WT1: Wilm's tumor susceptibility gene 1
XLT: Extended length tracheostomy
XRT: X-ray therapy

Table of Contents

I. General Thoracic Surgery

1. Early stage lung cancer (Ia-IIb)
David D. Odell, MD, and Matthew J. Schuchert, MD

Concept
- Evaluation of the patient with a newly discovered lung nodule
- Indications for surgical resection of isolated pulmonary nodules
- Operative and non-operative treatment options for early stage NSCLC

Chief Complaint
"A 57 yo man is referred to your office after a 1.1 cm irregular nodule is discovered in the right upper lobe of the lung on a CT chest performed to evaluate for pulmonary embolism following a knee replacement."

Differential
Lung cancer (Non-small cell, small cell, carcinoma in situ), neuroendocrine tumor (carcinoid), hamartoma, granuloma, (sarcoid, histoplasmosis, coccidiomycosis, fungal, tuberculosis), infection (viral or bacterial pneumonia), metastasis, infarction, atelectasis

History and physical
The history should focus on the identification of cancer risk factors: tobacco exposure history, occupational exposures (asbestos or other chemical inhalation), and a thorough personal and family cancer history. While primary symptoms related to pulmonary malignancy are absent in > 80% of patients, careful questioning can still elicit findings in some patients. These may be separated into 2 groups, symptoms related to the primary tumor and symptoms indicative of metastatic disease. Primary tumor symptoms include cough, hemoptysis, recurrent respiratory infections, dyspnea and chest pain. Symptoms potentially referable to metastatic disease might include bone pain, myalgias, headaches, visual changes, anorexia, weight loss and fatigue.

Tests
Imaging evaluation
CXR
- Low cost and readily available
- Useful for tracking a process over time or for the assessment of advanced disease such as effusion
- Limited utility in TNM staging

Chest CT scan
- Valuable for accurate assessment of the primary tumor
- Valuable for hilar and mediastinal lymph node evaluation (sensitivity and specificity ranging from 65-80%)
- Generally should have a current CT chest (within 6 weeks) for any patient undergoing resection

PET scan
- Most useful for evaluation of the mediastinal compartment and assessment of metastatic disease.
- Superior to CT alone for lymph node assessment
- Good NPV, poor PPV due to a high rate of false positive results

PET-CT scan
- Excellent sensitivity but limited specificity (due to false positives)
- 43% false positive rate in the ACOSOG Z0050 trial
- Superior to either CT or PET individually

Bone scan
- Low cost and widely available
- Less specific than PET and largely falling out of clinical favor

Chest MRI
- Useful for characterization of chest wall involvement
- Test of choice if concern for spinal column or brachial plexus involvement
- Poor characterization of primary lung tumor

Bronchoscopy
- Used to assess for presence and location of endobronchial disease
- Washing and brushings may be used for diagnosis in cases where biopsy of a parenchymal lesion is not possible or present
- Should be performed preoperatively in all settings of potential pulmonary resection

Physiologic evaluation
Pulmonary function tests
- *FEV-1.* The volume of air expelled in 1 second. This is the single test with the best correlation to postoperative functional outcome. A minimum of 40% predicted postoperative function is needed for a patient to remain free of oxygen following resection. That typically correlates to the following spirometric values prior to resection:
  - 2 L for pneumonectomy
  - 1 L for lobectomy
  - 0.6 L for segmentectomy
- *DLCO.* Diffusing capacity for carbon monoxide. This test is a measure of capillary permeability and the efficiency of gas exchange across the alveolar membrane. Patients need a minimum 40% predicted postoperative function to tolerate resection.

3

- Determination of the predicted postoperative pulmonary (Ppo) function (either FEV-1 or DLCO) can be determined by assessing the proportion of lung to be resected. A standard formula for this is as follows:

Ppo-FEV1 = FEV1 x [(19 segments - number of segments to be resected)/19 segments]

Ventilation/perfusion studies

Patients with significant airflow obstruction, central tumors, areas of atelectasis, pleural disease, or prior lung resection may have alterations in ventilation and/or pulmonary blood flow which invalidate the assumptions made with simple spirometric pulmonary function testing. In this circumstance, a quantitative radionuclide ventilation/perfusion scan can better indicate the contribution to ventilation of the region of lung tissue that you intend to resect. For borderline cases, exercise capability may be assessed if there is concern for poor preoperative lung function. A patient who can walk up two flights of stairs likely has adequate reserve. Also, VO2 max less than 15 mL/kg/min is associated with high risk of postoperative adverse events.

Cardiac evaluation

The cornerstone of preoperative cardiac evaluation is obtaining a thorough history from the patient. All patients should have an EKG performed as a baseline prior to surgery. Patients with risk factors or physical exam findings concerning for cardiac disease should be referred to a cardiologist for preoperative evaluation and consideration of a stress test before proceeding with pulmonary surgery.

Index scenario (additional information)

"Following a complete evaluation, the primary nodule is FDG-avid with an SUV of 7.1. There is no evidence of mediastinal adenopathy on CT and no activity beyond the primary nodule on PET. The patient is otherwise healthy and has an FEV1 of 97% predicted and a DLCO 110% predicted."

Treatment/management

In general, the surgeon's primary task is identifying those patients with a disease state amenable to primary surgical resection who are physiologically able to tolerate the operation itself. Keeping these tenets in mind will help to clearly frame the preoperative evaluation. A detailed understanding of the TNM staging system put forth by the AJCC is important for any practitioner providing care for patients with NSCLC. Generally speaking, early stage cancers are those in which the primary tumor is confined within the lobar lung parenchyma and there is no evidence of mediastinal lymph node involvement or distant disease. The above imaging and diagnostic studies are valuable tools in helping to make this determination preoperatively.

Some preoperative measures that may decrease risk include: smoking cessation, optimizing nutrition and use of epidural anesthesia.

Surgical resection is the therapy of choice for patients with early stage (stage I and II) non-small cell lung cancer. Surgery also has an important role in the treatment of selected patients with locally advanced disease (stage IIIa), as will be discussed elsewhere. Lobectomy with mediastinal lymph node sampling or dissection is considered the surgical standard of care for early stage non-small cell lung cancer (NSCLC). This approach is based on the findings of a randomized, controlled trial conducted by the Lung Cancer Study Group (LCSG) which compared lobar and sublobar approaches to tumor resection. This trial showed a threefold reduction in local recurrence (6.4% vs. 17.2%) and a 30% overall survival advantage (p = 0.088), establishing lobectomy as the 'gold standard' surgical resection. To date, this remains the only completed randomized trial comparing lobar and sublobar resection. Sublobar approaches to lung cancer resection (wedge and/or anatomic segmentectomy) have again gained support on the basis of several retrospective series including patients unable to tolerate lobectomy. While the term "sublobar" is often used generically, there are two distinct forms of sublobar resection. Segmentectomy involves the resection of an anatomic ventilator unit, with the individual identification and control of the segmental arterial and venous circulation as well as the segmental bronchus. By contrast, wedge resection is a non-anatomic extirpation of a lesion and surrounding tissue. While there are few direct comparisons, the available literature indicates that among sublobar approaches, anatomic segmentectomy may be an oncologically superior operation.

Appropriate selection of patients is important if sublobar resection with curative intent is to be offered. The primary factors involved are: a) tumor size b) the ability to obtain an adequate resection margin and c) performance of a careful lymph node assessment at the time of the operation. Patients with small (< 2 cm), peripheral Stage I tumors have been demonstrated in selected institutional series to have long-term outcomes similar to lobectomy with segmental resection. Achieving an adequate surgical margin is also essential regardless of the resection technique chosen. In patients treated with sublobar resection, a margin distance greater than the diameter of the tumor has been shown to significantly decrease rates of local recurrence. However, a true survival advantage has not been shown. Finally, a careful analysis of the N1 (lobar and hilar) nodal stations is important for patients considered for sublobar resection. If N1 disease is encountered intraoperatively, a

5

lobectomy should be performed for full evaluation of the intralobar nodes and clearance of regional lymph node metastasis. While there is a great deal of interest in this area, level 1 evidence supporting sublobar resection is not available and the procedure should typically be reserved for those patients in whom a lobectomy could not be safely performed (i.e., the patient has inadequate pulmonary reserve).

Ablative therapies such as radiofrequency (RF) ablation and stereotactic radiosurgery (SRS) are also entering into the treatment paradigm for medically inoperable patients. Both of these techniques allow for imaging directed tumor ablation. Additionally, ablation is of limited utility in many central tumors due to proximity to major airways or vascular structures. Further, the ability to pathologically assess nodal involvement is lost and the potential for local recurrence is higher than that seen with surgical resection in many series. These therapies are typically reserved for those who are not candidates for surgical resection.

Operative steps
Lobectomy with en-bloc resection of N1 lymph nodes combined with mediastinal lymph node sampling or dissection remains the standard surgical procedure in patients with NSCLC. While nuances exist with the approach to each of the lobectomies, certain general principles are applied regardless of the lobe to be resected.

Positioning and incisions
- A double lumen endotracheal tube is placed and the position verified bronchoscopically both before and after turning the patient (the three segmental bronchi to the right upper lobe should be clearly visible through the tracheal lumen and the blue balloon cuff should be visible). For most cases a left endobronchial tube is sufficient, but make sure to pull it back prior to any left proximal bronchial resections. If you have issues with ventilation on the side you are working on, stop and have anesthesia perform a bronchoscopy and reposition the tube. Alternatively, a bronchial blocker may be used for lung isolation.
- The patient is placed in the lateral decubitus position with the operative side up. An axillary roll is placed and the arms are brought forward and positioned at a 90° angle from the anterior chest.
- The patient is secured to the operating table and the bed is then flexed to accentuate the interspaces.
- For open lobectomy, the typical incision is a posterolateral thoracotomy through the 5th interspace. VATS lobectomy typically is approached via a utility incision (3-4 cm) in the axilla at the 4th interspace along with 2-3 additional working ports

(7th interspace – anterior axillary line; 9th interspace posterior mid-clavicular line).

Mobilization and Hilar dissection

- On entry to the chest, a thorough inspection of the pleural surface is performed and any suspicious lesions are biopsied.
- If there is concern (clinically or due to imaging findings) for mediastinal lymph node involvement, mediastinal lymph node dissection and frozen section evaluation may be performed prior to proceeding with lobectomy.
- The inferior pulmonary ligament is identified and mobilized to the level of the inferior pulmonary vein.
- The pleural reflection is incised posteriorly to the level of the azygos vein on the right or the aortic arch on the left. This will allow for good access to and visualization of the bronchus.
- The pleural reflection overlying the anterior mediastinum is incised, taking care to identify and avoid the phrenic nerve. Once the pleura is opened, both the superior and inferior pulmonary veins are identified.

Vascular dissection and division

- The pulmonary vein to the lobe of interest is circumferentially dissected using a blunt technique. For the upper and lower lobes, this dissection is done anteriorly at the hilum. For the right middle lobe, this dissection is performed within the fissure itself. Once identified and dissected free, the vein may be divided with a linear stapler. If doing a right upper lobe or middle lobe make certain that you visualize the bifurcation of the upper and middle veins so that you do not convert a single lobectomy to a bilobectomy inadvertently.
- Following division of the vein, the pulmonary artery comes into view. Careful blunt dissection is used to identify the artery and its side branches. These are individually divided with a vascular stapling device after assuring that the pulmonary artery branches to the other lobe(s) are identified and preserved. RUL - truncus (apical-anterior branch) + ascending artery to the posterior upper lobe segment (near the fissure); RML - RML artery branching anteriorly off the ongoing artery; RLL - ongoing beyond the middle artery. Note that the superior segmental artery arises near the middle artery and may need to be ligated separately; LUL - apical-anterior branch + anterior branch + lingular branches (1-2); LLL - superior segmental + basilar trunk.
- The vessels may be approached and divided in either order (vein or artery first) depending upon what is easiest anatomically.

7

Bronchial division

- After vascular division, the bronchus and perhaps some remaining parenchymal tissue (if the interlobar fissure is incomplete) are all that remain. Parenchymal division can be accomplished at this time using an endovascular stapler with a thick tissue staple load. Several firings are typically necessary. The staple line is oriented to follow the direction of the native fissure, with the ongoing pulmonary artery used as a guide for the deep margin in upper lobe resections.
- The peribronchial lymph nodes from the diseased lobe are cleared to expose the bronchial resection margin.
- The bronchus is divided with a linear stapler. The stapler is closed on the bronchus and initially not fired. The anesthesiologist is asked to ventilate the lung on operative side to ensure the remaining lobes aerate normally. If there are questions regarding airway patency, a pediatric bronchoscope may be passed through the operative side of the double lumen tube to visually assess the proposed bronchial stump to assure the airways to remaining lung parenchyma are not compromised.
- After completion of the lobectomy, the specimen is removed directly if a thoracotomy was performed, or placed in a specimen bag and withdrawn through the access incision if a thoracoscopic approach was used.
- The bronchial stump closure may be tested for leak intraoperatively by filling the chest with water and ventilating the operative side to assess for bubbling through the staple line. In patients who underwent induction chemoradiotherapy or in whom poor wound healing might be expected, the bronchial stump may be buttressed using a tissue flap (pleura, pericardial fat, intercostal muscle, etc.).
- Chest tubes are then placed under direct vision to completely drain the post-lobectomy space and the chest wall closed in the typical manner.

Technical considerations with specific lobectomies
Right upper lobe
- The pulmonary artery is easily injured while developing the plane between the upper lobe bronchus and the artery itself as well as during division of the recurrent posterior artery as the artery is under some tension in both cases.
- The phrenic nerve is closely related to the apex of the hilum and can be injured when dividing the mediastinal pleura or when taking down adhesions in this region.

8

Right middle lobe
- The ongoing pulmonary artery runs through the fissure and branches to the lower lobe can sometimes be mistaken for the middle lobe branch. Develop this dissection thoroughly before dividing any arterial branches.
- The arterial branch to the middle lobe is also easily injured by traction once the bronchus to the middle lobe is divided.
- Division of the middle lobe bronchus can easily compromise aeration to the lower lobe. This should be checked carefully prior to stapling.

Right lower lobe
- The middle lobe pulmonary artery is easily injured due to excessive traction while dissecting the lower lobe pulmonary artery branches.
- The middle lobe bronchus can be narrowed or twisted when stapling the basilar branches of the lower lobe bronchus.
- The phrenic nerve is close to the anterior hilum and should be carefully identified.

Left upper lobe
- The aorta and aortic arch are immediately behind the pleural dissection plane used to expose the posterior aspect of the left upper lobe. Small aortic side branches may be encountered, especially if there is an inflammatory component to the tumor process.
- The left recurrent laryngeal nerve loops around the aortic arch before ascending back to the neck. This structure may be injured during mobilization of the apex of the lobe or during aorticopulmonary window lymph node dissection.
- There are multiple small branches of the pulmonary artery to the left upper lobe. Care must be taken to develop a dissection plane travelling immediately along the vessel in order to avoid injury/avulsion.

Left lower lobe
- The ongoing pulmonary artery is typically identified within the fissure. However, the lingular branch often originates at the level of the fissure and may be inadvertently divided if care is not taken to identify this vessel.

Potential questions/alternative scenarios
"Do all patients need neuroimaging prior to resection?"
Routine use of neuroimaging has fallen out of favor in the preoperative evaluation of patients with early-stage lung cancer due to the extremely low rate of occult intracranial metastasis. The current standard of care is a thorough history and physical exam. Neuroimaging (preferentially

MRI) is then pursued for those patients with neurologic symptoms.

"How do you select patients for mediastinoscopy?"

While some surgeons practice routine mediastinoscopy for all patients with either known or suspected lung cancer, this approach is no longer the norm. Selective use of mediastinoscopy has become more standard, especially as the sensitivity of imaging techniques has improved. However, select groups of patients still have clear indications for mediastinoscopy (or other forms of surgical mediastinal evaluation). The most straightforward scenario is the patient with pathologically enlarged lymph nodes (> 1 cm in short axis diameter on CT) or with increased FDG avidity on PET. Centrally located tumors and T2 or larger lesions represent a relative indication due to the higher incidence of concomitant mediastinal disease. Adenocarcinoma and large cell primary tumor histology are also felt by some to be indications for pathologic mediastinal evaluation.

"You are evaluating a patient with a left upper lobe NSCLC who has increased FDG uptake on PET in the AP window lymph nodes. The patient is otherwise fit for surgery. How will you proceed operatively?"

There are two potential options for the evaluation of the AP window lymph nodes in this patient. Traditionally, the level 5 and 6 nodes could be accessed via a Chamberlain procedure. However, in this patient who is a reasonable surgical candidate, a thoracoscopic approach would offer the benefit of being able to proceed to definitive resection in the same operative setting. The patient would be intubated with a double lumen endotracheal tube and positioned in the right lateral decubitus position as for a lobectomy. A thoracoscopic exploration of the chest would be quickly performed to rule out intrapleural disease and the AP widow lymph nodes excised and sent for frozen section evaluation. If positive, the patient could be treated with neoadjuvant chemotherapy and brought back for surgical resection at a later time. A more conservative approach would be to treat the patient with definitive CRT in the setting of level 5 or 6 N2 disease, although this conservative approach is falling out favor for single station N2 disease, particularly in the setting of a left upper lobe cancer with level 5 or 6 nodal involvement. If negative, one may safely proceed with lobectomy. Many surgeons favor resection of a left upper lobe cancer regardless of a positive level 5 or 6 lymph node, as the survival is similar in this setting to patients with N1 disease (which would also be resected). In this setting, some argue that preoperative sampling of level 5 or 6 nodes is not needed, as the results will not change the treatment plan. Mediastinal lymph node sampling, including level 5 and 6, should still be performed, as patients with positive nodes should be treated with adjuvant therapy.

"You are operating on a patient with a suspected central lung cancer, but there is no biopsy-proven malignancy. What is your intraoperative approach to diagnosis?"

The answer to this question is largely dependent upon the location of the lesion of interest. Consequently, you will typically have a good idea of your approach from review of the CT scan prior to beginning the operation. Peripheral nodules are typically amenable to wedge resection, allowing for a frozen section diagnosis to be made prior to proceeding with lobectomy. While waiting for frozen section results, mediastinal lymph node sampling can be performed so that the operation continues to progress. In the case of more central lesions, a core needle biopsy can be taken under direct visualization/palpation in most cases. Rarely, an abnormality is centrally located and intimately associated with the pulmonary vasculature, precluding biopsy. In this circumstance, lobectomy is the most minimal resection which can be accomplished safely.

"While you are preparing to divide the upper lobe pulmonary artery for a right upper lobectomy, the pathology lab calls with results on a previously sampled 4R lymph node. You learn that this is positive for malignancy. How does this change the operative plan?"

This circumstance is really one of the surgeon's own creation. While there is an 8-15% incidence of occult mediastinal lymph node metastasis reported in the literature, this situation is not typically encountered mid-operation. If there is concern preoperatively for mediastinal disease, a mediastinal node dissection and frozen section evaluation should be performed prior to any pulmonary dissection. This will preserve the ability to treat the patient with neoadjuvant therapy and revisit operative resection post-induction with undisturbed tissue planes within the lobe. However, if there is an unexpected finding on nodal disease once dissection has begun (occult nodal disease); most surgeons would proceed with lobectomy and complete mediastinal lymph node dissection, then refer the patient for adjuvant chemotherapy.

"While dissecting the anterior hilum, a rent is made in the pulmonary artery. What is your strategy for managing this complication?"

Pulmonary artery injury is the most feared complication of lobectomy. However, good preparation can minimize the chances for an adverse outcome. During lobectomy, a sponge stick should be immediately available on the field at all times in case of vascular injury. Whether the approach is open or thoracoscopic, this can be used to quickly apply direct pressure to the injured vessel, compressing it against the vertebral bodies and the mediastinum and providing temporary control of the situation. Once this maneuver has been successfully performed and the acute blood loss is under control, plans for repair can be made.

The most important step at this point is to organize the resources around you to help care for the patient. See if another surgeon or partner is around to lend another set of experienced hands to the effort. Instruct anesthesia to prepare for the possibility of significant blood loss (get appropriate blood products in the room). For proximal injuries, cardiopulmonary bypass may be required for repair and perfusion should be notified to bring a bypass circuit to the OR. All suture materials, instruments, vascular clamps, and other supplies that might be needed for repair should be made immediately available. During this time a wide thoracotomy is performed to provide full exposure to the area of injury.

Once the plan has been formulated, repair of the injury can be commenced. The first step in this process is attempting to achieve proximal and distal control of the vessel. The strategy here will depend upon the location of injury and will be different in every case. However, one safe approach to proximal control is to enter the pericardium and encircle the pulmonary artery at this level. This will provide a free dissection plane proximal to the injury. The pulmonary artery can be snared with a tourniquet at this point. In many cases, this may be all that is required and division of the injured artery can be completed with a stapler if it is an injury to a branch that needed to be resected anyway (perhaps with a suture closure on the specimen side to prevent ongoing bleeding as the operation is completed). If the main PA or ongoing PA is injured, a direct suture repair is often possible for smaller injuries. Hemostasis is temporarily achieved by snaring the proximal PA and any major branches feeding the vessel beyond the snare. Vessel loops or small atraumatic vascular clamps may be used for distal and side branch control. Larger injuries may be repaired using a patch technique after vascular control has been gained. Note that having obtaining control of the extra-pericardial proximal PA is never a bad idea for right sided resections, especially if there is concern for a difficult dissection.

"You perform an uncomplicated resection for a 2.5 cm RLL tumor. Final pathology revealed an adenocarcinoma with 2 of 7 hilar lymph nodes positive for malignancy. How will you counsel this patient?"
This patient has T1b, N1, M0 disease (Stage IIa). Adjuvant chemotherapy should be discussed with the patient. While the number of clinical trials addressing this question remains small, a meta-analysis of several trials including patients who underwent surgical resection and were then randomized to either cisplatin-based chemotherapy or observation was published in 1995 and remains the most widely accepted data available. This study showed a 13% reduction in the hazard ratio for death and an overall 5% increase in survival in the chemotherapy arm.

- Appropriate treatment for lung cancer, especially early stage cancers amenable to surgery, is dependent upon accurate preoperative staging.
- Remember to assess the post-resection pathology report in order to advise patients regarding adjuvant chemotherapy.
- If there is concern about the ability to attain an adequate surgical margin, remember to verify using intraoperative frozen section.
- Consider sleeve resection in the case of a proximal tumor which is not otherwise advanced.
- Thoroughly assess the patient's functional status preoperatively.
- Have a systematic approach to pulmonary resections with good knowledge of arterial and venous control as it applies to individual lobes.
- Have a firm understanding of staging and preoperative physiologic testing.

Suggested readings

- Goldstraw P, Crowley J, Chansky K, et al; The IASLC Lung Cancer Staging Project: Proposals for the revision of the TNM stage groupings in the forthcoming (seventh) edition of the TNM classification of malignant tumors. *Journal of Thoracic Oncology* 2:706-14, 2007.
- Chemotherapy in Non-Small Cell Lung Cancer; A meta-analysis using updated data on individual patients from 52 randomized clinical trials. Non-Small Cell Lung Cancer Collaborative Group. *British Medical Journal* 311:899-909, 1995.
- NCCN Clinical Practice Guidelines in Oncology: Non-Small Cell Lung Cancer ver. 1.2013 epub @ nccn.org.
- LoCicero J.: Surgical treatment of non-small cell lung cancer. Shields TW et al. (eds) *General Thoracic Surgery* (7th edition) ed. Lippincott, Williams & Wilkins, Philadelphia PA 2009.
- Ginsberg and Rubinstein. Randomized trial of lobectomy versus limited resection for T1 N0 non-small cell lung cancer. Lung Cancer Study Group. *Ann Thorac Surg.* 1995;60[3]: 615.

Notes

2. Advanced non-small cell lung cancer
Benjamin Wei, MD, and Betty Tong, MD

Concept
- Preoperative work-up and staging of patients with advanced lung cancer
- TNM staging system and how this is used to guide management
- Indications for induction (neoadjuvant) therapy, surgery, and adjuvant therapies
- Multimodal therapy of advanced lung cancer, including Pancoast/superior sulcus tumors and tumors with chest wall involvement
- Contraindications for surgical resection
- Palliative options for advanced lung cancer

Chief complaint
"You have been referred a patient, previously a heavy smoker, with a 6 cm solid mass at the apex of the right lung. He complains of right shoulder pain radiating down the arm and paresthesias. How do you evaluate this patient?"

Differential
Small cell lung cancer, Non-small cell lung cancer (Adenocarcinoma, squamous cell carcinoma, large cell NSCLC, carcinoid tumor - typical and atypical), pulmonary metastasis, infectious process (i.e., aspergilloma, mycobacterial infection, abscess).

History and physical
History should focus on symptoms suggestive of 1) chest wall invasion, 2) neurologic and/or vascular involvement of tumor, and 3) metastatic disease. These include 1) chest wall pain, 2) paresthesias, pain, numbness, swelling, coolness, or weakness of the ipsilateral extremity, and 3) fever, night sweats, weight loss. The patient's overall functional and cardiopulmonary status should also be assessed to determine if he would be a potential candidate for operative intervention in case further evaluation reveals this as an option. The medical history should include specific questions about other significant comorbidities, prior chest surgery or radiation, smoking history, and prior malignancies.

Remember to assess the patient's neurologic and vascular status. Superior sulcus tumors may result in Horner's syndrome, which consists of miosis, ptosis, and anhidrosis of the affected side of the face. Delineate any neurologic deficits, whether sensory or motor, of the extremity on the side of the mass. Similarly, evaluating the upper extremities for pulse strength and edema should be done.

Tests

- *PET-CT scan from skull base to mid-thigh*: to assess for mediastinal and metastatic disease.
- *Head CT with IV contrast or brain MRI*: to evaluate for intracranial metastases, for which PET-CT is not useful.
- *Pulmonary function tests*: to evaluate the patient's surgical candidacy.

Index scenario (additional information)

"Physical exam reveals diminished sensation on the ulnar aspect of the arm, but no weakness. Pulses are intact and there is no arm swelling. There is no Horner's syndrome. PET-CT reveals a 6 cm right upper lobe FDG-avid mass with an SUVmax of 15. The mass appears to invade the chest wall, including the first and second ribs on the right. The mediastinal lymph nodes are enlarged (> 1 cm in diameter), but demonstrate minimal FDG activity (SUV < 2.5). Pulmonary function testing demonstrates FEV1 and DLCO of 65% and 70% predicted, respectively. Brain MRI is unremarkable. What is the next step?"

Treatment/management

The neurologic complaints and findings on physical exam, as well as the location of the mass, suggest that further evaluation for brachial plexus involvement should be done. MRI is generally the best diagnostic modality for determining if the brachial plexus and/or spinal cord are involved. MRI, or CT scan with IV contrast, can also help if invasion of the subclavian vessels is a possibility.

"MRI/MRA of the chest shows that the mass is impinging on the T1 nerve root. There is no evidence of invasion into the vertebral foramen or involvement of the vasculature. How would you like to proceed?"

The evidence in this case suggests a Pancoast, or superior sulcus, tumor. T1 nerve root involvement does not preclude surgery. Generally speaking, involvement of the C8 nerve or above, or spinal cord is a contraindication to surgery. Resection of C8 causes Klumpke paralysis (affects the forearm and intrinsic muscles of the hand), which may be an unacceptable outcome to the patient. Based on the PFTs obtained, the patient's predicted postoperative FEV1 and DLCO would be > 40% predicted and he would be a candidate for right upper lobectomy. Invasion of ribs 1-2 necessitates an en bloc chest wall resection. Induction chemoradiation followed by surgery has been shown to provide the best chance for cure in this patient population (Rusch JCO 2007). However, those with mediastinal disease (N2 or N3) do not derive additional benefit from surgery over chemoradiation alone. In addition, oncologists and radiation oncologists generally will not initiate treatment without a tissue diagnosis. Therefore this patient needs 3 additional studies:

- *Percutaneous CT-guided needle biopsy*: to establish the diagnosis of malignancy.
- *Bronchoscopy*: to evaluate for possible synchronous lesions/mainstem bronchus involvement/abnormal anatomy; endobronchial involvement is another poor prognostic factor.
- *Mediastinoscopy*: to determine if the patient has N2 or N3 disease, in which case he would no longer be a candidate for surgical resection. Mediastinoscopy remains the gold standard for assessment of mediastinal lymph nodes, as there is a significant false positive and false negative rate for PET-CT. Endobronchial ultrasound (EBUS) guided biopsy is being used at some centers, but is operator dependent and continues to be evaluated. This may be an option for trainees with extensive experience with this modality, but a negative result with EBUS would still provide impetus for conventional mediastinoscopy barring a contraindication (ex. previous mediastinoscopy, tracheostomy) (Annema JAMA 2010).

"Percutaneous CT-guided biopsy reveals squamous cell carcinoma. Bronchoscopy is unremarkable. Mediastinoscopy with biopsies of stations 2R, 4R, 4L, and 7 shows no evidence of cancer. What stage is this patient clinically? What is your treatment plan?"
This patient has clinical stage IIB cancer. It is T3N0, T3 because of chest wall invasion and involvement of the T1 nerve root. It remains N0 because mediastinoscopy demonstrated no N2 or N3 involvement. There was no hilar lymphadenopathy on PET-CT that would make the patient N1, and therefore the patient is staged at N0. Here it is useful to briefly review the relevant staging of lung cancer:
Stage IIB: consists of T2bN1 and T3N0
Stage IIIA: consists of T1-3N2 and T3N1 and T4N0-1

For this patient with a superior sulcus tumor involving or impinging on the T1 nerve, the best strategy is to proceed with induction chemoradiation followed by planned surgical resection. Induction chemoradiation in this situation comprises a platinum-based doublet (ideally cisplatin + etoposide, but cisplatin + vinblastine or carboplatin + paclitaxel are also acceptable) administered concurrently with 45-50 Gy of radiation. A repeat PET-CT scan should be performed after induction therapy to determine if the patient has responded to the treatment, or on the other hand, if interval disease progression or development of metastases has occurred.

"The patient undergoes induction chemoradiation with cisplatin and etoposide, as well as 50 Gy of radiation therapy. Aside from some fatigue, he tolerates it well and has no significant side effects. Repeat PET-CT scan shows that the mass appears slightly smaller, 4.5 cm in diameter, suggesting a treatment response. There is no evidence of new distant disease."

Our plan is to proceed with surgical resection.

Operative steps

- Consider diagnostic thoracoscopy to evaluate for metastatic pleural disease prior to performing thoracotomy.
- Posterior approach (Paulson incision) most common – posterolateral thoracotomy with medial extension near parallel to both spine and edge of scapula.
- Consider harvesting intercostal muscle flap on way in for bronchial stump coverage in this patient with preoperative XRT.
- En bloc right upper lobectomy with chest wall resection.
    - Resect 1 rib above and 1 rib below those involved by the tumor – in this case ribs 1-3
    - At least a 2 cm margin laterally/medially
    - Can separate lung from chest wall with a wedge resection if needed
    - Isolate and divide hilar vessels to the upper lobe individually
    - Send specimen for frozen section to obtain negative soft tissue margins on the chest wall and the bronchus
    - Remember to perform a mediastinal lymph node dissection or sampling
- Reconstruction of chest wall if defect is anterior, large (> 5 cm), or potential for scapular entrapment exists. If small or the defect is covered by the scapula (but unlikely to be entrapped by it), you can leave the defect unreconstructed. Options include:
    - Biological acellular dermal substitute (e.g., Strattice, AlloDerm)
    - PTFE (2 mm thickness, easy to handle)
    - Prolene mesh alone
    - Prolene with methylmethacrylate sandwich (rigid, but harder to handle/implant)
    - Soft tissue flap with the help of plastic surgery (latissimus – for posterior/anterior locations, pectoralis/TRAM – for anterior locations only) may be necessary if the defect is very large.

"This patient recovers from surgery. Final pathological staging is ypT3N0. All margins are negative. What additional therapy does he need?"

This patient will need adjuvant chemotherapy, most likely with a cisplatin-based doublet (options include cisplatin + etoposide, cisplatin + vinorelbine, cisplatin + vinblastine; 2nd line for those who cannot take cisplatin = carboplatin + paclitaxel). If the patient has mediastinal lymph node metastases identified on final pathology (missed by preoperative mediastinoscopy), a boost of mediastinal irradiation should be considered.

Potential questions/alternative scenarios

"You have the same original scenario as above, but it appears that there is invasion of the subclavian vessels on preoperative imaging. What would you do now?"

Again, induction chemoradiation followed by surgery is the ideal strategy, but now the involved portion of the vessel needs to be resected. The anterior (Dartevelle) approach provides excellent exposure in this situation. This incision is L shaped, starting superiorly near the ear and following the anterior border of the sternocleidomastoid inferiorly, then crossing horizontally towards to the shoulder parallel to and below the clavicle. This horizontal part of the incision can be made lower (and accompanied by a partial sternotomy with anterior thoracotomy in the 2nd or 3rd intercostal space) as needed. The sternal head of the SCM and the inferior belly of the omohyoid are divided to expose the thoracic inlet. Once it is determined that the tumor is resectable, the medial portion of the clavicle is removed. The vein can be resected without reconstruction. Elevation of the extremity postoperatively minimizes edema as collateral venous networks develop to compensate for venous resection. If there is invasion of the subclavian artery, the section involved should be resected and reconstructed, either with a primary reanastomosis or PTFE interposition graft. Carotid-to-subclavian bypass can also be considered. With vascular reconstruction, postoperative anticoagulation is recommended for a period of 6 months. Chest wall resection and lobectomy then proceeds after vessel invasion has been dealth with.

"You have the same original scenario as above, but it appears that there is invasion of the T2 vertebral body. How would you approach this situation?"

Invasion of a vertebral body upstages the patient to a T4 cancer. Typically, this would be suggested by preoperative cross-sectional imaging. An MRI should be obtained to evaluate for spinal cord involvement. Assuming that the cord is not involved, resection of part of the vertebral body can be performed along with the lobectomy. The invasion of more than 2 vertebral bodies is a contraindication to resection. Induction chemotherapy or chemoradiotherapy should be part of the treatment strategy in these patients. Involvement of a spinal surgeon is critical for dealing with this uncommon scenario.

"What if this was not a superior sulcus tumor, but a mass that demonstrated chest wall invasion of ribs 4-5? Would you treat this patient differently? This patient has a T3N0 with chest wall invasion, but NOT a superior sulcus tumor."
If the patient's mediastinal lymph node staging is negative and the lesion appears technically resectable, you would forgo induction chemoradiation and take him to surgery for chest wall resection w/lobectomy. Principles for chest wall reconstruction, described above, also apply here. This patient would then undergo at minimum adjuvant chemotherapy, regardless of nodal status. Adjuvant radiation would be considered if the patient has either N2 or greater staging on final pathology or positive margins.

"How about if this patient had preoperative mediastinoscopy that demonstrated N2 disease? What would you do?"
This patient has stage T3N2 disease with chest wall invasion and should receive definitive chemoradiation. Patients who are T3 because of chest wall invasion and N2 do not derive any survival benefit from surgery (Rusch JTCVS 2000).

"You have a patient with a 1.7 cm peripheral left lower lobe tumor, clinical stage I. Surprisingly, however, mediastinoscopy shows that station 4L is positive. What stage is he and how do you treat him? What if station 7 is positive also?"
This patient is T1a by tumor size (< 2 cm) and N2 (cancer in ipsilateral mediastinal nodes), which is stage IIIA. Remember that any N2 patient (except for T4N2 which is stage IIIB) is stage IIIA. Treatment for N2 patients depends on the details of the patient's clinical condition and which mediastinal lymph nodes are positive. There remain institutional biases with regards to optimal treatment. Single-station, microscopically positive mediastinal disease in a patient with good performance status would generally be an indication for induction chemotherapy followed by repeat PET-CT scan to confirm that disease progression and/or distant metastasis has not occurred. If not, then, mediastinal restaging may be done, followed by pulmonary resection if the mediastinum has been cleared. While there are randomized trial data demonstrating improved survival for patients with N2 disease undergoing induction therapy followed by surgery versus surgery alone (Rosell Semin Oncol 1994; Roth Lung Cancer 1998), patients with persistent N2 disease do not benefit from resection (Bueno ATS 2000). Mediastinal restaging can be

done either thoracoscopically or via mediastinoscopy if it has not been done before. In a patient with bulky mediastinal disease (> 2 cm nodes), multistation disease, or those patients whose general health status is unfavorable/borderline for surgical resection, definitive chemoradiation would be a better choice.

"You have the same patient — 1.7 cm left lower lobe tumor, but 4R is positive. What stage are you dealing with now and how do you treat him?"
This patient is T1aN3 (N3 = cancer in contralateral mediastinal nodes), and stage IIIB. Any N3 disease (and T4N2) is classified as stage IIIB. These patients should be treated with definitive chemoradiation.

"Again, same patient — 1.7 cm tumor, but mediastinoscopy is negative — however postoperatively you discover that the patient actually has N2 disease. What do you do now?"
This patient was a clinical stage I patient who has been upstaged postoperatively to pathological stage IIIA. He did not receive preoperative chemotherapy. He should now receive both adjuvant chemotherapy (if a patient is anything beyond N0, he should be considered for chemotherapy) and radiation (N2 or N3 disease discovered postoperatively, as well as positive margins, are an indication for radiation – assuming that the patient has not been irradiated before).

"Your patient now has a 6 cm RUL tumor, resected by lobectomy. Final pathology report demonstrates that the hilar nodes are negative for malignancy. Lymph nodes at stations 2R, 4R, 4L, and 7 are negative from mediastinoscopy and mediastinal lymph node dissection at the time of thoracotomy. What stage are we dealing with and would you recommend that this patient receive adjuvant therapy?"
This patient is Stage IB (T2bN0). He is T2b because of size (tumor between 5-7 cm in diameter), and N0 because his ipsilateral hilar nodes are negative. Based on the subgroup analysis of CALGB 9633 demonstrating a survival benefit in adjuvant chemotherapy in patients with tumors > 4 cm in size, he should be considered for adjuvant chemotherapy. There is no indication for radiation therapy (Strauss JCO 2008).

"You are in the OR with a patient for seemingly straightforward left lower lobectomy for a 3 cm cancer, however upon exploring the chest you determine that the pericardium is involved. How do you proceed?"
If you can determine that the contents *inside* the pericardium (e.g., heart and great vessels) are not involved, proceed with en bloc resection of the lobectomy with involved pericardium. Factors that result in T3 staging, besides chest wall invasion, are size > 7 cm, main stem bronchus

involvement < 2 cm from the carina, resultant atelectasis of the entire lung, different nodules in the same lobe, and involvement of the diaphragm, phrenic nerve, mediastinal pleura, or pericardium. Patients with main stem bronchus involvement > 2 cm from the carina may be candidates for sleeve lobectomy (see separate section), or pneumonectomy if a parenchymal-sparing lung resection is not possible. Patients with atelectasis of the entire lung may benefit from preoperative laser ablation or debridement of tumor, followed by consideration for a bronchoplastic procedure or pneumonectomy depending on location of the tumor and ability to achieve negative surgical margins. The diaphragm, phrenic nerve, mediastinal pleura, and/or pericardium may be taken en bloc with the pulmonary resection if invaded by tumor. These patients do not generally need induction therapy, but do benefit from adjuvant chemotherapy.

"You are in the OR for that same left lower lobectomy for cancer, however palpating the upper lobe reveals an additional roughly 1 cm nodule. What do you do now?"
In this situation, performing a wedge resection or segmentectomy of the smaller nodule would be warrented.

"Frozen section reveals non-small lung cancer. What do you do now?"
Proceeding with the lower lobectomy, even if cancer is present in the 2nd nodule, would be reasonable for most patients. Mediastinal lymph node dissection should also be done. Performing an unanticipated pneumonectomy would not be prudent. This patient has T4 cancer. Depending on location, additional pulmonary tumor nodules with the same histology as the primary site may upstage a cancer to anywhere from stage IIB (T3N0) to stage IV. Assume that patients are N0 or N1 by mediastinal staging for the following:

- *Same lobe (T3)*: lobectomy, followed by adjuvant chemotherapy.
- *Different lobes, same lung (T4)*: lobectomy (for larger nodule) + sublobar resection (for smaller nodule), as lung function permits.
- *Contralateral lung, single nodule*: this may represent synchronous primaries or a lung cancer with contralateral metastasis. One strategy to manage these patients is to perform mediastinoscopy followed by resection of the smaller nodule in the first sitting if the mediastinoscopy is negative. If the mediastinoscopy is positive, assume M1 disease (the mediastinal nodal disease means the disease is in transit and the contralateral lung nodule is more likely to be a metastasis rather than a primary) and treat with chemotherapy. If mediastinoscopy is negative, treat as two synchronous primaries and resect the smaller nodule in the same sitting. A 2nd stage operation involves resection of the larger nodule. The amount of lung resected will depend on the patient's

lung function and which lobes are involved.

- *Contralateral lung, multiple nodules*: treat as M1 disease.
- *Additional tumor nodule, different histology as primary*: treat as synchronous primaries.

"Invasion of what other structures would also make this patient's cancer T4?"
Involvement of the heart, mediastinum, great vessels, esophagus, recurrent laryngeal nerve, vertebral body, or carina leads to T4 staging. T4 disease has historically been considered unresectable, and is treated with palliation in most cases. If a patient has a T4N0 or T4N1 cancer, he is stage IIIA, and one can consider resection in certain special circumstances as delineated below:

- *Vertebral body invasion*: obtain MRI to confirm absence of spinal cord involvement, then can consider induction therapy (chemo or CRT) followed by pulmonary resection with vertebral body resection.
- *Carinal invasion*: may be candidate for carinal pneumonectomy. If a patient is T4N2, he is stage IIIB and should receive definitive CRT.

"You are sent a patient for consideration of lobectomy for biopsy-proven NSCLC, however your imaging reveals numerous liver and bony metastases. What now?"
Metastatic disease is staged and treated in the following manner:

- *M1a*: metastatic pulmonary nodules to contralateral lung, pleural nodules, malignant pleural or pericardial effusion – palliation
- *M1b*: distant metastases - palliation, unless
  - *Solitary brain met*: may consider pulmonary resection for T1-2 N0 M1 disease after brain met is treated with radiation or surgery. Patients with nodal disease and brain metastases are not surgical candidates (Billing JTCVS 2001).
  - *Solitary adrenal met*: FNA to confirm adrenal met, then may consider pulmonary resection and adrenalectomy (Mercier JTCVS 2005).

"You perform a left upper lobectomy for clinical stage I cancer. Pathological analysis is consistent with stage I, so he does not receive adjuvant therapy. Surveillance CT scan reveals a LLL nodule consistent with recurrence 2 years later. How would you deal with the following scenarios of locoregional recurrence?"

- *In all cases*: PET/CT (skull base to mid thigh) to evaluate for distant metastatic disease.

- *Isolated parenchymal recurrence*: re-resection if possible, SBRT or XRT if not technically feasible; consideration of adjuvant chemotherapy
- *Endobronchial obstruction*: laser ablation, stent, PDT, brachytherapy, or XRT for palliation
- *Mediastinal lymph node recurrence*: chemoradiation (if no radiation previously)
- *SVC obstruction*: chemoradiation. XRT alone, stent
- *Oligometastatic disease*: chemotherapy

Palliation options
- *Localized symptoms due to primary cancer deemed unresectable*: XRT
- *Brain mets, bony mets*: XRT followed by chemotherapy
- *Disseminated disease*: chemotherapy

Genetic mutation targeted chemotherapy regimens for palliation
- *Non-squamous NSCLC*: test for ALK (tyrosine kinase), EGFR, KRAS mutations
    - *If ALK+*: crizotinib
    - *If EGFR+*: erlotinib ("Tarceva")
    - *If both ALK/EGFR negative, unknown, or treatment failure with above regimens*: cisplatin-based doublet +/- bevacizumab ("Avastin")
    - *KRAS+ cancers*: generally poor response to EGFR inhibitors and chemotherapy
- *Squamous cell carcinoma*: cisplatin-based doublet +/- bevacizumab (no testing for ALK/EGFR)

Pearls/pitfalls
- Do not operate on N3 disease.
- Do not forget induction chemoradiation in patients with superior sulcus tumors, if you are planning on bringing them to the OR
- Do not operate on patients with superior sulcus tumors *and* N2 disease.
- Remember to perform head CT or brain MRI on patients with stage II cancer and above.
- Send margins on pulmonary resections (bronchial always, chest wall as needed).
- Develop an individualized strategy to deal with N2 disease and bilateral lung masses, based on the patient's pulmonary function, clinical status, and overall performance status.

- Complete evaluation of locally advanced lung cancer includes skull base-mid thigh PET-CT, brain MRI or head CT with IV contrast, pulmonary function testing, bronchoscopy, and mediastinoscopy. CT should include IV contrast if the tumor may invade major blood vessels. MRI is indicated if brachial plexus or spinal cord invasion is possible. If induction or definitive non-surgical therapy is indicated, obtaining a tissue diagnosis is generally required.
- Superior sulcus tumors should ideally be treated with induction chemoradiation followed by lobectomy with chest wall resection.
- Reconstruct chest wall defects unless small or covered by scapula: options include PTFE, prolene, prolene with methylmethacrylate, and for larger defects, muscle flaps.
- Any patient with a tumor > 4 cm in diameter or staged N1 or greater on pathology should receive adjuvant chemotherapy following surgery.
- Stage IIB patients (T2bN1, T3N0) should generally be treated with surgery followed by adjuvant chemotherapy.
- Stage IIIA patients that are N2 should generally be treated with induction chemotherapy followed by mediastinal restaging, and lobectomy if downstaged (exception is T3N2 patients with chest wall invasion à definitive chemoradiation). Patients with N2 disease should also eventually receive mediastinal irradiation as well, whether they undergo surgery or not.
- Stage IIIA patients with bulky mediastinal lymphadenopathy and stage IIIB patients (T1-4N3,T4N2) should typically be treated with definitive chemoradiation.
- Nearly all stage IV patients should be treated with chemotherapy, and palliative XRT as needed.
- Certain patients with T4 or M1 disease (vertebral body invasion, carinal invasion, solitary metastases to adrenal or brain) may be candidates for surgical resection.

Suggested readings

- National Comprehensive Cancer Network Clinical Guidelines for NSCLC (www.NCCN.org).
- Rusch VW, Giroux DJ et al. Induction chemoradiation and surgical resection for superior
  sulcus non-small-cell lung carcinomas: Long-term results of Southwest Oncology Group Trial 9416 (Intergroup Trial 0160). JCO 2007; 25:313-8.
- Annema JT, van Meerbeeck JP et al. Mediastinoscopy vs. Endosonography for Mediastinal Staging of Lung Cancer. JAMA. 2010;304(20):2245-2252.

- Rusch VW, Parekh KR et al. Factors determing outcome after surgical resection of T3 and T4 lung cancers of the superior sulcus. JTCVS 2000119:1147-53.
- Rosell R, Maestre J. A randomized trial of mitomycin/ifosfamide/cisplatin preoperative chemotherapy plus surgery versusu surgery alone in stage IIIA non-small cell lung cancer. Semin Oncol 1994; 21:28-33.
- Roth JA, Atkinson EN et al. Long-term follow-up of patients enrolled in a randomized trial comparing perioperative chemotherapy and surgery with surgery alone in resectable stage IIA non-smal-cell lung cancer. Lung Cancer 1998;21:1-6.

Notes

3. Small cell lung cancer

Shair Ahmed, MD, and Allan Pickens, MD

Concept
* Staging small cell lung cancer
* Workup for SCLC
* Appropriate surgical management in SCLC
* Non-surgical management of SCLC

Chief complaint

"A 65 yo woman presents to your office for a second opinion 3 weeks after a right lower lobe wedge resection for a 9 mm right lower lobe lesion that had been previously biopsied via percutaneous CT guidance, which was non-diagnostic. A VATS wedge biopsy was then performed, with the final pathology revealing SCLC. Her surgeon immediately referred her for chemotherapy and radiation. However, she wants a second opinion. Her comorbidities include hypertension and coronary artery disease. She has a 40 pack-year smoking history."

Differential

Non-small cell lung cancer, small cell lung cancer, carcinoid

History and physical

The symptoms of small cell lung cancer and non-small cell lung cancer are very similar, especially when small cell lung cancer presents at an early stage. Smoking tends to be the most common etiology of SCLC, but is also associated with radon and uranium mining. Be aware of the association of small cell lung cancer and paraneoplastic syndromes, which include Cushing syndrome, SIADH, and Lambert-Eaton myasthenic syndrome. As SCLC frequently metastasizes to the brain, it is important to ascertain neurological symptoms.

Tests

* *Imaging.* It is extremely important to stage the patient as accurately as possible. Imaging includes whole body PET-CT looking for regional and distant metastases. MRI or CT of the brain should be ordered. The mediastinum should be assessed via cervical mediastinoscopy.
* *Labs.* If paraneoplastic syndromes are suspected, then the appropriate workup should be done.
* *Pulmonary function tests (PFTs).* Lung function needs to be assessed to determine the patient tolerance for pulmonary resection.

- *Bronchoscopy.* It is important to assess for endobronchial lesions that can potentially change management (for example whether to consider a sleeve resection).

Index scenario (additional information)

"The patient's history and physical reveal no evidence of paraneoplastic syndromes and a benign physical exam. On imaging, there is slight uptake along the staple line from the prior wedge resection; however there is no evidence of regional or distant metastatic spread. There are several sub-centimeter mediastinal lymph nodes that are not PET avid. MRI of the brain reveals no metastases."

Treatment/management

Given the scenario, this is early stage SCLC in a functional patient with non-limiting comorbidities. While the bulk of the literature dictates the patient receive platinum-based chemotherapy and radiation, there is a role for surgical resection and adjuvant chemotherapy/radiation for early stage SCLC (T1-2 N0 lesions). The patient should undergo a cervical mediastinoscopy (see Chapter 6, Mediastinal staging) and if there is no mediastinal disease, a completion lobectomy with lymphadenectomy is indicated. Postoperatively, the patient should receive platinum-based chemotherapy and radiation.

Potential questions/alternative scenarios

"The patient in the above scenario during mediastinoscopy was found to have mediastinal disease (positive N2 lymph nodes), how would you proceed?"

The procedure should stop at the mediastinoscopy and the patient should undergo definitive platinum-based chemotherapy and radiation therapy.

"A similar patient with minimal comorbidities presents with a diagnosis of SCLC by needle biopsy, how would you proceed?"

The pathology should be re-reviewed. If SCLC is confirmed by a second review from a different pathologist, the workup should proceed. If there are no metastases, resection is indicated followed by adjuvant chemotherapy and radiation. On occasion, final histology can reveal a mixed histology that includes non-small cell lung cancer, which is best treated with resection to reduce local recurrence (treat like NSCLC, not SCLC when mixed). In addition, carcinoid tumors can be frequently misdiagnosed as SCLC, so a patient with a suspicious non-metastatic early malignant lesion should be given the chance at surgical resection.

"A similar patient presents with unresectable small cell lung cancer (3 cm right lower lobe lesion, N2 disease, no brain metastases). How would you manage this patient?"

The patient should undergo chemotherapy with platinum-based agents (Cisplatin or carboplatin) along with radiation therapy (45-50 Gy). As the literature supports pulmonary resection followed by adjuvant therapy in early stage SCLC (defined as T1-2N0 or T1N1) with favorable 5-year survival, the ACCP guidelines state that chemotherapy and radiation is first-line treatment for SCLC. The ACCP guidelines support pulmonary resection for lesions < 3 cm that are node negative, as metastases is less likely in this subgroup. In addition, there is a growing body of literature that suggests prophylactic cranial irradiation confers increased median survival and lower rate of symptomatic brain metastases.

Pearls/pitfalls

- For the purposes of pulmonary resection in early stage SCLC, the ACCP guidelines support pulmonary resection in patients with lesions less than 3 cm in size and no nodal metastases.
- Histology can be misdiagnosing, especially percutaneous or endobronchial biopsies. Have pathology re-read. If early stage disease is present, always consider resection.
- Check for paraneoplastic syndromes, such as SIADH, Cushings and Lambert-Eaton myasthenic syndrome.
- Medical treatment includes platinum based-chemotherapy and radiation.

Suggested readings

- Goldstein SD, Yang SC. Role of surgery in small cell lung cancer. *Surg Oncol Clin N Am.* 2011 Oct;20(4):769-77.
- Simon GR, Turrisi A; American College of Chest Physicians. Management of small cell lung cancer: ACCP evidence-based clinical practice guidelines (2nd edition). *Chest.* 2007 Sep;132(3 Suppl):324S-339S.

Notes

4. Pneumonectomy and sleeve resection

Michael P. Robich, MD, and Daniel Raymond, MD

Concept
- Preoperative evaluation of patient
- Indications for advanced resections
- Conduct of the operation and pitfalls
- Managing complications

Chief complaint
"A 60 yo man, 60 pack-year smoker is referred to you following evaluation for a cough which culminated in the identification of a 4 cm left hilar mass. A whole body PET-CT has been performed and shows the mass with involvement of the distal left main pulmonary artery and an SUVmax of 11, but no evidence mediastinal adenopathy or distant metastases."

Differential
Primary lung cancer (small cell v. non-small cell), metastatic cancer to the lung, lymphoma, hilar adenopathy.

History and physical
Evaluate for evidence of pre-existing cardiopulmonary disease or prior history of malignancy. Look for evidence of local invasion or metastatic disease. The onus is on the surgeon to appropriately diagnose and stage the patient in order to select the most appropriate therapy. Hoarseness or chest pain can signify mediastinal/chest wall invasion and thus a locally advanced process. Palpable cervical adenopathy, new bone pain or new neurologic symptom would suggest metastatic disease. Evidence of pleural effusion or elevated hemidiaphragm may also suggest an advanced stage process.

Tests
- *Establish diagnosis*: with large, central lesions, preoperative biopsy is necessary prior to attempts at resection in order to exclude diagnoses that would be treated non-operatively, such as small cell lung cancer, lymphoma, and certain metastatic processes. This is not necessary for small, peripheral lesions with a high probability of cancer. Central lesions cannot be wedged for diagnosis and diagnostic pneumonectomy should be avoided.
- *Establish stage.* The current gold standard for clinical staging includes a PET-CT scan and brain imaging (MRI or CT with IV contrast). Endobronchial ultrasound (EBUS) and/or cervical mediastinoscopy is necessary to confirm clinical staging prior to

proceeding with pneumonectomy.

- *Pulmonary assessment.* Assessment for tolerance for pulmonary resection is essential. This is based on history of exercise tolerance and pulmonary function tests. For patients undergoing pneumonectomy, quantitative VQ scanning is advisable in order to determine the postoperative predicted pulmonary function. Common indicators of a patient's ability to tolerate a pneumonectomy include a preoperative FEV1 of > 2 L or predicted postoperative FEV1 > 800 cc. Additional testing can include arterial blood gas, 6 minute walk test, and cardiopulmonary exercise testing.

- *Cardiac evaluation.* Echocardiogram is advisable prior to pneumonectomy to evaluate right heart function and exclude evidence of pulmonary hypertension. Cardiac stress testing or evaluation by a cardiologist is advisable prior to considering a major resection.

Index scenario (additional information)

"PFTs reveal an FEV1 of 2.6 L (73%) and DLCO 68%. Stress echo showed no reversible defects. Bronchoscopy reveals a tumor involving the secondary carina on the left without extension along the main stem bronchus. Biopsy reveals a squamous cell carcinoma. There is no radiographic evidence of metastatic disease. PET-CT is reported as positive in the left hilar lymph nodes and EBUS evaluation of the mediastinal nodes is negative. How would you like to proceed?"

Treatment/management

Pneumonectomy would be indicated in this circumstance for curative resection of this patient's clinical stage II disease. The authors recommend beginning with a mediastinoscopy to assure accurate mediastinal staging and avoid false negative EBUS evaluation. The mediastinoscopy would allow you to rule out N3 disease and N2 disease in level 4 and 7 nodes, but not 5 and 6. It is not necessary to evaluate 5 and 6 once the others have been deemed negative unless there is a suspicious appearing AP window node on imaging.

Pre-operative discussion should be undertaken with the anesthesia team to address needs for appropriate IV access, arterial line, foley catheter, intraoperative fluid management, perioperative antibiotic prophylaxis, DVT prophylaxis and airway management. For a left pneumonectomy, the patient can be managed with a right-sided double lumen endotracheal tube, a left-sided double lumen tube, or a single lumen tube with a bronchial blocker. Any tube or blocker in the left side will need to be withdrawn prior to division of the left mainstem bronchus. A right-sided double lumen tube is ideal for left sided resection but can be tricky to place since you have to keep an orifice open to the RUL.

Obtain single lung ventilation and position patient in lateral decubitus position after appropriate access has been obtained. A posterolateral thoracotomy at the level of the 5th rib provides optimal exposure to the hilum. A muscle sparing approach can be utilized. The 5th rib may be resected or the 6th rib notched for improved exposure. VATS approach should only be used by those with extensive experience. VATS may be useful prior to thoracotomy to assure there is no evidence of pleural dissemination.

It is important to examine for evidence of disease spread and biopsy any suspicious lesions/nodes. Pleural dissemination, pericardial dissemination, invasion of the aorta, esophagus, or heart are contraindications to proceeding. Bulky, multi-station mediastinal adenopathy is a relative contraindication although unlikely with thorough preoperative evaluation. Chest wall, pericardial, diaphragm or limited vena cava involvement can be resected en bloc. Prior to embarking on pneumonectomy a final attempt should be made to determine if a lesser resection, including sleeve resection, is possible.

Operative steps
Left pneumonectomy
- Incise the mediastinal pleura circumferentially around the hilum, reflect phrenic nerve anteriorly with minimal manipulation, and takedown the inferior pulmonary ligament.
- Begin with circumferential dissection and isolation of the superior and inferior pulmonary veins.
- Continue dissection cephalad from the superior pulmonary vein and circumferentially isolate the main pulmonary artery. Avoid injury to recurrent laryngeal nerve (avoid cautery under the aortic arch).
- Following isolation of the main pulmonary artery, place an umbilical tape or clamp.
- Temporary (~1 minute) occlusion of the PA can show how the patient will tolerate shunting of all blood flow to a single lung. Look for signs of intolerance, i.e., tachycardia and/or hypotension. If hypotension occurs, assure appropriate location of clamp (make sure not too proximal, obstructing the main PA) and consider TEE evaluation. If clamp reposition does not remedy the situation and RV dysfunction is identified, abort the procedure.
- If extra length of PA is needed, one can divide the ligamentum arteriosum (watch for the recurrent laryngeal nerve) or open the pericardium (from below the inferior PV to above the PA) to expose the origin of the PA.

- Divide the PA. If adequate length, a vascular stapler can be used. If inadequate length, divide the PA between 2 vascular clamps and oversew with 5-0 prolene. Place anchoring sutures on the ends of the PA prior to division of the vessel to prevent the divided vessel from slipping through the proximal clamp.
- Divide the pulmonary veins with a vascular stapler.
- Expose the left main bronchus to the level of the carina and remove level 4 and 7 lymph nodes. Avoid injury to the recurrent laryngeal nerve.
- Traction applied to the distal airway can facilitate dissection of the proximal main stem to allow for division just distal to the carina.
- Once the stapler is applied check airway pressures to look for impingement of remaining airway.
- After removing the specimen, obtain hemostasis and check for leak a from the bronchial stump.
- Reinforce the bronchial stump to prevent BPF, which is more important on the right, as the left bronchus will often retract into the mediastinum. Options for bronchial reinforcement include pericardial fat, pericardium, pleura, or azygos vein flaps. Alternatively, consider intercostal muscle or serratus anterior flaps in cases of gross infection or previous radiation.
- Complete mediastinal lymphadenectomy.

Right pneumonectomy
- More physiologically taxing and prone to complications.
- Approach is similar to left side, with a few differences.
- Azygos vein needs to be reflected superiorly to expose the proximal right mainstem bronchus.
- The superior pulmonary vein may be divided first to provide better exposure to the right PA as long as the surgeon has assured tolerance for resection.
- Buttressing of the bronchial stump is necessary to minimize the risk of postoperative BPF.

Management of the pneumonectomy space
Options include:
- Chest tube attached to pneumonectomy balanced drainage system (not pleuravac).
- Intrapleural catheter (usually a 8-12 Fr soft tube with a 3-way stopcock).
- No drain. (The authors prefer a small intrapleural catheter placed in a cephalad to caudad direction through the 3rd or 4th intercostal space, anterior axillary line. The authors remove 600-800 cc of air from the pleural space once the chest is closed and the catheter is

then removed).

- Postoperative CXR is examined for mediastinal shift. Air can be added or removed to balance the mediastinum if utilizing a catheter or with angiocath inserted through lateral chest wall if no drain utilized.
- Tube usually removed on POD 1 or 2 if mediastinum remains stable. If a chest tube was utilized, the tube tract should be closed carefully to prevent pleurocutaneous fistula and retrograde infection.

Potential questions/alternative scenarios

"The morning after a left pneumonectomy the patient develops progressive hypotension. What is your management?"

The differential for postoperative hypotension is broad and a systematic approach should be utilized. The physician assessing the patient should consider bleeding, hypovolemia secondary to volume restriction, myocardial ischemia, arrhythmia, epidural-related pressure changes, hypoxia, and mediastinal shift. If a chest tube is being utilized, output is certainly an excellent indicator of bleeding. If not, a stat CXR may reveal a rapidly filling pneumonectomy space, implying bleeding, or significant mediastinal shift that may be impairing cardiac preload (treated by instilling air into the pneumonectomy space to shift the mediastinum back towards the midline). Evaluation of hemoglobin may be helpful, although acute bleeding may not result in an immediate hemoglobin drop. Evaluation of an EKG and cardiac enzymes should be utilized to investigate cardiac events. Epidural-related hypotension can be addressed acutely with a volume challenge and temporary cessation of the epidural. Volume challenges may be used judiciously due to concerns regarding post-pneumonectomy pulmonary edema. Hypoxia should be excluded with pulse oximetry and supplemental oxygen should be titrated.

"Three days after a right pneumonectomy a patient is noted to have a new left lower lobe infiltrate, cough, frothy sputum, and respiratory failure. How will you proceed?"

The mortality rate for pneumonectomy is reported to be 3-12% with a 15-75% rate of complications. The most common complications are respiratory failure, pulmonary edema, pneumonia, empyema, arrhythmias, MI, PE and BPF. This scenario is describing a BPF in the perioperative setting. Early BPFs occur within one month postoperatively and are usually due to technical errors involving closure of the bronchial stump. Late BPFs occur later than one month and are typically attributed to inadequate healing of the bronchial stump. Incidence of BPF after pneumonectomy is reported to be from 1-10% with a mortality of 30-50%. Immediate management includes positioning the patient operative side down and head elevated to avoid contamination of the remaining lung, tube thoracostomy to drain the pleural space, and broad spectrum antibiotics. Emergency reoperation with repair, coverage of the bronchial stump with a well-vascularized flap, and washout of the pleural space is required. The patient should be treated aggressively for postoperative pneumonia and observed carefully for development of empyema.

"A patient 6 weeks post left pneumonectomy presents to clinic with fever and new onset cough productive of blood-tinged sputum. CXR reveals a declining air-fluid level in the left hemithorax. What's your management?"

This patient is presenting with a delayed or late BPF. The first steps are to medically stabilize the patient, administer broad spectrum antibiotics, and place a chest tube to drain the pleural space. Bronchoscopy and surgical exploration should then be undertaken to evaluate the bronchial stump and the postpneumonectomy space once the patient has been stabilized. If no obvious BPF is identified, the pleural space should be washed out, debrided, and drained if there is gross contamination. A Clagett window procedure is the next step and should be undertaken after 3-4 week of closed drainage to allow the mediastinum to stabilize. If the BPF presents late, the mediastinum may already be stabilized and the interval to operation may be shorter. In rare circumstances, no contamination is identified and the chest may be washed out and closed. If there is a visible BPF, the acute management is the same with closed drainage to allow the mediastinum to stabilize. If the fistula closes, a Clagett window closure can be attempted. If the BPF persists, attempts at closure can be made with muscle flaps or omentum once the patient has recovered totally from their initial surgical intervention and subsequent evaluation reveals no evidence of recurrent cancer.

"On preoperative imaging it appears control of the PA will be difficult. How can you approach this tumor?"

Intrapericardial control of the pulmonary artery can be obtained through a posterolateral thoracotomy. Alternatively, median sternotomy can be performed to gain control of the intrapericardial PA. Both right and left pneumonectomy can be performed via sternotomy.

"The tumor invades the chest wall, pericardium, adventitia of the aorta, superficial muscle of the esophagus, or focal area of SVC. How will you proceed?"

Tumor involving the chest wall, pericardium, focal vertebral body involvement and focal SVC involvement may be resected en bloc by surgeons with appropriate experience. Most surgeons would consider aortic or esophageal invasion a contraindication to proceeding. Clips should be placed to guide future radiotherapy if margins are close.

"The tumor involves the proximal vagus nerve on the left. How will you manage this?"

The nerve should be resected en bloc with the specimen. The patient should then be considered for vocal cord medialization in the immediate postoperative period.

"An active 57 yo woman is referred to you with a 19 mm carcinoid tumor in the origin of the right upper lobe bronchus. How would you approach the resection?"

After complete history and physical, radiographic staging and cardiopulmonary testing as for all pulmonary resection candidates you must decide on a resection strategy. A bronchoplastic resection, such as sleeve resection, is a reasonable consideration in this case to spare the right middle and lower lobes. This type of operation was originally developed for patients who could not tolerate pneumonectomy, but the indications have expanded and certain patients can benefit from a limited resection.

Common indications for sleeve include:

- Lesions involving main or lobar bronchi close to the main bronchi
- Benign or low grade tumors (carcinoid being the most common)
- Bulky peribronchial lymph node involvement
- Tumors in the lateral aspect of the lower trachea or carina

Contraindications:

- Locally advanced T4 tumors
- Patients with N2 or N3 disease
- Inability to achieve negative margins

It is important to fully assess the extent of the tumor on bronchoscopy to determine if a sleeve resection will be feasible. The lesion can be biopsied and mucosa proximal and distal to the lesion can be sampled to assess for local spread. Decreased bronchial motion with respiration has been described as a sign of tumor extension.

Right upper lobe bronchial sleeve resection

- Formulate a plan with anesthesiology to ensure a successful ventilation strategy. For sleeve resections on the right, a left-sided double lumen tube should be utilized and vice versa.
- Preoperative bronchoscopy is mandatory.
- *Incision*: posterolateral thoracotomy in the 5th interspace; harvest 5th intercostal muscle during entry and carefully preserve the vascular pedicle.
- Posterior mediastinal pleura is opened to expose the right mainstem, trachea, and esophagus.
- Divide the azygos vein.

- Assess for local invasion and resectability. Excessive lymph node dissection should be avoided.
- Dissect and divide the pulmonary veins, arteries, and fissures as usual.
- Sharply divide the distal mainstem **bronchus** and proximal bronchus intermedius perpendicular to the long axis. Get frozen section to assure negative margins (minimum: 5 mm negative margin for high-grade carcinomas and 3 mm for low grade).
- Release inferior pulmonary ligament to decrease tension. Infrahilar pericardial release can provide more length if needed. Also a mediastinoscopy can be used to release tension.
- Create an end-to-end anastomosis. Interrupted absorbable suture with knots outside the airway to decrease granuloma formation are preferable in the cartilaginous portion of the airway. Interrupted or running sutures may be used in the membranous portion. Check for leak by submersion and ventilation to 30 cm water pressure and cover anastomosis with vascularized tissue. Intercostal flaps should be placed primarily between the anastomosis and the pulmonary artery. Complete encirclement of the anastomosis could result in later stenosis if the muscle flap calcifies. Azygos vein, pericardial fat pad, and parietal pleura can provide alternative sources for coverage.

Potential questions/alternative scenarios

"Postoperative day 8 after a right upper lobe sleeve lobectomy a patient develops fever and respiratory failure. Bronchoscopy shows necrosis and focal dehiscence of the anastomosis. CXR shows increase in the airspace on the operative side. How will you manage?"

Complications after sleeve lobectomy include sputum retention and secondary atelectasis, bronchovascular and bronchopulmonary fistula, and anastomotic failure (stricture and breakdown). Anastomotic breakdown is reported to occur in about 1% of patients. If there is a large air leak, intubation of the left mainstem bronchus will prevent significant ongoing tidal volume loss. If the leak is moderate to small, both lungs can be ventilated, assuming there is adequate drainage of the right pleural space. Therefore tube thoracostomy and administration of broad spectrum antibiotics should be the next step after intubation. Further management depends on the timing and size of the dehiscence. Early dehiscence (not clearly defined, but occurring in the early postoperative period) may be treated with debridement, additional mobilization of the remaining lung/hilum, and reanastomosis with tissue coverage in select cases. For dehiscences 5 mm or less, simple chest tube drainage may be all that is needed, particularly if there was tissue coverage of the anastomosis and there is minimal air leakage. For larger dehiscences and those with smaller defects but ongoing significant air leak or pleural contamination, consideration should be given to completion pneumonectomy. Anastomotic strictures may occur late and can typically be treated with balloon dilation. In rare cases, debridement of the stricture may be needed with methods such as Nd:YAG laser.

"Postoperative day 14 the previous patient develops hemoptysis. How will you manage?"
Anastomotic failure can ultimately lead to development of bronchovascular fistula. This patient should be urgently brought to the operating room with preparation for large-volume bleeding. The patient should be carefully intubated with a left sided double lumen ETT, which is bronchoscopically guided into position to avoid anastomotic disruption. If blood or clot is identified at the anastomosis and a bronchovascular fistula is suspected, emergency completion pneumonectomy utilizing sternotomy for proximal pulmonary arterial control should be performed. There is typically no role for angiography and embolization in this potentially fatal setting.

"How do you handle a bronchial size mismatch during the end-to-end bronchial anastomosis?"
Traveling further between bites on the larger sized bronchus should fix small size mismatches. Alternatively, a longitudinal wedge can be cut from the larger bronchus to allow tapering and better size match. Telescoping is an advanced technique that can be discussed by those with experience.

"How do the outcome for sleeve lobectomy compare to pneumonectomy for NSCLC?"
Recent data have shown 30-day mortality for sleeve lobectomy to be approximately 5%. 5- and 10-year survival after sleeve have been reported to be 40% and 30%, respectively. Several large series have shown a 5-year survival rate of approximately 40% for pneumonectomy as well. Sleeve lobectomy is associated with superior 5-year survival rates in some series, decreased operative mortality, and comparable complication rates when compared to pneumonectomy. Factors decreasing long-term survival following a sleeve lobectomy include incomplete resection and increasing nodal involvement. In one series of 249 patients reported by Kim et al, locoregional recurrences with sleeve lobectomy occurred in 32.6% of patients versus 8.5% in pneumonectomy. There was no significant difference in overall survival at 5 years.

Pearls/pitfalls

- Careful preoperative assessment is vital to select appropriate patients for pneumonectomy.
- Always attempt lesser resection when possible especially in patients that are not candidates for pneumonectomy.
- Occlude PA prior to division to ensure pneumonectomy will be tolerated. Do not divide pulmonary veins prior to this occlusion test.

Suggested readings

- Shields TW, LoCicero, Ponn RJ (eds). Sleeve Lobectomy. Pneumonectomy and its Modifications. General Thoracic Surgery. Pennsylvania: Lippincott, Williams & Wilkins. (5th edition).
- Predina JD, Kunkala M, Aliperti LA, et al. Sleeve lobectomy: current indications and future directions. Ann Thorac Cardiovasc Surg. 2010 Oct;16(5):310-8.

Notes

5. Pulmonary carcinoid

Shair Ahmed, MD, and Allan Pickens, MD

Concept
- Classification and presentation of carcinoid tumors (typical vs. atypical)
- Diagnostic options
- Management of typical vs. atypical carcinoid, peripheral vs. central, N0-N2 mediastinal disease
- Special circumstances

Chief complaint
"A 38 yo woman is referred to your office for evaluation of an incidental lung lesion seen on chest CT during a recent workup for trauma. She denies any complaints of cough, shortness of breath or pleuritic chest pain. On chest CT, the lesion is located centrally in the right lower lobe, measures 1.2 cm, and has a smooth homogenous appearance with well-demarcated borders."

Differential
Mucoepidermoid tumors, large cell neuroendocrine tumor, non-small cell lung cancer, small cell lung cancer

History and physical
The symptoms of carcinoid tumors depend on location, whether peripheral or central. Peripheral lesions tend to be asymptomatic and found incidentally. Central lesions present with symptoms such as cough, recurrent pneumonia, and hemoptysis. Rarely can patients present with carcinoid syndrome, which consists of diarrhea and episodic flushing. The vast majority of patients presenting with carcinoid syndrome will have advanced disease due to liver metastases. Bronchial carcinoids can present with paraneoplastic syndromes as well, most notably Cushing's syndrome. The most common source of ectopic adrenocorticotopic hormone (ACTH) is bronchial carcinoid tumors. Patients who present with pulmonary carcinoid tumors are typically younger than patients with NSCLC (median presentation in 40's, ~20 years earlier than NSCLC. Also, bimodal peaks in age distribution at 35 and 55 years).

Tests
- *Imaging.* Chest CT with IV contrast is needed to evaluate the characteristics of the lesion as well as assess the mediastinum for lymphadenopathy. Determine the location of the lesion (whether peripheral or central), the characteristics of the lesions (typically homogenous and well demarcated), and evaluate the hilum and

mediastinum for nodal disease. Carcinoids are metabolically inactive and on PET-CT have very little uptake. However, PET-CT is useful as lesions that have low uptake are more likely to be carcinoid as opposed to lesions with high uptake, which tend to be small cell or non-small cell lung cancer. An octreotide scan may be useful if there is concern for distant metastatic disease (more likely with central tumors, N2 disease, or carcinoid syndrome).

- *Labs.* If carcinoid syndrome is suspected, then proceed with measuring urine 5-hydroxyindoleacteic acid (5-HIAA) with a 24 hour collection (in addition to imaging, which will reveal liver mets in most cases). If Cushing's syndrome symptoms exist, then measure serum ACTH.

- *Pulmonary function tests (PFTs).* Lung function needs to be assessed to determine tolerance of a pulmonary resection depending on the clinical scenario. This is crucial for central tumors that may require a pneumonectomy or sleeve lobectomy.

- *Bronchoscopy.* Patients with central lesions may have visible disease that can be seen endobronchially. The central tumors are smooth and rounded; they are often red to reddish brown and covered with bronchial mucosa. Adequate sampling can yield the diagnosis of carcinoid. Endobronchial carcinoids tend to be hypervascular, therefore during biopsy be prepared to handle possible bleeding.

Index scenario (additional information)

"The patient's history and physical reveal no symptoms and no comorbidities. The mass on CT is 1.2 cm, homogenous, well demarcated and centrally located in the right lower lobe with no hilar or mediastinal lymphadenopathy. Bronchoscopy showed no endobronchial lesion. The patient's PFTs revealed an FEV 1 of 82% of predicted and DLCO of 60% of predicted. How would you proceed?"

Treatment/management

Diagnosis for this situation is based on clinical suspicion given the age of the patient and image findings. Needle biopsy is commonly non-diagnostic in the case of carcinoid and treatment is based primarily on clinical presentation. In this situation, the patient is young, without comorbidities, and has good pulmonary reserve; the patient will likely tolerate a pulmonary resection for diagnostic and therapeutic purposes. Intraoperative frozen section cannot differentiate between typical and atypical carcinoid.

Operative steps

Goals – explore, perform lobectomy.

- Double lumen ETT, adequate IV access, arterial line, foley catheter.
- Thoracoscopic approach (VATS)/versus open depending on comfort - (see Chapter 1, Early stage lung cancer (Ia-IIb) for additional details).
- Take down the inferior pulmonary ligament, send station 9 lymph nodes for permanent.
- Identify and dissect inferior pulmonary vein, locate and preserve the right middle lobe vein; once clearly identified, transect the inferior pulmonary vein.
- Dissect right lower lobe pulmonary artery; transect the right lower lobe pulmonary artery.
- Dissect the right lower lobe bronchus, careful to be distal from the bronchus to the right middle lobe. Ensure the preserved lung reinflates prior to transecting the right lower lobe bronchus.
- Complete the fissure between the right middle and right lower lobe.
- Ensure complete lung expansion and leave chest tube posteriorly and to the apex.

Potential questions/alternative scenarios

"The patient in the above scenario presented with a central lesion, however was found to have hilar lymphadenopathy. How would you proceed?"

Patients with a central carcinoid and hilar adenopathy are more likely to have an atypical carcinoid and should undergo mediastinoscopy before resection. This is also consistent with the ACCP guidelines for central lesions and N1 nodal disease. If the patient does have N2 disease, then they should undergo further imaging to work up for distant metastases including brain MRI, CT abdomen/pelvis, +/- PET CT, and/or octreotide scan. Neoadjuvant treatment with re-assessment for resection can be considered, although the modalities available for restaging are suboptimal. For this reason, some advocate resection after induction therapy with or without restaging.

"A 70 yo patient presents with a central pulmonary lesion with characteristics suggesting carcinoid and mediastinal lymphadenopathy by imaging. How would you proceed?"

Patients age > 50 with a central pulmonary lesion are more likely to have atypical carcinoid. In this situation, mediastinoscopy is indicated, which can yield the diagnosis of atypical carcinoid on final path (not frozen) if there is indeed lymph node involvement. Further imaging for distant metastases is warranted. Although the literature is not definitive, preoperative chemotherapy and radiation may also be considered (using regimen for small cell lung cancer, platinum-based chemotherapy) before proceeding to resection.

"A 65 yo man presented with a pedunculated endobronchial lesion on diagnostic bronchoscopy, CT chest reveals no extra-bronchial extension of the mass and no hilar or mediastinal disease. How would you manage this patient?"
Endobronchial resection is an option in this select group of patients who have isolated endobronchial pedunculated typical carcinoid. Endobronchial resection is not an option for atypical carcinoid, as these lesions are likely to have further extension. However, if this method is utilized, the patient requires extensive long-term follow-up including bronchoscopy, CT, and EBUS. It may cause significant structuring from scar tissue needing further intervention. Endobronchial resection can also be used to manage symptomatic patients in a palliative manner for whom surgical resection is contraindicated.

Pearls/pitfalls

- Typical carcinoid defined as tumor with neuroendocrine features, < 2 mitotic figures per 10 high power fields (hpfs) and no evidence of necrosis.
- Atypical carcinoid has 2 to 10 mitotic figures per 10 hpfs with evidence of necrosis or architectural disruption.
- Indolent, well-demarcated homogenous lesions are characteristic of carcinoid.
- Bi-modal distribution, with peaks age 30-39 and 50-59.
- Metabolically inactive, will usually not be detected on PET.
- Bronchial carcinoids do not present with carcinoid syndrome unless metastatic.
- Mediastinoscopy for hilar or mediastinal disease, if mediastinal disease present, pursue metastatic workup before resection.
- Resection for typical carcinoid is mainstay of treatment, even if N2 disease present given good long term survival.
- If chemotherapy needed, use regimen for small cell lung cancer (platinum-based).

Suggested readings

- Detterbeck FC. Management of carcinoid tumors. *Ann Thorac Surg.* 2010 Mar;89(3):998-1005.
- Simon GR, Turrisi A; American College of Chest Physicians. Management of small cell lung cancer: ACCP evidence-based clinical practice guidelines (2nd edition).*Chest.* 2007 Sep;132(3 Suppl):324S-339S.

- Wirth LJ, Carter MR, Jänne PA, Johnson BE Outcome of patients with pulmonary carcinoid tumors receiving chemotherapy or chemoradiotherapy. *Lung Cancer.* 2004 May;44(2):213-20.

Notes

6. Mediastinal staging

David D. Odell, MD, and Jonathan D'Cuhna, MD

Concept
- Indications for mediastinal evaluation
- Operative approaches to mediastinal staging
- Limitations of individual techniques
- Potential complications of mediastinoscopy and management

Chief complaint
"A 54 yo man with a 30 pack-year smoking history is referred to you by his primary care physician after a 4.3 cm right upper lobe mass was discovered on chest CT that was obtained to evaluate a 'persistent pneumonia'. A subsequent CT-guided biopsy of this lesion was pathologically consistent with adenocarcinoma. CT scan shows evidence of medistinal lymphadenopathy."

Differential
Mediastinal lymph node metastasis (N2 or N3 disease), reactive lymphadenopathy (due to a concomitant congestive heart failure or pulmonary infectious process), prior granulomatous disease (especially in patients with exposure history for tuberculosis, histoplasmosis, coccidiomycosis or other caseating infections), sarcoidosis, secondary lymphatic malignancy (lymphoma).

While the pathologic diagnosis of the primary tumor has been established in this scenario, staging is not complete. Prior to resection, an evaluation of the mediastinum for lymphatic involvement must be undertaken in addition to an assessment for distant metastatic disease. Lymphatic metastases may be seen in the setting of the radiographically normal mediastinum. In addition, adenopathy may be seen in several alternative clinical scenarios.

History and physical
A focused history should be taken to evaluate the candidacy of the patient for curative lung resection. A careful smoking history should be taken in all patients evaluated for lung cancer and current smokers should be strongly encouraged to quit smoking 2-3 weeks prior to surgical intervention, if possible. History of recent upper respiratory tract infection or pneumonia may increase the likelihood of reactive mediastinal adenopathy. Any prior history of surgical intervention in the neck or chest as well as prior chest radiation should be carefully reviewed as these issues may increase the difficulty of surgical staging.

A thorough physical exam should be performed with special attention paid to palpation of the cervical and supraclavicular lymph nodes. Neck extension should be evaluated to enhance understanding of the ability to position the patient for mediastinoscopy. Finally, careful auscultation of the carotid arteries should be performed. The finding of a bruit should prompt a formal duplex evaluation prior to any surgical staging procedure.

Tests

Preoperative testing in patients undergoing mediastinal staging for pulmonary malignancy centers on 3 main goals:
The first is to establish a clinical stage.
- CT or PET-CT (evaluate the thorax and upper abdomen for distant metastases)
- MRI or CT with contrast of the brain if neurologic symptoms are present

The second is to rule out any hazards to mediastinal staging.
- *CT chest*: aortic and head vessel calcification or aneurysmal disease
- *Carotid duplex*: for a patient with a bruit

The third is to assess the patients ability to tolerate any form of lung resection.
- Pulmonary function testing
- EKG (+/- formal cardiac evaluation depending upon patient age and clinical risk)

Index scenario (additional information)
"You counsel the patient that prior to surgical resection, a complete staging evaluation is necessary. He undergoes a PET-CT which demonstrates increased FDG avidity in the 4R and 7 nodal stations. The nodes are 1.4 cm in size at each of these stations, but normal on the contralateral side."

Treatment/management
Most surgeons agree that pathologic lymph node sampling is clearly indicated for nodes > 1 cm in short-axis diameter on CT or for any nodes with positive uptake on PET (typically an SUV > 2.5). T2 (> 3 cm) or greater tumors represent a relative indication as the rates of concomitant mediastinal disease are higher with these cancers. Adenocarcinoma and large cell primary tumor histology are also felt by some to be indications for pathologic mediastinal evaluation.

While cervical mediastinoscopy remains the gold standard, several methods of tissue-level mediastinal evaluation are available to the surgeon. Cervical mediastinoscopy allows access to level 2, 4, and 7 lymph node stations and can be done with an extremely low risk of morbidity and mortality. Potential complications include injury to adjacent vascular structures (discussed below), the recurrent laryngeal nerves (especially on the left), and esophageal or airway injury from biopsy attempts.

Endobronchial ultrasound (EBUS) guided fine needle aspiration affords the ability to sample nodal stations 2, 3, 4, 7, 10, and 11. Several studies have shown that EBUS provides accurate (> 97%) mediastinal staging. The use of rapid on-site pathologic evaluation to verify sample adequacy is helpful. The positive predictive value of the test is nearly 100% in most trials, while the negative predictive value has shown more variability. This has led some authors to recommend mediastinoscopy following a negative EBUS evaluation in patients with a high pre-test probability for mediastinal lymph node metastasis. Endoscopic ultrasound has also been used in mediastinal staging as an adjunct to mediastinoscopy and offers access to the level 5, 7, 8 and 9 lymph node stations.

Tumors of the left upper lobe commonly have initial lymph node metastases to the aorticopulmonary window lymph node (levels 5 and 6). These stations are not accessible by mediastinoscopy or by EBUS. This is one of the few scenarios in which resection can be considered in the setting of N2 disease (level 5 and 6 are level 2 nodes). The reason for this is that studies have shown that survival is similar for patient who undergo resection with N1 disease and those who undergo resection for a left upper lobe tumor and positive level 5 or 6 lymph nodes. The surgeon has a few options here. A conservative approach would be to confirm N2 involvement of the level 5 or 6 lymph nodes by biopsy (VATS or Chamberlain) and if positive, refer the patient for induction CRT. Another would be to give induction therapy without the biopsy, restage with PET-CT, and proceed with resection if there is no evidence of disease outside the primary and level 5 or 6 nodes. Finally, one may choose to proceed with resection and mediastinal lymph node dissection, followed by adjuvant CRT. On the other hand, if 5 and 6 appear abnormal in the setting of a right-sided tumor, which would indicate N3 disease, then it certainly needs to be sampled preoperatively.

The traditional approach to sampling this nodal basin is the Chamberlain procedure (anterior mediastinotomy), discussed below. Thoracoscopy also allows for an excellent ipsilateral nodal evaluation, including hilar lymph nodes. This approach has the added benefit of allowing for an evaluation of the primary tumor. Most often frozen section staging is performed before proceeding to resection in the same operative setting.

Thoracoscopic mediastinal lymph node evaluation is typically aimed at levels 4R and 7 from the right chest and levels 5, 6, and 7 from the left chest. Additional procedures for staging are necessary if there is concern regarding other nodal stations not accessed from the chest in patients undergoing primary VATS staging. Finally, staging of the ipsilateral hemithorax may be accomplished via thoracotomy, though this approach has fallen out of favor as a primary staging modality given the associated morbidity and efficacy of a VATS approach.

Operative steps

Mediastinoscopy

- General anesthesia in hospital-based setting.
- Supine positioning with a transverse scapular roll to elevate the chest and allow extension of the neck. The patient should be positioned with the head as high as possible on the operating room table to maximize extension. The surgical field should be prepped to include both the neck and entire anterior chest/upper abdomen in case emergency conversion to sternotomy is required.
- Incision is made transversely 1-2 cm above the sternal notch. The platysma is divided transversely. The strap muscles are separated vertically in the midline. The dissection is carried in the midline down to the pretracheal fascia.
- Incise the fascia with sharp scissors and enter the avascular pretracheal space.
- Blunt finger dissection along the anterior trachea into the mediastinum. One should be able to reach the carina, as well as the R and L mainstem bronchi.
- Establish vascular landmarks (innominate artery, arch of the aorta, R main PA) by digital palpation.
- Insert the mediastinoscope and follow the dissected pretracheal plane.
- Keeping the trachea and bronchi in view with the mediastinoscope is important to maintain orientation.
- Complete the dissection to the level of the carina by advancing the scope and performing blunt dissection with a suction device. Bluntly dissect along the right and left main stem bronchi, which will also help to maintain orientation.
- Lymph nodes are identified and individually dissected free from surrounding tissues using the suction device. Samples of nodal tissue are taken with a large cup laryngeal biopsy forceps. The upper paratracheal stations are typically sampled first, followed by the lower paratracheal stations. The subcarinal space is sampled last as this is most prone to bleeding.
- Level 2 nodes are above the innominate vein, level 4 are below the innominate vein and level 7 are within the subcarinal space.

- After sampling is complete, the scope is withdrawn as the region is inspected for bleeding. The skin incision is then closed in layers.

Anterior mediastinoscopy (Chamberlain procedure)
- Incision over the 2nd rib at the junction with the sternum. Some surgeons use a vertical incision so as to allow the extension of the dissection to another interspace if needed. The 2nd costal cartilage is removed to allow access.
- The pleura is pushed laterally using blunt dissection until the AP window lymph nodes are reached.
- Many surgeons insert a mediastinoscope through the interspace to facilitate dissection, rather than removing the costal cartilage.

Potential questions/alternative scenarios
"Will you plan to proceed to resection if there is no nodal metastasis demonstrated on frozen section?"
Either immediate or delayed resection is a reasonable choice. Some surgeons advocate a staged approach, with mediastinoscopy performed in a separate setting from the definitive resection for patients who present a higher operative risk due to medical comorbidities. In this setting, the staging procedure affords the opportunity to evaluate the patient's response to general anesthesia. Confidence in your pathology team is important when making decisions based on frozen section. Delaying surgery following mediastinoscopy has the potential to make the mediastinal lymph node sampling/dissection more complicated when one returns during the formal resection.

"In assessing the 4R lymph node station on mediastinoscopy, a dark structure is seen but you are unsure if this is a lymph node."
Do not biopsy any structure that is not clearly identified as a lymph node. The azygos vein and R pulmonary artery are both potentially mistaken for lymph nodes in the 4R position. Proceed with further gentle suction dissection around the node. If you are still unable to determine that the structure is not vascular, a long 21 gauge spinal needle may be used to aspirate the structure through the mediastinoscope.

"During mediastinoscopy, biopsy of a clearly defined lymph node in the subcarinal space results in significant bleeding, obscuring vision."
When the source of bleeding is clearly known to be a node or a small vessel within a nodal packet, the situation is best managed by passing a 1" gauze packing strip into the mediastinum via the mediastinoscope. Alternatively or additionally, one may pack operating room sponge(s) into the mediastinum for additional counter-pressure. The packing is allowed to remain in place for 2-10 minutes and then withdrawn. Selective use of electrocautery under direct vision may also be helpful in

controlling bleeding from nodal vasculature. Use of electrocautery should be avoided when taking lymph node biopsies from the 4L station to avoid injury to the left recurrent laryngeal nerve.

"While attempting to take a biopsy of the 4R lymph node station, a copious amount of blood fills the mediastinoscope, immediately obscuring vision. Simultaneously, the patient becomes hypotensive." In this scenario, a major vascular injury has occurred. Immediate understanding of the situation and mobilization of the appropriate resources is necessary to achieve a favorable outcome. To achieve temporary vascular control, one should pack the mediastinum with gauze via the mediastinoscope (as described above). The operating room team, anesthesia, and perfusion should be alerted regarding your concerns. Blood for transfusion should be brought to the operating room. Intravenous access should be optimized during this window of meta-stability. The surgeon should also call for additional surgical support as having additional sets of hands is key. In this biopsy location, the two structures most likely to be injured are the azygos vein and the right main pulmonary artery. Either of these vascular injuries will require immediate open operative intervention. When uncertain, a median sternotomy offers the most flexibility in dealing with vascular injuries given the ability to initiate cardiopulmonary bypass. Median sternotomy is preferred for injuries to the aortic arch, innominate artery, main pulmonary artery, and the superior vena cava. Even the azygos vein can be repaired via sternotomy. Consideration may also be given to proceeding to lobectomy rather than repair, especially if the tumor itself involves the right upper lobe. Selection of the appropriate operative approach for repair will depend upon the surgeon's assessment of the most likely area of injury.

Regardless of the incision, the primary operative goal is to quickly achieve vascular control. For proximal injuries, this may require cardiopulmonary bypass. Generally, assume the injury is worse than you think, as this is often the case. Further, you must be prepared as sometimes the injury may extend as you try to repair it. Once the incision is made, the injury is visually assessed and a plan for control and repair is formulated. Hilar injuries often require intrapericardial access for adequate proximal control (see Chapter 1, Early stage lung cancer (Ia-IIb). Vascular clamps are placed proximally and distally to the injury and repair/resection is then performed in a controlled manner.

"The bleeding source is localized to the right main pulmonary artery. After entering the pericardium, you are unable to get control of the injury proximally." While many pulmonary vascular injuries can be adequately controlled and exposed for repair with local dissection, proximal injuries will

typically require support with cardiopulmonary bypass for repair. Local control is established with direct pressure until a cardiopulmonary bypass circuit is available. Give full dose heparin and then place a proximal aortic cannula and two-stage venous cannula via the right atrium. Once ACT is within reasonable range (ideally > 480), initiate CPB. This will afford good decompression for repair. It is not necessary to arrest the heart in most circumstances to repair injuries to venous structures or the pulmonary arteries.

"An injury to the aortic arch is suspected, what will be your approach to assessment of the injury and repair?"
The initial goal is to attain control of bleeding in this situation. This may be accomplished by aggressively packing the mediastinum with gauze as described above. Rarely, this maneuver is not effective and either digital compression via the mediastinoscopy incision or emergency sternotomy may be required. If the injury is to the innominate artery, then perform a median sternotomy, give 10,000 units of heparin, obtain proximal and distal control, and repair directly or with a graft interposition.

Any injury to the aortic arch should be repaired with the assistance of cardiopulmonary bypass and may require circulatory arrest depending upon the extent of the injury. Once the bleeding is controlled, a careful assessment of the injury is necessary in order to plan the operation. The typical location of injury is along the undersurface of the aortic arch. Median sternotomy allows for direct visualization. TEE evaluation is invaluable to assess for the presence of aortic dissection and in some cases to localize the injury itself and guide cannulation. If the injury is focal, repair with pledgeted suture may be appropriate. However, care must be taken to rule out the presence of a dissection if a limited local repair is performed. If the injury is too extensive or your suture does not stop the bleeding, then give heparin and initiate CPB. Hopefully the injury is proximal to where you can safely cannulate and clamp. It this is true, then there should not be a need for circulatory arrest. If you can't clamp and cannulate distal to the injury then cannulate wherever you can on the ascending or arch, keep digital pressure on the injury, get venous access (2 stage RA vs. bicaval) and start cooling. Once you get to 20°, circ arrest and repair with or without graft material as needed. Recannulate the graft/ascending aorta and start warming. If there is a dissection this gets more complicated as a formal dissection repair will be required (see Chapters 47-48, Iatrogenic aortic dissection and Type A aortic dissection).

- Mediastinal metastasis may be found in as high as 10% of patients with a negative PET CT.
- Radiographic definition of pathological adenopathy is > 1 cm in short axis diameter.
- Recurrent laryngeal nerve injuries occur most commonly on the left and are usually a result of traction during dissection, not direct biopsy. 5-10% of patients may have hoarseness following mediastinoscopy.
- In addition to the complications highlighted above, mediastinoscopy has the following additional complications: tracheobronchial tree tear, esophageal tear, recurrent nerve injury, pneumothorax, thoracic duct injury, mediastinitis, venous air embolism, stroke, and tumor implantation.
- Contraindications (relative) to mediastinoscopy are as follows: Tracheostomies or laryngectomy, large goiter with calcifications, aneurysm or heavy calcification of the aortic arch or innominate artery, previous violation of the pretracheal plane by process such as mediastinitis, superior vena cava syndrome.

Suggested readings

- Goldstraw P, Crowley J, Chansky K, et al; The IASLC Lung Cancer Staging Project: Proposals for the revision of the TNM stage groupings in the forthcoming (seventh) edition of the TNM classification of malignant tumors. *Journal of Thoracic Oncology* 2:706-14, 2007.
- Pearson FG, The use of mediastinoscopy in the selection of patients for lung cancer operations. *Annals of Thoracic Surgery* 30:205-7, 1980.
- Detterbeck FC, Jantz MA, Wallace M, Invasive mediastinal staging of lung cancer. ACCP evidence-based clinical practice guidelines. (2nd edition) *Chest* 132 (3 Suppl): 202S-220S, 2007.
- Ahmad US, Blum MG. Invasive diagnostic procedures. General Thoracic Surgery (7th edition) ed. Shields TW et al. Lippincott, Williams & Wilkins, Philadelphia PA. 2009.

Notes

7. Pulmonary metastasectomy

Fatuma Kromah, MD, and Dennis Wigle, MD

Concept

- Knowledge of primary tumors that metastasize to the lung
- Presentation of a patient with pulmonary metastasis
- Diagnostic evaluation
- Criteria for surgical intervention
- Contraindications and limitations to pulmonary metastasectomy
- Technical aspects of metastasectomy
- Pitfalls in pulmonary metastasectomy
- Non-surgical management

Chief complaint

"A 41 yo woman who is a former smoker is referred to you with a history of surgical resection and adjuvant chemotherapy 3 years prior for a locoregionally advanced colon cancer. She is now referred to you after a CT scan revealed bilateral pulmonary nodules, an enlarged subcarinal lymph node, and a mass in the posterior right hepatic lobe. What are your differential diagnoses and how would you proceed?"

Differential

- Metastatic colon cancer to the liver and lung
  - Colorectal cancer pulmonary metastasis fast facts
    - 20% metastases at the time of initial diagnosis.
    - 5-year survival in untreated metastatic disease: < 5-10%.
    - 5-year survival after pulmonary metastasectomy: 39-56%.
- Primary lung cancer with metastasis to the liver
- Synchronous primary lung and liver cancers
- Primary liver cancer with metastasis to the lung
- Metastatic colon cancer and primary lung cancer
- Benign lesions

NOTE: Other primary tumors that metastasize to the lung with some published pulmonary metastasectomy survival rates

- Sarcomas
  - Soft tissue sarcoma
    - 3-year survival without metastasectomy: 2%.
    - 3-year survival with metastasectomy: 23%

- Osteogenic sarcoma
  - Favorable diagnostic factors: less than two metastases and disease-free interval (DFI) > 24 months.
- Breast carcinoma
  - 5-, 10-, 15-year survival with pulmonary metastasectomy: 38%, 22%, and 20% respectively.
- Head and neck cancer
  - 5-year survival rates after metastasectomy: 29% to 59%
- Renal cell carcinoma
  - 5-year survival with pulmonary metastasectomy:
    - 42-45% after complete resection
    - 8-22% after incomplete resection.
- Germ cell cancer
  - 5-year survival with pulmonary metastasectomy for testicular germ cell cancer: 68%.
- Melanoma
  - 5-year survival with incomplete resection: 13%
  - 5-year survival with pulmonary metastasectomy: 21%
- Gastric
  - 5-year survival with chemotherapy: 2%
  - 5-year survival with pulmonary metastasectomy: 33%.
- Endocrine tumors
  - 5-year survival with pulmonary metastasectomy: 61%
- Gynecologic tumor
  - Uterine cancer 5-year survival rate with metastasectomy: 53%.
  - Cervical cancer 5-year survival rate with metastasectomy: 0-52%.
- Hepatocellular carcinoma
  - 5-year overall survival (OS): 40.9%.

History and physical

Patients presenting with pulmonary metastases are asymptomatic 75% to 90% of the time with lesions found incidentally during staging and follow-up of the primary malignancy. In obtaining a history, one should inquire about symptoms like hemoptysis that may be caused by centrally located lesions, cough suggesting endobronchial involvement, pain as a result of pleural involvement or chest wall invasion, and dyspnea which may be suggestive of airway obstruction or pleural effusion. Assessing the patient's cardiac and pulmonary functional status is vital in determining candidacy for surgical intervention. Inquiry of cancer risk factors like tobacco usage should be made with smoking cessation counseling as needed. Additionally, a thorough history to include the patient's comorbidities, prior surgeries (especially any prior thoracic surgeries), and family history of cancer should be obtained. It is also important to ensure that there are no symptoms related to recurrent colon cancer.

"This patient's history and physical exam is otherwise unremarkable except for a prior smoking history (20 pack-years) and the abdominal surgical scars. Her performance status is ECOG score zero (good functional status). What tests or studies should be obtained?"

Tests
- *CXR*: may be initial imaging identifying the suspicious lesion(s).
- *Computed tomography scan*: gold standard for pulmonary metastases. 4-5 mm helical CT scans detect 20% more nodules than conventional CT scan and result in 12% increase in the number of definite nodules detected. Suggested timing for obtaining CT scan is within 4 weeks of metastasectomy.
- *PET-CT scan*. PET may be positive in only 67.5% of metastatic pulmonary nodules and is not sensitive for evaluation of lung nodules in the metastatic setting. PET mediastinal staging has a sensitivity, accuracy, and negative predictive value of 100%, 96%, and 100%, respectively, versus 71%, 92%, and 95% for CT scan alone.
- *Bronchoscopy*: important for central lesions with possible endobronchial invasion.
- *Endobronchial ultrasound (EBUS) and mediastinoscopy*: used only if there is suspicious mediastinal lymphadenopathy. If the mediastinum is positive, the survival benefit of metastasectomy decreases significantly and it is arguable if one should proceed with resection.
- *Pulmonary function testing (PFT)*: is required for assessing performance status and ability to tolerate surgery (see Chapter 1, Early stage lung cancer (Ia-IIb), on lung cancer regarding PFT criteria for resection).

Index scenario (additional information)
"The CT scan characteristics of the lesions were highly suspicious for metastasis so a biopsy was not performed. The patient undergoes chemotherapy. Follow-up CT scan shows stable pulmonary nodules and decrease in the size of the liver metastasis with internal necrosis. What would you do next?"

Treatment/management

Since the pulmonary lesions are stable, it is decided the patient will undergo abdominal surgery first and subsequently the pulmonary metastasectomy. The patient undergoes a right hepatectomy. The hepatic lesion is consistent with colon metastasis. One month postoperatively, a repeat CT scan showed no new intra-abdominal metastases. There is a new 1.5 cm lymph node adjacent to the SVC and pulmonary vein in addition to the bilateral pulmonary nodules. You decide on simultaneous bilateral pulmonary metastasectomies with video assisted thorascopic surgery (VATS) for wedge resections and mediastinal lymphadenectomy.

Operative steps

- General anesthesia with double-lumen endotracheal tube
- Lateral decubitus position with flexion of bed
- VATS incisions and examination of the lung and chest cavity
- Identification of the pulmonary nodules by visualization and digital palpation
- Wedge resections with 1 cm margins using endoscopic stapler and ensuring that excessive lung parenchymal tissue is not resected
- Placement of wedged lung into a protective bag and removal from the chest cavity to prevent droplet spread or contamination
- Specimen should be sent for frozen section to make sure that the lesion is not a primary lung cancer (particularly since the patient has a smoking history)
- Mediastinal lymph node dissection
- Obtain hemostasis, place chest tube, and re-expand the lung under direct visualization
- Close incisions
- Reposition patient in lateral decubitus position on opposite side and repeat as above

"The final pathology report comes back and further examination of the dissected lymph nodes shows one lymph node positive for metastatic cancer. Is there a role for lymph node dissection during pulmonary metastasectomy?"

The reported incidence of mediastinal nodal metastases: 5%-28.6% for all cell types. Lymph node metastases at the time of pulmonary metastasectomy have an adverse effect on prognosis. Three-year survival with negative lymph nodes has been shown to be 69%, compared with 38% for patients with positive lymph nodes. Complete mediastinal lymph node dissection improves staging and can guide treatment. This area is somewhat controversial, as many surgeons do not routinely perform a mediastinal lymph node sampling or dissection at the time of metastasectomy. However, if there are FDG-avid mediastinal lymph nodes or enlarged lymph nodes (> 1 cm in the short axis), then mediastinal lymph dissection is certainly warranted.

"What are the selection criteria for pulmonary metastasectomy?"
Patients may be considered for pulmonary metastasectomy if there is proven control of the primary tumor (no recurrence or residual disease at the primary site) with complete R0 resection, ability to resect all metastatic disease, and sufficient cardiopulmonary reserve for the planned resection. Re-resection can be considered in selected patients. Ablative techniques (SBRT, RF ablation) can be considered when the patient is not a surgical candidate (inadequate physiologic reserve, refuses surgery) and the lesion(s) is amenable to complete ablation. Patients with resectable synchronous metastases can be resected synchronously or using a staged approach.

"What surgical options and approaches are there for bilateral pulmonary metastases?"
The surgical approach used for metastasectomy is based on the principle of performing a complete resection with preservation of lung tissue (in case of future metastasectomy). Standard therapy is wedge resection with a negative 1 cm margin. Deeply located or central lesions may require anatomic resection: segmentectomy, lobectomy, or, rarely, pneumonectomy. Approaches include:

- *Sternotomy.* Allows for simultaneous exposure, visualization, examination, and palpation of bilateral lungs. Issues with sternal wound healing after radiation. Difficult access to the posterolateral left lung.

- *Sequential thoracotomies.* Allow healing and recovery from the first surgery before performing the next. Optimal time for contralateral resection is unclear, however most recommend a repeat chest CT for surgical planning prior to the subsequent resection.

- *Bilateral thoracotomies (clamshell).* Allows access to both hemithorax during the same operation. Internal mammary arteries are sacrificed. Increased morbidity versus unilateral approach.

- *Video-assisted thoracic surgery (VATS).* Less pain and shorter hospital stay. Studies have shown comparable 5-year overall survival rates and median survival for thoracotomy and VATS. Lose bimanual tactile ability, potentially resulting in higher rate of missed metastases.

"The patient presents to you one year after her pulmonary metastasectomy with a CT scan of the chest that now shows new right-sided pulmonary nodules suspicious for colon metastases. Is there any evidence to support performing multiple metastasectomies for recurrent pulmonary metastases? How is survival affected?"

Multiple attempts to re-establish intrathoracic control of metastatic disease can be justified in carefully selected patients, but the magnitude of benefit decreases with each subsequent attempt. 5-year survival for patients undergoing 2 metastasectomies is 60%, 3 metastasectomies is 33%, and 4 or more metastasectomies is 38% (all-comers, not just colon metastases). From the time a recurrence is declared unresectable, 2-year survival is 19% (median 8 months).

"What if the patient has insufficient cardiopulmonary reserve to tolerate surgery or has had multiple prior surgeries? Alternatively, what if the patient is a surgical candidate but declines surgery? What alternative treatments are available?"

- *Stereotatic body radiation therapy (SBRT).* Safe, tolerable, and effective local treatment option in select patients.
- *Radiofrequency (RF) ablation.* Inclusion criteria are: lesions < 5 cm in diameter, inoperable non–small cell lung cancer, and no more than four secondary lesions bilaterally. The feasibility depends on factors including the presence of an "access window" and proximity to hilar structures. Uncorrectable coagulopathy is an absolute contraindication for RF ablation. Complications of RF ablation include pneumothorax, pleural effusion, hyperpyrexia, infection, and hemorrhage.
- *Neodymium:yttrium-aluminum garnet laser (Nd:YAG).* Treatment with Nd:YAG laser may facilitate complete resection of multiple bilateral
centrally located metastases, is lobe sparing, and can improve long-term survival.
- *Isolated lung perfusion.* An alternative chemotherapeutic delivery method that allows high local doses with reduced incidence of systemic toxicities.

Pearls/pitfalls

- Metastesectomy should not be performed unless there is sufficient evidence to support local control of the primary tumor site.
- Pulmonary metastatic lesions should be amenable to complete resection to consider metastasectomy.
- Good prognostic indicators for pulmonary metastasectomies are resectability, disease-free interval greater than 36 months, and solitary metastases in select patients.
- Overall survival can be improved in multiple histologic tumors.

- A video-assisted approach for pulmonary metastasectomy in select patients offers comparable survival benefit compared to open procedures.
- Mediastinal staging is essential in identifying patients who are not disease-free and who may require additional treatment, as the presence of lymph node metastasis has an adverse effect on prognosis.
- Pulmonary metastasectomy can be performed concomitantly, sequentially, or staged without a change in survival.
- Local ablative therapy is a safe and effective modality. These techniques are proving to be a satisfactory alternative to surgery with an increasing role in non-surgical candidates and those who do not want surgery. The alternatives should be addressed from a multidisciplinary approach.

Suggested readings

- Pastorino U, Buyse M, Friedel G, et al. Long-term results of lung metastasectomy: Prognostic analyses based on 5206 cases. *J Thorac Cardiovasc Surg 1997;113:37-049.*
- Ercan S. Nichols FC. Trastek VF. Deschamps C. et al. Prognostic significance of lymph node metastasis found during pulmonary metastasectomy for extrapulmonary carcinoma. *Annals of Thoracic Surgery 2004 May;77(5):1786-91.*
- Jaklitsch MT, Mery CM, Lukanich JM, et al. Sequential thoracic metastasectomy prolong survival by re-establishing local control within the chest. *J Thorac Cardiovasc Surg 2001;121:657-67.*
- National Cancer Comprehensive Network Guidelines Version 1.2013 Colon Cancer.
  Accessed September 23, 2012.
  http://www.nccn.org/professionals/physician_gls/PDF/colon.pdf.
- Erhunmwunsee L, D'Amico TA. Surgical Management of Pulmonary Metastases. *Ann Thorac Surg. 2009;88:2052-2060.*

Notes

8. Pleural effusions and empyema

Nakul Vakil, MD, and Daniel Raymond, MD

Concept
- Diagnosis of pleural effusions
- Initial management
- Fluid analysis
- Operative management
- Pitfalls and alternative solutions

Chief complaint
"A 70 yo man on the medical service is referred to you because of an increasing right-sided pleural effusion and shortness of breath."

Differential
The differential for shortness of breath is broad. However, a history and physical as well as review of imaging will suggest if the SOB is most likely caused by the effusion or another etiology (cardiac, pulmonary embolism, etc). The differential for an effusion includes cardiogenic, infectious, malignant or hepatic (hepatic hydrothorax) causes.

History and physical
Dyspnea is the most common complaint associated with an effusion. Chest auscultation (decreased breath sounds, dullness to percussion, etc.) can help establish a diagnosis. Presence of systemic signs of infection (fevers, WBC elevation) can lead one to suspect an empyema/parapneumonic effusion. Heart sound auscultation and assessment of JVD/lower extremity edema could suggest a cardiac etiology. Abdominal exam revealing caput medusa or ascites may suggest hepatic pathology (hepatic hydrothorax). A known, prior, or suspected neoplasm, chest pain and prior smoking/asbestos exposure may suggest a malignant etiology.

Tests
- *CXR.* Plain AP or PA/lateral will identify the effusion. Traditional teaching is to obtain a decubitus film to rule out loculations. This may not be needed with the availability of ultrasound/CT scanning. Typically, there will need to be at about 200 cc of fluid to see blunting of the costophrenic angle on a plain film.
- *Ultrasound (U/S).* U/S can provide information regarding loculations, the distance between the effusion and chest wall, and depth of the effusion itself.

- *Chest CT.* CT scan provides additional information on the lung tissue, mediastinal lymph nodes and upper abdominal pathology which may differentiate pleural versus non-pleural processes. CT scanning will also provide information on thickness of pleura, pleural nodularity, anatomy of loculated fluid, and entrapment. Contrasted CT scans are superior at identification of adenopathy and differentiating atelectatic lung from pleural masses.

Index scenario (additional information)

"The patient has been hospitalized over the past several days for urosepsis. His unilateral right effusion has recently increased and is accompanied by low grade fevers and an increasing oxygen requirement. He is already on antibiotics for the resolving urosepsis. CXR shows a moderate right-sided effusion."

Treatment/management

Thoracentesis is typically the first step after radiographic evaluation of an effusion. Thoracentesis often confirms a suspicion based on H&P and imaging. It is both diagnostic (exudative versus transudative, cytology, gram stain and culture) and can be therapeutic in cases of certain effusions. Thoracentesis can be done: 1) using real time ultrasound, 2) with ultrasound marking of the chest wall for guidance of subsequent thoracentesis, 3) one to two rib spaces below the area of dullness to percussion, or 4) with CT guidance. The traditional teaching is to drain less than 1500 cc initially or to stop drainage when the patient has chest discomfort or coughing in order to avoid re-expansion pulmonary edema. Thoracentesis should generally be avoided in patients on mechanical ventilatory support because of a higher risk of pneumothorax and difficult positioning -- these patients are better candidates for tube thoracostomy. The gross appearance of aspirated fluid may suggest the process at work. Bloody aspirates are associated with trauma or malignancy; purulence suggests an empyema, and milky appearance suggests a chylothorax. Less obvious distinctions can be made based on the pleural fluid analysis.

Fluid is typically sent for culture, cytology, cell count with differential, LDH, Glucose, protein, and pH. Additional tests can be ordered when esophageal or pancreatic etiologies are suspected such as amylase. Although there are others, Light's criteria is the classic way of making this determination based on pleural fluid characteristics. It has a very high sensitivity but is less specific. Exudates are defined as: pleural to serum protein ratio > 0.5, pleural to serum LDH ratio > 0.6, and a pleural LDH > 2/3 the upper limits of the laboratory's normal serum LDH value. Different strategies are employed for benign versus malignant effusions.

Benign effusions

Transudative

Most benign transudative effusions are caused by congestive heart failure and/or renal failure and tend to be bilateral. These should be medically managed with treatment of the underlying cause. Nephrotic syndrome and hepatic hydrothorax are less common causes. These too should be managed with attention to the underlying process. Recurrent symptomatic effusions can be ameliorated with thoracentesis. Tube thoracostomy is not recommended in hepatic hydrothorax.

Exudative

Management of exudative effusions is more complex. Parapneumonic effusions are those exudative effusions associated with a pneumonia or other lung infections. The evolution of an exudative effusion is from an exudative phase with negative bacterial studies and free-flowing fluid, to a fibropurulent phase (positive bacterial studies) and frequently with loculation, and finally to a chronic, organized phase with a pleural rind.

- Uncomplicated parapneumonic effusions generally do not need drainage (other than what was achieved already by thoracentesis). These can be managed with appropriate antibiotics. Most of these resolve on their own, but a small percentage progress to empyema. If the patient is symptomatic (i.e., dyspneic), the effusion should be drained.
- The presence of purulence or positive bacterial studies necessitates drainage. This can be done with tube thoracostomy or image-guided (US or CT) placement of small bore drains. If this fails, one can consider fibrinolysis through an existing tube (i.e., intrapleural administration of tPA). Failure is defined as incomplete drainage of the empyema or incomplete expansion of the lung. Failure of tube thoracostomy, presence of a trapped lung, or a persistent effusion (greater than two to three weeks where there is likely to be a significant inflammatory process) necessitates either thoracoscopic or open decortication.
- Uncomplicated post-cardiotomy exudative effusions can almost always be managed medically or with thoracentesis. Surgery is for the few who develop lung entrapment.
- Patients who fail surgical treatment of the empyema or those with bronchopleural fistulae may need open pleural drainage by a cavernostomy (Eloesser flap or Clagett window).

Malignant effusions

Metastatic disease to the pleura affects pleural fluid reabsorption and/or production. Moderate to large symptomatic effusions can be managed initially with thoracentesis (also diagnostic) and with pleurodesis or an indwelling pleural catheter, as malignant effusions tend to recur.

- *Pleurodesis*: only possible when there already is pleural apposition (i.e., cannot work in cases of lung entrapment). This can be done either through an existing catheter or thoracostomy tube, or during a VATS procedure.
- *Indwelling pleural catheter*. This is an option for patients who lack pleural apposition and in those whom the risks of an operative intervention (decortication) outweigh the benefits (e.g., PleurX Catheter).

Potential questions/alternative scenarios

"Thoracentesis reveals purulence and an exudative effusion by Light's criteria. The empyema is only partially drained on post-procedure imaging. Records indicate he has had this effusion for three weeks."

First, the fluid should be sent for culture and IV antibiotics should be tailored appropriately. The patient's effusion has likely progressed to the fibropurulent or chronic, organized phase. If the patient is not septic and is hemodynamically stable, taking a more conservative approach (non-operative) is reasonable. A non-contrast CT of the chest will be helpful to determine if there are extensive loculations or the presence of a thick rind. If there are minimal loculations and no rind, placement of one or two chest tubes may allow for complete drainage of the pleural space. If there are significant loculations, then the surgeon has a couple of options. One or two chest tubes can be placed and fibrinolysis attempted with tPA administration through the tubes. If only one or two pockets of undrained fluid remain, image-guided (either CT or US) thoracentesis or placement of smaller pleural catheters may provide adequate drainage. If this fails, proceed to the OR for VATS or open drainage. Alternatively, since the chance of complete drainage is lower in the presence of significant loculations, it is reasonable to proceed to the OR for drainage and disruption of loculations at the first encounter rather than prolonging things with multiple chest tubes. Rarely is a complete decortication needed at this stage, but be prepared for the possibility of finding a thicker rind than anticipated. Moreover, if the patient has persistent fevers or starts becoming septic, then earlier operative intervention is required. Success may be higher with an open then VATS procedure, although it is very reasonable to start with VATS.

"You are referred another patient who has recovered from a left-sided pneumonia. He was noted to have a parapneumonic effusion at the time of infection, which was drained by thoracentesis once. His repeat CXR 2 weeks later shows clear lungs, but a persistent left-sided effusion. This is again drained by thoracentesis and pleural fluid cultures are negative. After drainage of the effusion, the lung does not re-expand fully. A non-contrast CT does not show any loculations. The patient gets progressively more short of breath over the next 3 days and

the effusion has reaccumulated. How would you manage this patient?"
The patient likely has a fibrothorax First a bronchoscopy should be performed to make sure there is no mucus plugging that is preventing ventilation of the atelectatic lung. Assuming the airways are clear, then it can be assumed the lung is not expanding due to an entrapped lung. Treatment is decortication. Thoracoscopic treatment may not be successful as this is likely a long standing process; it can be attempted with a low threshold to convert to open thoracotomy.

Operative steps

Decortication

Thoracoscopic or open approaches are reasonable, however success with thoracoscopic approaches decreases with duration of effusion and presence of a chronic empyema. Objectives of decortication are 1) Wide drainage - break up loculations, drain residual fluid, leave well placed drainage tubes 2) Lung expansion - separate the pleural peel from the visceral pleura along the entire pleural surface (including the diaphragmatic pleural surface) in order to establish complete lung expansion.

- Double lumen intubation, 2 large bore IV's, foley.
- Position the patient in the right decubitus position with the left side up and isolate the lung.
- A posterolateral thoracotomy in the fifth intercostal space will provide adequate exposure. If a VATS approach is to be taken, care must be taken to avoid placing the initial port too low in the chest, as there will be volume loss from the atelectatic lung and the diaphragm will be higher than usual. The remaining ports are placed under direct thoracoscopic vision.
- Care must be taken when entering the chest, as the lung may be adherent to the parietal pleura.
- Once in the chest, residual fluid should be drained and sent for gram stain and culture.
- The pleural peel, or rind, must then be meticulously dissected away from the visceral pleura of the lung; avoid tearing into the parenchyma. Doing so will result in air leaks postoperatively, necessitating prolonged chest tube drainage.
- Decorticating the lung may result in significant bleeding from the lung surface due to the extensive inflammation. Blood transfusion may be needed if this is excessive.
- The lung must be freed up circumferentially, including the diaphragmatic surface of the lung.
- Once the lung has been freed up, the chest is irrigated and the atelectatic lung is then ventilated. Areas that do not expand fully may need additional decortication. Full lung re-expansion is crucial for a successful decortication.

- Multiple chest tubes are placed to assure adequate drainage and the chest is closed.
- Bleeding from the lung surface typically subsides with full lung re-expansion and pleural apposition, but it is not uncommon for there to be some persistent oozing for a few hours postoperatively. Make sure clotting factors are replaced as needed. Get as much hemostasis as possible prior to leaving the OR
- The patient should be extubated as soon as possible to reduce air leaks. At times some positive pressure may be warranted for adequate lung expansion of residual segments.
- Chest tubes remain until all air leaks have resolved and drainage is minimal.

"A 67 yo man with recent STEMI treated with multiple drug eluting stents, EF of 30%, on Plavix, and renal failure now presents one month after a pneumonia that was complicated by a parapneumonic effusion treated with thoracostomy tube drainage. His chest CT shows an effusion with multiple locules of gas and a thick pleural peel, consistent with an empyema. There are also multiple pockets of fluid that are not easily accessible by percutaneous drainage. He is septic, but blood pressures are stable on minimal pressor support. He has been on broad spectrum antibiotics for 2 days. You feel that he needs drainage and decortication, but are concerned that he is too high risk to tolerate this. What are some alternative options."

An Eloesser flap represents a quicker and safer operation for a very ill and debilitated patient who may not tolerate a full decortication. One needs to ensure that the lung is in fact trapped and will not collapse based on timing (> 3 weeks), imaging alone (thick rind), or imaging pre- and post-drainage (lung stays entrapped). Resect a segment of 2 to 3 ribs in the dependent portion of the chest. Suture the skin to the thickened pleural rind or the ribs to keep the site open. The cavity can be irrigated daily and the chest packed with wet to dry gauze. Once the patient is medically stable, nutritionally replete, the cavity begins to granulate in, and significant air leaks have resolved, then a VAC dressing may be applied. Alternatively the space can be filled with tissue (muscle or omental flap) to obliterate the space once the empyema cavity has been cleared of infection.

"You are consulted on a patient with metastatic breast cancer who is severely debilitated. She was admitted with complaints of dyspnea and was found to have a moderate left pleural effusion, which was drained by thoracentesis. Cytology was positive. Her post-drainage CXR shows full lung re-expansion and her symptoms are significantly improved.

She wants to know if you can do anything to prevent this from happening again."

This patient is a good candidate for pleurodesis given that the lung has fully expanded and the high likelihood of recurrence. Chemical irritants (sclerosants) cause pleural inflammation, eventually causing fusion of the visceral and parietal pleura if there is good pleural apposition. Adequate pleural drainage is needed for at least 48-72 hours after the sclerosing agent is administered to prevent reaccumulation of fluid and separation of the pleural surfaces. Options include sterile talc, doxycycline, or bleomycin. These agents can cause significant discomfort due to the inflammation they cause and adequate analgesia is required. Talc can be administered through a chest tube (but not smaller pleural catheters) at the bedside or through small incisions (VATS or open) in the operating room. Doxycycline or bleomycin can be administered via chest tube or smaller pleural catheters. If pleurodesis is unsuccessful in this debilitated patient with metastatic disease, then placement of a permanent indwelling pleural catheter (e.g., PleurX Catheter) is another option.

"You are referred a patient with metastatic esophageal cancer who is severely debilitated. The patient has a right-sided malignant effusion that has been drained by thoracentesis multiple times in the past. The most recent post-drainage CXR is read as a right hydropneumothorax. How would you manage this patient?"

This patient has an entrapped lung with a space that will re-accumulate. In other words, there is no pneumothorax. These patients cannot be successfully managed with pleurodesis, as pleural apposition is needed for this to be successful. Severely debilitated patients may not tolerate a thoracotomy for palliation of symptoms and survival in this type of metastatic cancer may be limited. In this case, the patient may be best served by a long term indwelling, tunneled pleural catheter that can be placed with or without VATS (Pleurex).

"You are consulted on a patient with a history of Child's class B cirrhosis and ascites. He has had multiple prior thoracenteses for a recurrent, transudative, right pleural effusion. The patient now has severe shortness of breath and opacification of the right chest on portable CXR despite drainage only 2 days ago. How would you proceed?"

This is likely a hepatic hydrothorax. Treatment is continued serial thoracenteses for relief of symptoms and aggressive treatment of portal hypertension, including diuresis and consideration for TIPS. Chest tubes should be avoided in cirrhotic patients with hepatic hydrothorax due to concerns for development of pleurocutaneous fistulae, as chest tube output will remain significant until the underlying disease process has been treated.

65

- *Light's criteria for exudative process*: pleural to serum protein ratio > 0.5, pleural to serum LDH ratio > 0.6; highly sensitive, less specific.
- Pleurodesis is an option only when there is pleural apposition, consider decortication or indwelling catheter drainage in cases of lung entrapment. Pleurodesis (versus repeated tapping) should be considered for malignant pleural effusions in patients with pleural apposition and life expectancy greater than 1-2 months.
- Most parapneumonic effusions do not require tube thoracostomy drainage. It is indicated for effusions that cause dyspnea or for those with purulence or positive bacterial studies.
- In cases of benign effusion, the goals of tube thoracostomy are drainage of fluid and full lung expansion, if this fails then one should consider VATS or open decortication. VATS or open decortication should be first line treatment in well established effusions which are unlikely to benefit from local therapy.
- Avoid chest tubes in patients with hepatic hydrothorax.

Suggested readings

- British thoracic society pleural disease guideline 2010 – a quick reference guide. *Thoracic Society Reports.* 2(3): 20.

Notes

9. Infectious lung disease

David Mauchley, MD, and John Mitchell, MD

Concept
- General work-up for a patient with a pulmonary infection
- Bacterial pulmonary abscess
- Aspergilloma
- Zygomycosis
- Multidrug-resistant tuberculosis

Chief complaint
"You are called by one of your internal medicine colleagues to evaluate a 75 yo woman admitted for presumed community acquired pneumonia. Since admission 24 hours ago, she has had persistent fevers and productive sputum despite IV antibiotic therapy. You have been consulted because she has additionally developed hemoptysis in the last few hours."

Differential
Community acquired pneumonia, tuberculosis, invasive fungal infection, pulmonary abscess, bronchiectasis, malignancy (post-obstructive infection)

History and physical
Typical symptoms of the majority of pulmonary infections include cough, dyspnea, sputum production, and pleuritic chest pain. Timing and duration of these symptoms is important to determine whether this is an acute or chronic problem. A patient with a bacterial pulmonary abscess would likely have had symptoms for a shorter period of time than a patient with recurrent infections in the setting of bronchiectasis. The immunologic status of the patient is also very important when evaluating a patient with complicated lung infection. Immunosuppressed patients (previous transplant, chemotherapy, long term steroid use) are more likely to suffer from invasive *Aspergillus* infection. A history of structural lung disease (bullous emphysema, fibrotic lung disease, cavitary tuberculosis, sarcoidosis with bullae) makes the diagnosis of mycetoma (*aspergillus, histoplasma, blastomyces, coccidioides*) more likely.

Typical physical exam findings in patients with lung infections include fever, tachycardia, and tachypnea. Crackles on auscultation are also common. In the setting of a parapneumonic effusion, breath sounds may be diminished or absent on the affected side. Evaluation of dentition can be of some use in patients with suspected bacterial pulmonary abscess, as aspiration of anaerobic organisms from oral infections can lead to abscess formation.

Tests

- *Imaging.* PA/lateral CXR can identify the location of consolidation in the event of pneumonia. There might also be evidence of a pulmonary abscess or parapneumonic effusion on plain film. Chest CT will give more detailed anatomic information and should be ordered in the event that the plain films do not offer a definitive diagnosis.

- *Labs.* Any patient hospitalized with a pulmonary infectious problem that requires surgical consultation should have a complete blood count, basic electrolytes, renal and hepatic function tests, and a coagulation panel sent. In febrile patients, blood cultures, urinalysis, and urine culture should be obtained. All patients with a suspected pulmonary infection should have a sputum culture sent. If a pulmonary resection is being entertained, preoperative spirometry and diffusion capacity can be used to estimate perioperative risk. If surgery is indicated, a type and screen or crossmatch should be ordered depending on the complexity of operation and likelihood of major blood loss.

- *Identification of organisms.* In order to successfully treat a pulmonary infection, it is helpful to accurately identify the precipitating pathogen. Sputum should be collected in any patient suspected of having a pulmonary infection, but these samples are negative 50% of the time in cases where the presence of infection has been proven in other ways. Furthermore, many sputum samples come back contaminated with normal respiratory flora, making them useless. There are a number of other more invasive means of obtaining an accurate diagnosis.

  - *Fiberoptic bronchoscopy.* This method allows direct sampling of the infected part of the lung. Collection of bronchoalveolar lavage samples from this area helps eliminate contamination with normal respiratory flora.

  - *Endobronchial ultrasound.* In rare cases where samples of pulmonary parenchyma are needed for definitive sampling. Fine needle aspirates can be taken under ultrasound guidance.

  - *Transthoracic needle aspiration.* Performing an aspiration or biopsy of a suspected area of infection eliminates the possibility of contamination with respiratory flora considerably. This technique is particularly helpful when obtaining samples from an abscess cavity or pleural effusion/empyema.

"The patient's history and physical reveal that her symptoms of cough, malaise, and fever have been going on for approximately one week. Her hemoptysis started yesterday and is ultimately what brought her to the hospital. Over the last month she has noticed that she has developed some difficulty swallowing and frequently chokes when eating. She is previously healthy and is on no medications. Her WBC is elevated at 25,000 and the rest of her labs are normal. Sputum, blood and urine cultures are pending. CT scan shows a 5 x 6 cm cavity in the superior segment of her right lower lobe with an air-fluid level and surrounding parenchymal consolidation."

Treatment/management

Given her history, there is high suspicion for a bacterial pulmonary abscess, particularly with the recent aspiration symptoms. Furthermore, pulmonary abscesses frequently will develop in the superior segments of either lower lobe because of their dependent locations. The posterior segments of the upper lobes are also frequently involved for the same reason. Treatment of a bacterial pulmonary abscess is medical initially and involves antibacterial therapy, chest physiotherapy/postural drainage, and nutritional support. Antibiotic coverage should start broad and be narrowed based on culture results. If aspiration is suspected or the patient recently has significant dental work, anaerobic coverage should be initiated. The most commonly involved organisms are: Peptostreptococcus, Bacteroides, Staph aureus, Strep pneumo, Haemophilus, Klebsiella, Mycobacteria. Antibiotics are generally continued for 6-8 weeks.

Differentiating a simple bacterial pulmonary abscess from an infected cavitary lung carcinoma can be challenging. If there is any question of malignancy, flexible bronchoscopy can be performed to rule out an obstructing tumor or other foreign body and as a way to obtain a tissue sample if possible. Additional culture specimens can be obtained at the same time to help target the offending organism. If the bronchoscopy is unrevealing and there is still high suspicion for malignancy, transthoracic biopsy of the thickest part of the cavity's wall may lead to a diagnosis.

For those abscesses that show no signs of draining internally on bronchoscopy, external catheter drainage may be required. This is typically performed by interventional radiology and is necessary in the minority of bacterial pulmonary abscess cases (i.e., persisting fevers, abscess is not receding or is getting bigger despite appropriate antibiotics). Catheter drainage has greatly decreased the need for surgical intervention in these cases. Catheter placement through areas of suspected pleural symphysis is optimal to minimize leakage into the pleural space.

Surgical intervention is only required in approximately 10% or less of lung abscesses. The indications for surgery are:

- Persistent infection secondary to bronchial obstruction from foreign body or tumor
- A multidrug-resistant pathogen
- Large abscess greater than 6 cm
- Massive hemoptysis
- Rupture of abscess cavity with resultant empyema/bronchopleural fistula
- Cavitary malignancy, or inability to rule out malignancy

Typically, surgical management is limited to excision of the involved parenchyma. Most commonly, this requires a lobectomy or segmentectomy depending on the size of the cavity. These cases may be attempted with a video-assisted thoracoscopic (VATS) approach, but the adhesions associated with the abscess cavity may make the resection difficult. A double lumen endotracheal tube should be utilized to prevent potential spilling of purulent debris into the contralateral lung. Use of autologous tissue buttressing

of the bronchial stump is suggested only in difficult to treat (i.e., multidrug resistant) infections. In cases where there is concern for residual pleural space, rotation of latissimus or omental flaps can be used to fill the thoracic cavity. If rupture of the abscess cavity has occurred prior to surgical intervention, decortication in addition to resection may be required.

Cavernostomy is reserved for patients in whom antibiotic therapy and percutaneous drainage have failed, and are too unstable to tolerate a resection. After drainage and debridement of the cavity, the space should be filled with a vascularized soft tissue flap and closed. The alternative to this is to marsupialize the cavity to the atmosphere via limited rib resection. This should be reserved for the most critically ill patients as the morbidity from the resultant wound is not trivial. One last situation where cavernostomy may be the best approach is in the patient who would require a pneumonectomy to adequately resect their cavity. Pneumonectomy in the setting of lung abscess carries very high morbidity and mortality rates. The rate of both bronchopleural fistula (BPF) formation as well as empyema without BPF are much higher in this situation.

Potential questions/alternative scenarios

"You are asked to see a 35 yo man who is one year status post kidney transplant who has fevers, cough, and a 4 cm by 4 cm cavitary lesion in his right upper lobe."

The immunosuppression that is required for the kidney transplant makes a fungal infection much more likely. Abscess cavities secondary to histoplasma or blastomycosis are possible, but aspergilloma is more likely. An aspergilloma is a conglomeration of Aspergillus hyphae, fibrin, mucus, and cellular debris. They may occur in immunocompetent patients with structural lung disease such as bullous emphysema, fibrotic lung disease, cavitary tuberculosis, or sarcoidosis with bullae. In immunocompromised patients, the aspergillus will rapidly destroy lung parenchyma and create a cavity. Often they are asymptomatic until they cause hemoptysis, but can cause pulmonary symptoms such as cough and pleuritic chest pain. The classic CT scan finding is a ball of tissue within a cavity that does not entirely fill the space, leading to the radiologic description of an "air crescent sign." Diagnosis can be verified with sputum culture or serum antibodies specific to aspergillus.

Surgical therapy is indicated in any patient with aspergilloma and hemoptysis, and is also indicated in the following circumstances due to poor prognosis: Increasing size of aspergilloma on imaging, immunosuppression, increasing aspergillus-specific IgG, and HIV infection. In those with hemoptysis, preoperative embolization of feeding bronchial arteries can temporize the bleeding, but surgical resection is recommended at this point because the aspergilloma will invariably recruit new blood supply. Surgical therapy often requires lobectomy, but in cases of small lesions may only require a sublobar resection. These operations tend to be quite difficult due to the dense vascular adhesions associated with the cavity.

"You are asked to see a 55 yo man who was admitted to the MICU with diabetic ketoacidosis (DKA), fevers, and respiratory failure. Over the course of the last 12 hours, his oxygen requirement has gone up from 40% to 60% and he has a rapidly expanding right sided infiltrate on CXR. CT scan shows a dense infiltrative process localized to the right upper lobe and part of the middle lobe with possible involvement of the chest wall."

The combination of findings above are concerning for a zygomycosis (previously known as mucormycosis) infection. Pulmonary zygomycosis is most commonly seen in poorly controlled diabetics, specifically those who present to the hospital in DKA, and neutropenic patients, such as those undergoing bone marrow transplantation. Patients with pulmonary zygomycosis typically present with fevers and pulmonary infiltrates refractory to antibiotics. The progression of disease is often very rapid and it will spread across anatomic boundaries. It is not uncommon to see invasion of the chest wall, pericardium, and other surrounding structures.

Treatment of pulmonary zygomycosis involves three key components: reversal of underlying condition (ketoacidosis, neutropenia), antifungal therapy, and surgical debridement. Antifungal treatment consists of high-dose amphotericin B (1-1.5 mg/kg per day) and is continued until all signs of infection have resolved. Operative intervention is indicated in patients who have disease limited to one lung. All involved lung parenchyma should be resected in addition to involved chest wall tissue. Patients with pulmonary zygomycosis who undergo aggressive surgical debridement have a significant survival advantage to those who are treated medically. However, overall prognosis remains poor as many of these patients are marginal surgical candidates due to the rapid progression of infection and their underlying comorbidities.

"A 48 yo man with known multidrug-resistant tuberculosis (MDR-TB) is referred to your clinic for possible surgical resection of persistent disease. He has been on medical treatment for several months and remains sputum culture positive. On CT scan he has a 9 cm by 13 cm cavity in his right upper lobe that has been slowly increasing in size over this time period."

MDR-TB is defined as a strain of TB that is resistant to at least isoniazid and rifampin. Despite this resistance, the majority of MDR-TB cases will not require surgical intervention, although resection of persistent parenchymal disease in these patients is clearly associated with improved outcomes. Surgery is usually needed to treat the complications of MDR-TB infection. The most common of these complications include:

- Massive hemoptysis
- Bronchopleural fistula
- Empyema
- Bronchiectasis or destroyed lung
- Broncholiths
- Aspergilloma

Preoperative evaluation of these patients should focus on optimizing the patient's baseline physical status to reduce the chances of morbidity and mortality. The nutritional status of a patient with MDR-TB is often compromised and may require enteral tube feeds preoperatively. Routine cardiac and pulmonary function testing should be performed, although in the case of a patient with cavitary disease or destroyed lung, resecting the diseased lung will not often alter overall pulmonary function. To further elucidate this in patients with borderline spirometry and diffusion capacity, a VQ scan can be helpful.

The most common parenchymal resection for MDR-TB is lobectomy, followed by pneumonectomy. In the patient described above, removal of his right upper lobe will greatly increase his chances of obtaining a negative sputum culture as the cavity serves as a reservoir of bacteria that are isolated from circulation and antibacterial medications. Approach to resections for MDR-TB is typically through a posterolateral thoracotomy, although a video-assisted approach can be used for lesions that are surrounded by lung parenchyma. In cases involving the pleura, an extrapleural dissection may be needed to remove the lung without causing soilage of the pleural space. The bronchial stump should be covered with muscle or omentum in patients with a positive preoperative sputum smear, significant drug resistance, or polymicrobial contamination (remember to preserve an intercostal flap at the time of thoracotomy). When adhesive disease involves the hilum, it can be easier to gain intrapericardial control of the pulmonary vessels. In pneumonectomy cases that result in significant contamination of the pleural space, it is advisable to leave an intentional Eloesser flap to prevent postoperative empyema. This space may then be closed several weeks later with instillation of modified antibiotic solution (Clagett procedure).

Pearls/pitfalls

- Surgical resection is rarely required for infectious lung disease.
- When required, surgical resection is limited to involved parenchyma. This often will require a segmentectomy or lobectomy.
- Resection for infectious lung disease can feasibly be performed via VATS, however vascular adhesions can complicate the dissection and there should be a low threshold for conversion to an open procedure.
- Cavitary malignancy should always be ruled out in the setting of a suspected pulmonary abscess that is not responsive to conventional therapy.
- Aspergilloma, and other fungal infections, are rare in immunocompetent patients without structural lung disease.
- When performing a resection for infection with multidrug-resistant organisms, it is advisable to cover the bronchial stump with a vascular tissue pedicle.

Suggested readings

- Passera, E. et al. Pulmonary Aspergilloma: Clinical Aspects and Surgical Treatment Outcome. *Thorac Surg Clin*. 2012; 22: 345-61.
- Jaroszewski, D. et al. Diagnosis and Management of Lung Infections. *Thorac Surg Clin*. 2012; 22: 301-24.

- Merritt, R. et al. Indications for Surgery in Patients with Localized Pulmonary Infection. *Thorac Surg Clin*. 2012; 22: 325-332.
- Weyant, MJ. et al. Multidrug-Resistant Pulmonary Tuberculosis: Surgical Challenges. *Thorac Surg Clin*. 2012; 22: 271-276.

Notes

10. Hemoptysis

Matthew D. Taylor, MD, and Christine L. Lau, MD, MBA

Concept
- Differential for hemoptysis
- Initial patient stabilization
- Indications for OR
- Treatment according to etiology

Chief complaint
"A 67 yo man is admitted to the medical intensive care unit (MICU) with acute respiratory distress. An urgent thoracic surgery consultation is requested for 'airway bleeding.'"

Differential
Chronic inflammatory disease (most common cause of hemoptysis - bronchiectasis, cystic fibrosis, aspergillosis, and TB), tracheoinnominate fistula (usually occurs 1-2 weeks after tracheostomy), neoplasm (massive hemoptysis associated with tumor erosion into pulmonary vasculature, most commonly seen with squamous carcinoma of the right or left main stem bronchus), diffuse lung diseases (SLE, Wegener's granulomatosis, polyarteritis nodosa, Takayasu's arteritis, may cause alveolar hemorrhage leading to hemoptysis), trauma (penetrating chest injuries, deceleration injuries), pulmonary embolism (can result in infarction, hemorrhage, and subsequent necrosis), arteriovenous fistula (rare AV malformations usually congenital in origin, represents 2% of all cases of massive hemoptysis), cardiovascular disease (associated with elevated pulmonary venous pressures - mitral stenosis or congenital heart disease). The differential should also include oropharyngeal tumors or oropharyngeal trauma, as well as upper GI causes (esophageal, gastric) that may be mistaken for hemoptysis.

History and physical
Note that the first priority is to assess and protect airway, breathing, and circulation as outlined below under treatment/management. Do not proceed to history and physical nor tests until the primary survey has been addressed. Once stabilized, obtain a medical history focusing on possible infectious causes, tracheostomy, malignancy, trauma, underlying cardiovascular disease, and chronic inflammatory diseases. Ask about any history of upper GI problems. Also inquire about coagulopathies, history of easy bleeding, and any anticoagulant medications.

Physical examination in the unstable patient is outlined below under treatment/management. Once stabilized, proceed with the secondary survey which confirms airway, breathing, and circulation. Verify that vitals and saturations are stable. Assess the patient's mental status, cardiovascular exam, and distal pulses. Examine the oropharynx for evidence of trauma or masses. A nasolaryngoscope may be useful for evaluation of the nares and oropharynx. Look for stigmata of liver disease (caput medusae, ascites). Place an NG tube with lavage to rule out active UGI bleeding.

Tests

Below is a list of tests that will be relevant to the patient's management. They can be ordered during or after the primary survey and patient stabilization. These tests aim to elucidate the etiology of the bleed as well as the patient's overall state of health.

- *Bronchoscopy (diagnostic and therapeutic).* Define the location of the bleeding source. Should be the first step in management and work-up of hemoptysis. Rigid or flexible depending on the scenario (see below). Have dilute epinephrine ready as a lavage, since this may help vasoconstrict smaller, superficial areas of bleeding.
- *CXR*: parenchymal disease, air fluid levels (abscess).
- *Basic labs*: CBC, complete metabolic panel, ABG, and coagulation studies.
- *CT chest with IV contrast (for the stable patient only).* Rule out lung mass, tracheal lesions, or cavitary lesions.
- *PFTs (for the stable patient only).* Determine ability to tolerate lung resection if needed.
- *Echo, stress testing (for the stable patient only).* Evaluate cardiovascular fitness in patients at risk of cardiovascular disease prior to any pulmonary resection.

Index scenario (additional information)
"This patient is currently coughing up 2 cups of clotted blood while you are evaluating him. His oxygen saturation is 86% on 10 L of oxygen. Hematocrit is 19. He has no tracheostomy. He is tachypneic. What is your next step in management?"

Treatment/management
Primary survey and initial stabilization:

A - *Airway* - This patient in his current state warrants a definitive airway via a single lumen endotracheal tube (ETT) using rapid sequence intubation (succinylcholine, etomidate, cricoid pressure).

B - *Breathing* - Confirm that the ETT is allowing adequate ventilation as assessed by auscultation, O2 saturation, and ABG. Bronchoscopy is crucial to clear initially formed clot that may accumulate in the trachea to allow adequate ventilation and determine the affected area, otherwise asphyxiation and death is sure to ensue. If the bleeding is profuse and inhibiting ventilation, advance the ETT into the unaffected mainstem bronchus (flexible bronchoscopy will be needed to make this determination) and inflate the cuff, then reassess. This should allow you to catch up from a ventilatory and hemodynamic standpoint. It may help to reposition the patient with the affected lung side down (dependent) to prevent aspiration of blood into the unaffected lung.

C - *Circulation* - Large bore IV access, resuscitation with blood products, and correction of coagulopathy. Note that blood loss of > 600 mL in 4 hours is associated with a 71% mortality. Blood loss of > 1 L in 24 hours is associated with a 58% mortality. Continue with a quick secondary survey as described above with any adjunctive tests that are reasonable to order. In this case a CXR, labs, NG tube, and flexible bronchoscopy (if not already done) are reasonable. It is useful to have irrigation, low dose epinephrine as a lavage, and suction available at the time of flexible bronchoscopy. Pull the ETT back to the trachea above the carina. Advance the scope, irrigate, suction and evaluate the area of interest as well as the other lobes as tolerated.

"You have been able to stabilize the patient from a hemodynamic and ventilatory standpoint. You notice bleeding coming from the RLL bronchus. It is persistent. A CXR showed an air fluid level in the RLL. NG tube lavage was clear. Coagulation factors were corrected. ABG shows a HCT of 26% after transfusion. How do you wish to proceed?"
In a patient who is hemodynamically stable, easily ventilated with a controlled airway, and only minor or moderate hemoptysis, it may be reasonable to take a slightly less aggressive approach. Sedatives and anti-tussives will help to minimize coughing and recurrent bleeding. Bronchodilators should be avoided, as they have a vasodilatory effect on the pulmonary vasculature. Hypertension should also be controlled. Imaging with a CT angiogram or angiography may provide useful information that will help determine the next subsequent steps in treatment.

In this scenario it is difficult to adequately evaluate and treat the right lower lobe lesion through the flexible bronchoscope at the bedside. There is known identified ongoing hemorrhage. The most prudent and efficient course of action is to proceed to the OR suite for rigid bronchoscopy.

Operative steps
Rigid bronchoscopy

- In a patient with uncontrolled bleeding without a controlled airway, rigid bronchoscopy is warranted. A rigid bronchoscope has a larger diameter, facilitating suctioning and instrumentation. These interventions are limited by the smaller diameter of the flexible bronchoscopes, which is why rigid is preferred in emergency cases with large-volume hemoptysis. A jet ventilation circuit will be needed. This patient already has a single lumen ETT in place. Flexible bronchoscopy and large bore catheter suctioning is performed to clear the airway of as much blood as possible. Jet ventilation and rigid bronchoscope are readied and the patient is extubated and the rigid scope is passed as follows:

- A teeth guard is placed on the upper teeth. The left hand of the surgeon is placed palm down and grasps the upper teeth. The rigid bronchoscope is slid between the index and thumb and acts as a fulcrum as the scope is passed distally. Anesthesia or an assistant can help to expose the vocal cords with a laryngoscope, sweeping the tongue away and lifting the epiglottis. The beveled tip of the rigid scope should be anterior and will help to lift the epiglottis as well. Once the cords are seen through the rigid scope, it is rotated 90° to allow the tip to pass through the cords.

- A large bore suction catheter is passed through the rigid scope and the airway is cleared of as much clot as possible to visualize the carina/determine right from left.

- The main stem of the unaffected lung is intubated and jet ventilation is carried out until oxygen saturations are stable and within normal range.

- The rigid scope is then pulled back and the main stem bronchus of the affected lung is intubated with the rigid scope. Additional suctioning is carried out until the source of bleeding is identified or O2 saturations being to decline. The affected lobar or segmental bronchus is then treated with ice-cold saline lavage (1 liter) with 1 mg of epinephrine (mixed prior to lavage) in the bleeding orifice for 10-15 seconds. This facilitates clot clearance and has the potential to slow or stop the bleeding altogether.

- It is necessary to alternate between intubation (with the rigid scope) of the unaffected lung, followed by ventilation and recovery, then intubation of the affected lung, followed by treatment.

- A flexible bronchoscope may be passed through the rigid scope to better visualize areas of bleeding. This also allows passage of a Fogarty embolectomy balloon into an affected segmental bronchus to prevent ongoing bleeding into the remaining lung if ice-saline lavage is unsuccessful. A bronchial blocker may be used to occlude a lobar or main stem bronchus. These measures (balloon occlusion) may be useful if temporizing measures are needed while arrangements are made to proceed with operation, transfer to the angio suite, optimize hemodynamics, or if reversal of coagulopathy is needed.

- If bleeding is from any orifice except the right upper lobe, the rigid bronchoscope may be wedged for selective lavage. The flexible scope allows good access to the upper lobe and can be wedged for lavage. Wedging the rigid scope in the right upper lobe is difficult, but for bleeding from all other lobes, the rigid scope provides optimal access for lavage and other treatments.

Potential questions/alternative scenarios

"After performing saline/epinephrine lavage, the patient continues to bleed uncontrollably. What is the next step in management?"
As explained above, one option is to place a Fogarty embolectomy balloon catheter into the segmental orifice or a bronchial blocker into the lobar or main stem bronchus of the bleeding source to control the bleed and ongoing soilage of the lung. The bronchus of the unaffected lung is then intubated, a tube exchanger in passed through the rigid scope, and a single lumen (or double lumen tube if the unaffected side happens to be the left) is passed over the tube exchanger into the unaffected bronchus after the rigid scope has been removed. The patient should then be transferred to angiography for bronchial artery embolization with single lung ventilation. Bronchial artery embolization is successful in 90% of cases. Bronchial artery embolization is ideal for situations where there are multiple sources of bleeding. Embolization may also play a role for temporizing ongoing hemoptysis until a more definitive surgical plan is devised.

"Attempts at bronchial artery embolization have failed. What is your next plan of action?"
This constitutes failure of non-surgical options. The next step would be pulmonary resection of the bleeding source which in this case involves the RLL. Traditional incisions/exposures can be used for this form of pulmonary resection. Operative mortality for this indication is approximately 10%. It is clearly not ideal to perform a right lower lobectomy in the emergency setting, but it is necessary if all other options have failed. The conduct of the procedure follows the same outline described under pulmonary resections in the lung cancer chapters with the exception that the tissue will be much more inflamed, friable, and bloody. Lymph node sampling/dissection is not required unless cancer is suspected. If bleeding is coming from the right or left and one is not able to locate the source (lobar or segmental bronchus) by bronchoscopy or angiography, a pneumonectomy may be required if it is

truly a life threatening situation and exsanguination/asphyxiation appears imminent.

"The patient has successful arterial embolization for massive hemoptysis. The etiology of the patient's hemoptysis is an aspergilloma with a cavitary lesion. How do you wish to proceed?"
The patient should be treated with IV antifungal therapy (i.e., Amphotericin) for at least a week followed by reassessment of clinical status, CXR and CT scan. If the patient has not had a recurrence of bleeding nor evidence of sepsis, and the imaging shows a stable cavitary lesion with or without regression, then continue conservative management as long as possible. In the meantime it is not unreasonable to get PFTs and cardiovascular workup as indicated in the event that a resection is warranted. If the patient has a recurrence, becomes sicker, or the abscess fails to improve after 2-3 weeks of therapy, then consider percutaneous drainage with infusion of intracavitary Amphotericin B. If her clinical condition fails to improve, then resection may be warranted. Note that any recurrent bleed will be handled just as outlined above in the index scenario. If you need to resect, you will want to do this on an elective or urgent basis rather than as an emergency. Also note that prior to any resection a malignancy should be ruled out (see Chapter 9, Infections lung disease).

"The patient's pulmonary function tests indicate that he would not tolerate resection. What is the next plan of action?"
CT-guided intracavitary amphotericin paste has been successful in preventing recurrent hemoptysis and for obliterating the cavitary site.

"A 65 yo obese man with a history of COPD and colon cancer develops profuse bleeding from a tracheostomy. The tracheostomy was placed 1 week ago for respiratory insufficiency after an open colectomy. What is the next step in the management of this patient?"
You would proceed as outlined above for the index scenario with a few alterations. First maneuver would be to attempt to overinflate the tracheostomy cuff to tamponade bleeding. If this maneuver is not successful, the tracheostomy tube is removed. Endotracheal intubation is performed while a finger is inserted through the tracheostomy stoma to provide manual compression of the innominate artery to the posterior table of the sternum. The patient is then taken urgently to the OR where a sternotomy is performed and the fistula is repaired. The repair involves resection with primary repair, resection with interposition graft (unless infected), or ligation of the innominate artery (assuming an intact circle of Willis) (see Chapter 23, Tracheal strictures and fistulae).

"A 68 yo man with a known tracheal mass (presumed squamous cell carcinoma from outside reports) presents with hemoptysis. You stabilize the patient in the ICU as outlined above and are able to pass an ETT with bronchoscopic guidance just beyond the lesion. You clear the airways with the bronchoscope and note no distal bleeding source. Once stable, you pull the tube back to irrigate and visualize the bleeding source and note the presence of an irregular mass occupying 50% of the circumference at the mid trachea and extending about 2 cm in length. The mass is very friable with multiple bleeding points. How do you proceed?"

You approach this patient just as you did the index case above. Here you are lucky that you could get the tube beyond the lesion. If there was any difficulty in doing this, you should not pull the tube back and "peek" at the lesion, but rather go directly to the OR for rigid bronchoscopy. In the current scenario you were able to get a sense of the characteristics of the mass, but will not be able to control the bleeding safely with a flexible bronchoscope at the bedside. Proceed to the OR for rigid bronchoscopy. Your primary objective is to obtain hemostasis. A biopsy of the lesion may stir up more bleeding, but can be entertained if the bleeding has subsided and there is a safe region to biopsy. This patient will need a complete workup prior to any sort of tracheal resection. If the bleeding does not stop, then proceed to angiography for embolization. This is not an ideal option since you would like to preserve as much vascularity to the trachea as possible for your resection and anastomosis.

If you were unable to get the ETT past the lesion, suction as much clot as you can, leave the tube proximal or remove, and hand ventilate as you go to the OR for a rigid bronchoscopy. This is clearly a very dangerous situation that requires immediate attention and transport to the OR. You have no other way of getting access. Refer to chapter 24 on tracheal tumors for staging and treatment options for constricting tracheal masses.

Pearls/pitfalls
- *Initial stabilization of patient*: correction of coagulopathy, IV access, intubation with positive pressure ventilation.
- Treatment for massive hemoptysis
  - *Bronchoscopy*: iced-saline/epinephrine lavage, laser coagulation, topical coagulants, endobronchial blockade, and single lung ventilation strategies.
  - Bronchial artery embolization.
  - Surgical resection of bleeding source.

Suggested readings

- Wigle DA, Waddell TK. Investigation and management of massive hemoptysis. Patterson GA, Cooper JD, Deslauriers J, Lerut AEMR, Luketich JD, Rice TW, and Pearson FG (eds). *Pearson's Thoracic and Esophageal Surgery*. Philadelphia: Churchill Livingstone 2008:507-27.
- McNamee C, Conlan A. Massive hemoptysis. Lewis MI and McKenna RJ, (eds). *Medical Management of the Thoracic Surgery Patient*. Philadelphia: Saunders 2009:174-80.

Notes

11. COPD, emphysema, and spontaneous pneumothorax

Mara B. Antonoff, MD, and Traves D. Crabtree, MD

Concept

- Differential diagnosis for spontaneous pneumothorax
- Surgical management options for emphysema/ bullous disease
- Considerations of candidacy for lung volume reduction surgery
- Conduct of lung volume reduction operative procedures
- End-stage emphysema and basic lung transplant considerations

Chief complaint

"A 51 yo man presents to the emergency department complaining of sudden onset of shortness of breath and pleuritic chest pain. Chest x-ray demonstrates right-sided hyperlucency with absence of pulmonary markings."

Differential

The diagnosis of pneumothorax is revealed by the X-ray findings. Potential etiologies include: trauma, iatrogenic injury, primary spontaneous pneumothorax, or secondary spontaneous pneumothorax from underlying conditions such as bullous diseases/chronic obstructive pulmonary disease (COPD), connective tissue disorders, malignancy, cystic disease, catamenial disease, or infection.

History and physical

A very limited history and exam should occur after the diagnosis of large pneumothorax, with tube thoracostomy performed early. A focused history should be obtained in order to rule out traumatic/iatrogenic sources and to elucidate any underlying lung disease as potential etiology of a secondary spontaneous pneumothorax. If underlying pulmonary processes are present, questions should focus on severity of disease and overall fitness for operative intervention. A focused exam should be performed, with emphasis on return of breath sounds bilaterally, adequacy of pulmonary excursion, work of breathing, and stigmata of chronic pulmonary disease, such as clubbing.

Tests

- *CXR*: mandatory in all.
- *Chest computed tomography (CT)*: identify blebs and delineate surgical anatomy, particularly in patients with underlying lung disease, prior chest surgery, or possible loculations.
- *Pulmonary function testing*: assess forced expiratory volume in 1 second (FEV1) and diffusion capacity in the lung of carbon monoxide (DLCO).

Index scenario (additional information)

"This patient has a PMH significant for COPD and long-standing smoking history. He describes a similar episode of spontaneous pneumothorax treated with right-sided chest tube 6 months prior. The patient reports periodic DOE and generalized limitations in activity due to SOB. Chest CT reveals re-expansion of the right lung with chest tube in place and several large apical blebs, right greater than left, with fairly normal underlying lung parenchyma. The patient has a continuous, large air leak."

Treatment/management

The pneumothorax was adequately treated/ temporized with chest tube placement. Indications for surgical intervention include recurrent pneumothoraces, persistent air leak following tube thoracostomy, failure of lung re-expansion, extensive underlying parenchymal disease that puts the patient at higher risk for recurrence, or patients with limited health care access in the event of recurrence (i.e., pilots). Recurrence rates for primary pneumothoraces range from 16-52%, and, for secondary pneumothoraces, range from 40% to 56%; this risk can be reduced dramatically by operative bleb resection. In conducting bleb resection, it is imperative that one also performs adjunct procedures to enhance lung apposition to the chest wall, including pleurectomy or mechanical/chemical pleurodesis. Bleb resection with pleurectomy results in a recurrence rate of 1-5%. Pleural abrasion is technically less demanding and has a recurrent pneumothorax rate of approximately 2%. Mechanical pleurodesis and pleurectomy both carry an elevated risk of hemorrhagic complications compared with chemical pleurodesis. Chemical pleurodesis may be performed intraoperatively or via chest tube and is most commonly performed using talc, with doxycycline used alternatively (autologous blood [blood patch] and bleomycin have also been described). Instillation of talc slurry or other sclerosing agents via the chest tube tends to have a pneumothorax recurrence rate of 8-25%, while use of aerosolized talc with video-assisted thoracic surgery (VATS) has a reported recurrence rate of 5% to 9%. It is important that the lung be fully expanded for pleurodesis to be effective, as the pleural surfaces must be in apposition for obliteration of the pleural space to occur. It is also important to note that pleurodesis is often done with reservation in young patients or patients who may require additional surgery given the difficulty of chest re-entry. It is thus important to consider all variables when deciding pleurodesis.

VATS has served as a favorable option replacing posterolateral thoracotomy as an operative approach for this disease process. With a minimally invasive approach, one can obtain good visualization and carry out the procedure with less pain and shorter length of hospital stay.

Bleb resection, pleurectomy, and pleurodesis can be performed in a single setting.

Operative steps

- General endotracheal anesthesia with double-lumen endotracheal tube; large-bore intravenous access, arterial line (as clinically indicated), foley catheter.
- Lateral decubitus positioning.
- VATS approach unless contraindicated.
- Take care upon entering chest to avoid injury to underlying lung and perform complete adhesiolysis in order to gain adequate visualization.
- Attempt to identify leaking bulla (which may be challenging in an isolated lung). A brief period of low-volume ventilation on the affected side may facilitate localization.
- Resect leaking bulla, if it can be identified. Use sequential firings of an endoscopic stapler; consider buttressed staple loads, however minimal evidence to support use. If a bleb cannot be clearly identified, some advocate an apical wedge resection regardless.
- Reinflate underlying lung under direct vision and be prepared to perform a toilet bronchoscopy if unable to re-expand.
- Consider using spray sealant on the staple line to minimize the risk of prolonged postoperative air leak.
- Perform apical pleurectomy, scoring pleura along the rib with electrocautery and peeling downward with grasper. Be sure to avoid aggressive pleurectomy in area of recurrent laryngeal nerve (RLN), phrenic nerve, and sympathetic chain.
- Mechanical pleural abrasion with folded cautery scratch pad. (Here, too, be careful to avoid injury to RLN, phrenic nerve, or sympathetic chain).
- *Chemical pleurodesis*: 1-2 spray bottles (4 grams per bottle) of aerosolized talc, allowing contents to disperse around thoracic cavity.
- Leave a chest tube and place to -20 cm H_2O in operating room to rule out bleeding, then switch to water seal, which has shown to have better results in the immediate postoperative period. Chest tubes are typically left in place for 48 to 72 hours to allow for pleural symphysis to develop. Resolution of any air leaks is also necessary prior to tube removal.

Potential questions/alternative scenarios

"What if this same patient were referred to you in an outpatient setting for his chronic symptoms (in the absence of the pneumothorax)? What surgical options might be considered for management of severe, symptomatic emphysema?"

Based on the findings of the National Emphysema Treatment Trial, lung volume reduction surgery (LVRS) has been shown to be efficacious, safe, and durable in the management of *select* patients with disabling emphysema refractory to maximal medical therapy. Patients should be enrolled in preoperative pulmonary rehabilitation, which may improve some patients to the point that they will no longer require surgery, optimize some persistently symptomatic patients preoperatively, and identify patients too unfit to undergo operative intervention. Additional medical optimization should include oxygen and bronchodilators as indicated. Spirometry should be performed, and FEV1 and DLCO used to quantify the extent of airflow obstruction and gas trapping. Radiographic evaluation (non-contrast chest CT) is used to identify patients with characteristics most favorable for lung volume reduction surgery. Patients with severe, heterogeneous, upper-lobe predominant disease tend to have the greatest improvements in exercise tolerance, spirometry, and quality of life postoperatively. In addition, long-term survival is also improved in patients with heterogeneous, upper-lobe predominant disease and a low maximal work load during exercise testing who undergo LVRS compared to medical therapy.

Outcomes tend to be more variable and less promising among patients with homogeneous or non-upper-lobe predominant emphysema, for this reason these patients are typically treated with medical therapy alone. Patients should not be considered for LVRS if they are currently smoking (or are < 6 months tobacco-free) or if they have a concurrent malignancy, advanced age, or other medical contraindications to operative intervention. Previous thoracic surgical procedures are relative but not absolute contraindications for LVRS.

"What if this patient had a homogeneous distribution of emphysematous changes? When should patients with end-stage emphysema be considered for lung transplantation?"

Patients with a homogeneous distribution of emphysema on CT have had less successful outcomes with LVRS, such that it is not recommended in individuals with such anatomic disease distribution. For these patients, lung transplantation remains a viable option. Other relative indicators which might suggest that a patient will be better served by lung transplantation than with LVRS include: oxygen dependence > 6 liters/minute at rest, FEV1 or DLCO < 20% of the predicted value, $PaCO_2$ > 55 mmHg, and pulmonary hypertension. Long-term survival following lung transplantation for end-stage emphysema is poorer than that of patients transplanted for cystic fibrosis, alpha-1 antitrypsin deficiency, and primary pulmonary hypertension. *However*, survival following lung transplantation for COPD has been shown to be comparable to survival following LVRS, and transplant remains an appropriate consideration for patients failing maximal medical management and unlikely (based on anatomic considerations) to benefit from LVRS.

Pearls/pitfalls

- Patients with secondary spontaneous pneumothorax are more likely to have prolonged air leaks and to have recurrent pneumothoraces; consideration should be given to operative management of such individuals.

- A VATS approach can be highly effective in the management of emphysema/bullous disease. Greatest efficacy is achieved by performing bleb resection, apical pleurectomy, and mechanical and/or chemical pleurodesis.

- LVRS serves as a potential operative strategy in patients with severe emphysema refractory to medical management. Good outcome is predicted by heterogeneous disease (mostly apical blebs) and symptomatic COPD.

- Patients with homogeneous disease, significant oxygen dependence at rest, FEV1 < 20% of the predicted value, $PaCO_2 > 55$ mmHg, and pulmonary hypertension may not have optimal outcomes with LVRS. In these individuals, careful consideration may be given to lung transplantation.

Suggested readings

- Chambers A, Scarci M. In patients with first-episode primary spontaneous pneumothorax is video-assisted thoracoscopic surgery superior to tube thoracostomy alone in terms of time to resolution of pneumothorax and incidence of recurrence? *Interactive Cardiovascular and Thoracic Surgery*. Nov 17 2009;9(6):1003-1008.

- Criner GJ, Cordova F, Sternberg AL, Martinez FJ. The National Emphysema Treatment Trial (NETT): Part I: Lessons Learned about Emphysema. *American Journal of Respiratory and Critical Care Medicine*. Oct 01 2011;184(7):763-770.

- Criner GJ, Cordova F, Sternberg AL, Martinez FJ. The National Emphysema Treatment Trial (NETT): Part II: Lessons Learned about Lung Volume Reduction Surgery. *American Journal of Respiratory and Critical Care Medicine*. Oct 16 2011;184(8):881-893.

Notes

12. Thoracic trauma

Sagar S. Damle, MD, and Michael J. Weyant, MD

Concept
- ATLS Resuscitation
- Differential diagnosis for possible injuries
- Diagnostic tests
- Conduct of care with prioritization of injuries
- Specific operative interventions for particular injuries

Chief complaint
"A 35 yo man is brought into the ED after a gunshot wound to the left chest. His vital signs are reportedly stable with volume resuscitation in the field. He is reportedly awake, but dazed and confused."

Differential
Penetrating injuries to lung, heart, esophagus, chest wall. Also, blunt force injuries to lung, esophagus, and heart. Note that hemodynamically significant cardiac injuries are discussed in Chapter 46, Cardiac trauma.

History and physical
Focus on the critical steps of ATLS resuscitation. Remember that during ATLS protocols, diagnosis and treatment are done simultaneously during primary survey, which serves as your history and physical. Define the pattern of injury (i.e., anterior "box", posterior "box" – see Chapter 46, Cardiac trauma). Remember the steps: A-B-C-D-E then secondary survey. Airway: confirm patient has adequate airway, especially if patient has large degree of subcutaneous emphysema. Intubate early for airway stability. Breathing: Confirm adequacy of oxygenation/ventilation. Look for chest wall deformities, entry/exit wounds sites, and flail movement of chest wall. Evaluate for extent of crepitus and/or chest wall hemorrhage. Get CXR. Also remember to CONFIRM result of therapy - did repeat CXR demonstrate evacuation of hemothorax? Most lung injuries will not lead to severe inability to ventilate and oxygenate patient. However, if the patient has a central airway injury from trauma, consider mainstem intubation or double-lumen ventilation during your "B" assessment. Cardiovascular: Examine for pulses and hemodynamic stability. Listen to heart sounds and check for JVD. Remember the penetrating injuries near great vessels or heart, and blunt force, may lead to pseudoaneurysms, cardiac trauma, etc. without direct injury. Perform FAST and rule out tamponade. If equivocal, place central venous catheter and evaluate CVP. D and E will not be covered in this topic.

Tests

- *Labs.* Usual trauma labs are useful. Particularly important to obtain ABG and Type & Cross.
- *X-rays.* "BIG 3." Lateral C-spine, CXR and pelvis. Clearly we will be most concerned with CXR with particular attention to: pneumothorax, hemothorax, mediastinal shifting, apical cap, multiple rib fx, scapula fx, 1st rib fracture, loss of aortic knob/contour, and left effusion without rib fracture. Although a CXR is a quick test, it often lacks sensitivity and specificity.
- *FAST or E-FAST.* Particularly useful will be the subxiphoid view and bilateral hemithoraces, if done. Ideal for evaluating for possible tamponade in ED. Remember that repeat FAST also has a tremendous value as some fluid pockets will develop later.
- *CTA chest.* Especially useful to rule out great vessel injury. Patient should be hemodynamically stable to undergo CT. Do not send tenuous patient to the scanner. CT is of particularly higher yield in patients with high-impact mechanisms or CXR findings suggestive of injury (apical cap, 1st rib fx, scapula fx, multiple rib fx, loss of aortic knob etc.). CT is also useful for transmediastinal GSWs to outline tract and evaluate for possible collateral damage. Echocardiography (TEE) and angiography have limited, if any role, in evaluation of traumatic thoracic injuries with today's CT technology.

Index scenario (additional information)

"The patient is awake but has labored breathing. During his initial primary survey, he is intubated and 2 large bore IVs are placed and he is started on NS resuscitation. He is noted to have an entry wound in the left axilla and an exit wound in the right 4th ICS in the anterior axillary line. In addition, he has a large abrasion over the lateral left chest wall, consistent with a sledge hammer blow. While getting trauma X-rays, he is hypotensive with tracheal deviation to the left. A right chest tube is placed with return of a large amount of air and 300 cc of blood. CXR does not demonstrate any retained bullet fragments, but does demonstrate multiple fractured ribs on the left and a large amount of subcutaneous air, as well as bilateral hemithoraces and near-complete collapse of the left lung. After placing a left-sided chest tube, there are large air leaks with > 1000 cc of blood return from the left tube upon initial insertion. Although he seems to stabilize somewhat, over the next 30 minutes, the left chest tube output is 600 mL and there is severe blowing air leaks in the right chest tube. How would you proceed?"

Treatment/management

Again, life-saving treatment is done during primary survey. During airway evaluation, if one suspects a high airway injury, consideration can be made for mainstem intubation. However, ideally, rapidly performed bronchoscopy should be done or available, as well to diagnose. Unfortunately, bronchoscopic findings of airway injuries may be subtle and can be easily missed. Also, availability of a bronchoscope in the ED can be variable. During evaluation of adequacy of breathing and oxygenation/ventilation, chest tubes should be placed liberally with suspected thoracic trauma. Evaluate for amount, type, and persistence of drainage. After intervention, make certain to re-evaluate patient for improvements after each therapeutic intervention. During cardiac evaluation, perform FAST initially and REPEAT at intervals to assess for accumulation of fluid, especially in patient who goes from stable to unstable. Have a low threshold to place large IVs and potential central access for CVP evaluation and more rapid resuscitation. If patient is in extremis or loses vital signs in ED, consider ED thoracotomy for stabilization. If hemodynamics are transiently stabilized, but decompensation continues, rapidly transport patient to the OR for operative intervention. If the patient's chest tube output remains low and hemodynamics are stable, consideration should be given for CTA to evaluate the bullet tract and associated injuries.

Operative steps

- Operative approach will vary based on injury.
- *Positioning.* Supine with patient prepped from chin to toes (standard trauma prep/drape). Although a lateral decubitus position would be possible, it limits one's ability to gain access to the abdominal cavity or contralateral hemithorax. Avoid suggesting this positioning.
- *Anesthesia considerations.* Double-lumen intubation, while ideal, is typically not possible due to trauma situation and airway edema. Consider alternatives for lung isolation including main stem intubation and bronchial blockers.
- *Incision.* The most versatile approach will be a thoracotomy with the patient in a supine position. This allows the possibility to extend the incision into the contralateral chest for treatment of contralateral injuries (i.e., clamshell). In addition, the clamshell also allows excellent exposure to the heart and great proximal great vessels. For this scenario, perform clamshell thoracotomy from the beginning as there is significant hemorrhage from the left chest and persistent pneumothorax on the right. The sternum can be quickly divided transversely with either a sternal saw or heavy scissors. Be cognizant of the internal mammary arteries (i.e., ligate).

- After incision, control life-threatening bleeding with pressure, clamps, etc. as needed and available.
- If poor or limited venous access, place right atrial cannula for rapid infusion.
- In this scenario, bronchoscopy should be performed to evaluate for central airway injury., which typically can be addressed with either segmental resection (if extensive damage or tissue loss) or primary closure (if limited damage).
- Also in this scenario, address source of bleeding in the left chest with appropriate therapy. Bleeding from bullet tract in lung can be addressed with tractotomy and oversewing of bleeding vessels. Tractotomy is performed by placing the anvil of a GIA stapler in the bullet tract and opening the lung parenchyma with stapler to the periphery of lung. Great vessel injuries must be addressed with proximal/distal control and either primary repair (rare) or interposition graft (vein or graft).

"In the operating room, you perform a clamshell thoracotomy to gain access to both chests. You note the bullet tract entering the left lung with profuse bleeding coming from the tract. The bullet appears to have traversed the mediastinum behind the great vessels. You note an injury to the trachea. How would you proceed?"

It appears that at the moment, there is reasonable control of the airway. If the ETT is too high and the tracheal injury is making it difficult to ventilate the patient, advance the ETT gently with a combination of fiber optic bronchoscopy and direct palpation. Once the airway control is established, even temporarily, address the bleeding from the lung with a tractotomy. Next, turn attention back to the tracheal injury. Unroof the mediatinal pleura overlying the trachea for a reasonable distance from the right chest. Identify the injury and freshen the edges. If at possible, primary repair should be performed. If a near-circumferential injury, one may need to perform a segmental resection and primary anastomosis (see Chapters 23-24, Tracheal strictures and fistulae and Malignant lesions of the trachea). Of note, the distal trachea, as well as the right *and* left mainstem bronchi can be relatively easy to reach from the right chest. Since most injuries occur posteriorly, this provides good access for repair. More proximal tracheal injuries must be approached from the neck, typically with a collar incision (discussed in Chapter 24, Malignant lesions of the trachea). The distal trachea can also be reached via sternotomy. After opening the anterior pericardium, the SVC is mobilized laterally to the patient's right and the ascending aorta/arch to the patient's left. The posterior pericardium is then opened to gain access to the airway.

"Is there anything else you would do?"

Airway injuries and transmediastinal GSW are often associated with other injuries. Especially in this case, one MUST evaluate the esophagus. Therefore, prior to closing chest, perform EGD. If any questions, explore area around the esophagus near bullet track. Repair primarily if there is healthy tissue. Widely drain and buttress with well-vascularized tissue.

Potential questions/alternative scenarios

"After placing the left-sided chest tube, you note greenish fluid coming from the chest tube. Does this change your evaluation and/or operative approach?"

Clearly this should raise the suspicion of a diaphragmatic injury and probably gastric or small bowel injury (either from the trauma or from iatrogenic injury from your chest tube placement since stomach or bowel is in the chest). Acute diaphragmatic ruptures can be approached through the abdomen or through the chest. In this scenario, the chest would be ideal since there is now contamination of the pleural space. A low left thoracotomy (6th or 7th intercostal space, imaging can help to determine the optimal entry site) will be needed. The visceral organ perforation is repaired and then returned to the abdomen. Since there has been minimal scarring, primary repair of the diaphragm is usually feasible. There will typically be a rim of diaphragm that remains along the ribs. Horizontal mattress (+/- pledgets, if infected using felt pledgets is not advised) stitches using non-absorbable suture are placed to bring the free edge of the diaphragm to the costal rim of diaphragm. If the defect is large and some of the diaphragm muscle is destroyed, debridement is required and a patch (i.e., PTFE, Gortex, Alloderm) may be needed. A biologic mesh would be ideal the setting of contamination, such as described here. If there were no contamination in the chest, the herniated viscera can be reduced from the abdomen and the repair performed in similar fashion from below. In this scenario, the chest should be washed out and multiple chest tubes left to avoid the late complication of an empyema.

Diaphragmatic injuries are one of the most commonly missed traumatic injuries. These injuries may be small and not easily seen on initial trauma imaging. Ruptures such as these may become symptomatic with time as the intraabdominal content eventually find their way into the chest. Chronic diaphragmatic ruptures are typically approached from the chest, as reduction of the herniated viscera may required lysing of adhesions or the contents may become incarcerated. The diaphragm also becomes less pliable in the setting of chronic rupture and primary repair may not be accomplished without tension, in which case a patch is needed.

"Soon after arrival in the ED, the patient becomes suddenly hypotensive and unresponsive. The nurses are unable to palpate a pulse."

Although controversial, this is an indication for an ED thoracotomy. Institutional protocols will vary, the basic steps involve a large anterolateral thoracotomy, typically in the 6th ICS. All dissection is done with a scalpel or scissors. Next, the pericardium is opened widely anterior and longitudinal to the phrenic nerve and the heart is delivered into the left chest. The pleura is incised over the distal aorta and a cross-clamp is applied. At this point, cardiac massage can begin as well as damage control or repair of cardiac trauma or lung trauma (refer to Cardiac Trauma).

"After initial evaluation of the patient, he is noted to have only a tangential gunshot wound without penetration into the thorax. However, on CXR, he is noted to have multiple rib fractures and some 'haziness' in the right lung fields. He states that he feels short of breath, but he is oxygenating well. What is your approach to treat him now?"

Do not fall into the trap of the stable patient and jump into your planned chest tube. He should still undergo ABCDE of ATLS. However, he clearly needs a right-sided chest tube to evacuate potential clot.

"On repeat CXR after chest tube placement, he continues to have some 'haziness' in the right hemithorax. What now?"

Confirm that the patient is stable and that the chest tube is functioning properly with tidaling and drainage. If the patient is stable, consider obtaining a CT scan to evaluate for retained hemothorax vs. diffuse pulmonary contusions. If the CT demonstrates retained blood, there are two options. One is to place a second chest tube and the other is to plan for a VATS cleanout once he is stable, usually within 24-48 hours. Either approach is reasonable; however, a second chest tube is often not sufficient and may not avoid a trip to the operating room. Some data suggests that early VATS offers early time to discharge and less chest tube days than a second chest tube. Early evacuation of hemothoraces is also easier, as the blood/clot is typically still liquified. Delays in evacuating the hemothorax may result in organization of the clot and formation of a pleural rind, which then would require evacuation of the hemothorax as well as a more time consuming decortication. Particularly in the setting of trauma, retained hemothoraces may become infected, again arguing for early evacuation and washout of the chest.

If there is in fact no retained hemothoraces, which can easily be assessed on CT, one must be concerned about pulmonary contusion. Multiple rib fractures should raise the suspicion of underlying pulmonary contusion.

Adequate pain control is of paramount importance in the setting of multiple rib fractures to avoid splinting and promote adequate ventilation. Pain from multiple rib fracture and underlying pulmonary contusion should be treated aggressively with an epidural, intercostal nerve blocks, or a PCA. Judicious fluid management may be helpful in the setting of pulmonary contusion, but may not be prudent in the setting of polytrauma. There should be a low threshold for intubation and mechanical ventilation in the setting of multiple rib fractures and extensive pulmonary contusion, particularly in the setting of flail chest.

"Instead of being shot, the patient was stabbed with a long ice pick. His vitals are otherwise stable, but his CXR demonstrates a small left hemopneumothorax. What is your approach."
ABC's first. Clearly, you do not want to remove the object in the ED. Urgently prep the patient and OR for operative thoracotomy. Dual-lumen ventilation is ideal. Have blood readily available.

"You note the ice pick enters the left chest in the lower axilla and you make a posterolateral thoracotomy. Upon entering the chest, the lung is deflated and the ice pick traverses the superior segment of the lower lobe and appears to enter the aorta. What is your operative plan?"
Luckily, the situation is controlled, for the most part. Ideally, we should get proximal and distal control of the aorta before removing the ice pick. However, this is not always possible. Another option is to dissect out the lateral aspect of the aorta where the ice pick enters and place a side biting clamp around it. With the side-biter ready to go, remove the ice pick and side-bite the aorta. Remember to give a little heparin as well, if the patient will tolerate it. Then, dissect the adventitia, identify the hole and repair it. This repair may require a few interrupted sutures or a patch. Be sure to have perfusion and circuit in the room in the event there's a need for cardiopulmonary bypass. Cannulation might include distal descending aortic with left atrial for partial bypass or femoral venous and arterial.

"Your assistant removed the ice pick but inadvertently lacerates the aorta. There is torrential bleeding. After occluding the aorta with your hand, you notice that there is a piece of aortic wall on the ice pick and a nearly circumferential hole in the aorta. Now what?"
Again, plan to get proximal and distal control. Then, resect the damaged portion of the aorta and perform a primary repair. Use of cardiopulmonary bypass, circulatory arrest or partial left heart bypass will depend on the location and severity of the injury as well as any associated dissection flap.

"The ends of the aorta will not come together."
Place an interposition graft of Dacron and wash the chest out thoroughly.

Pearls/pitfalls

- Be wary of the "stable patient." Many intrathoracic injuries (tamponade, tension ptx, ongoing hemothorax) will present with a "stable" picture, but decompensation occurs quickly. All thoracic injuries, especially those to "the anterior box" require complete evaluation before declaring the patient stable for observation.
- Do not deviate from ATLS protocols and get side-tracked.
- Operative planning should be done taking into account all possible scenarios.

Suggested readings

- Bastos R, Baisden CR, Harker L et al. Penetrating thoracic trauma. *Semin Thorac Cardiovasc Surg.* 2008:20:19-25.
- Bastos R, Calhoon JH, Baisden CE. Flail chest and pulmonary contusion. *Semin Thorac Cardiovasc Surg.* 2008:20: 39-45.
- Carpenter AJ. Diagnostic techniques in thoracic trauma. *Semin Thorac Cardiovasc Surg.* 2008:20: 2-5.

Notes

13. Malignant pleural mesothelioma

Shawn S. Groth, MD, Marcelo C. DaSilva, MD, and

David J. Sugarbaker, MD

Concept
- Discuss the preoperative testing to determine resectability for patients with malignant pleural mesothelioma (MPM)
- Discuss the indications and critical surgical steps for extrapleural pneumonectomy (EPP) and extended pleurectomy/decortication (EPD)
- Discuss the postoperative management and complications after EPP and EPD

Chief complaint
"A 65 yo man is referred to you by his primary care physician for evaluation of right pleural thickening and nodularity. As part of a workup for a two month history of dyspnea, a chest x-ray was obtained four weeks ago which revealed a right pleural effusion. A thoracentesis was performed with 1000 cc of cloudy, serous fluid being drained. Cytology was negative for malignancy. A non-contrast chest CT was obtained that demonstrated diffuse pleural thickening and nodularity of the right hemithorax and resolution of the effusion."

Differential
The differential for pleural thickening and pleural nodules includes benign etiologies, such as mesothelial hyperplasia, benign pleural plaque, benign solitary fibrous tumor of the pleura, lipoma, mesothelial cyst, adenomatous tumor, and schwannoma. Malignant causes include primary pleural tumors such as malignant pleural mesothelioma, malignant solitary fibrous tumor, pleural thymoma, sarcoma (liposarcoma, leiomyosarcoma, rhabdomyosarcoma), pleuropulmonary blastoma, small cell carcinoma of the pleura, and desmoid tumor. Neoplasms with pleural metastases may also present in this fashion with primaries such as primary lung cancer, extrathoracic carcinomas, extrathoracic sarcomas, melanoma, and germ cell tumors being the most common.

History and physical
A focused history should inquire into common presenting symptoms for MPM (i.e., dyspnea, chest pain, fevers, cough, hemoptysis, and anorexia), asbestos exposure, family history of MPM, chest radiation, and an assessment of the patient's functional status. Nutrition is a vital aspect of caring for all cancer patients; inquire about weight loss, anorexia, and dietary intake. A focused physical examination should include a general assessment of the patient's physiological and nutritional

status. Auscultate and percuss the chest to assess diminished breath sounds, chest wall excursion (contraction of the hemithorax often suggests chest wall invasion), and palpable chest wall masses (including previous biopsy sites). Assess for cervical, supraclavicular, and axillary adenopathy. Examine the abdomen for masses and/or ascites (signs of peritoneal involvement).

Tests
Tissue diagnosis
- *Approach.* The first step is to obtain tissue for diagnosis. Only 30% to 50% of MPM patients are diagnosed by thoracentesis and cytology. The authors prefer a thoracoscopic biopsy of the pleura, which provides a definitive diagnosis with a high degree of accuracy and minimal risk. In most instances, this can be done as an outpatient procedure.
- *Histological subtypes.* The primary MPM histological subtypes are epithelioid, sarcomatoid, and biphasic (which is composed of at least 10% epithelial and sarcomatoid elements). Pure sarcomatoid and biphasic tumors carry the worse prognosis.
- *Pathology review.* The diagnosis of MPM should be confirmed by an experienced pathologist. In addition to hematoxylin and eosin staining, the diagnosis of MPM is based on immunohistochemical features (antibodies to calretinin, keratin antibody AE1/AE3 - a product of Wilm's tumor susceptibility gene 1 (WT1)). Antibodies to CEA, Leu-M1, and TTF1 suggest NSCLC. Antibodies to calretinin and WT1 are consistent with epithelioid MPM, whereas sarcomatoid MPM has nuclear pleomorphism and stains strongly for keratin.

Pretreatment staging
- *CT.* A noncontrast chest CT is the primary imaging modality for diagnosis, staging and post-treatment surveillance of MPM. Common CT findings in MPM include: pleural thickening, involvement of the fissure, pleural effusion, contraction of the involved hemithorax and mediastinal shift. Once the diagnosis is established, it is useful to assess for mediastinal adenopathy, mediastinal invasion, chest wall invasion, transdiaphragmatic involvement, and contralateral disease.
- *PET/CT.* The authors also routinely obtain an integrated PET/CT scan. It increases the sensitivity to detect mediastinal lymph node metastases, subtle chest wall involvement, and occult extrathoracic disease. The baseline SUVmax has prognostic significance and, if neoadjuvant chemotherapy is given, is a useful metric to follow on post-treatment imaging.

- *MRI.* A gadolinium-enhanced chest MRI is a useful adjunct to chest CT to assess for chest wall, transdiaphragmatic, mediastinal, and contralateral invasion. We obtain a chest MRI for all of our patients.
- *Mediastinal lymph node biopsy.* All potential candidates for resection should undergo EBUS-TBNA, EUS-FNA, or cervical mediastinoscopy for histologic assessment of N2 disease. Those with N2 disease should undergo neoadjuvant chemotherapy.

Physiological fitness
- Appropriate candidates for surgery should have a good functional/performance status (i.e., Karnofsky performance status of 70 or greater), normal hepatic function, normal renal function (CrCl > 60 mL/min), and adequate cardiopulmonary reserve.

Assessment of cardiopulmonary status
- *Oximetry.* For all patients, we assess their oxygenation saturation (by pulse oximetry) at rest and with activity (i.e., during a 6 minute walk test). It provides an invaluable and inexpensive assessment of their pulmonary function.
- *Pulmonary function tests (PFTs).* All patients should have formal PFTs. For patients with COPD or pulmonary fibrosis, assess DLCO as well. Patients with poor underlying pulmonary function (postop predicted FEV1 < 40% or DLCO < 40%) are not candidates for resection.
- *Quantitative VQ scan.* All potential candidates for resection should have a quantitative VQ scan. Such an assessment is used to calculate the postoperative predicted (PPO) FEV1 (FEV1 x % perfusion to non-affected lung) to ascertain whether or not the patient could tolerate a pneumonectomy without an undue risk for respiratory complications. Patients with a ppoFEV1 below the following values are not candidates for resection: EPD, < 1.0 L; left EPP, < 1.0 L; right EPP, < 1.2 to 1.4 L. The relative perfusion to each lung is also important for determining candidacy for a resection. For instance, a patient with a ppoFEV1 of 1.2 L and a relative perfusion of 10% to the affected lung is less likely to have complications than a patient with a ppoFEV1 of 1.2 L and a relative perfusion of 50%. In such patients, other parameters should be taken into consideration when determining medical operability.
- *Transthoracic echo (TTE).* All patients should undergo a TTE to assess LV and RV function, underlying valve disease and to estimate PA pressures (from the degree of TR). Patients with an estimated PA pressure of 30 mmHg and a right atrial pressure roughly 1/3 systemic are not candidates for resection.

- *Cardiac stress test.* All patients with an active cardiac condition should undergo preoperative stress testing. Consider preoperative testing in patients with at least one cardiac risk factor and a functional capacity of 4 metabolic equivalents or less.

Index scenario (additional information)

"The patient underwent pleuroscopy and biopsy of a parietal pleural nodule; final pathology demonstrated the presence of epithelioid MPM. He then underwent a PET/CT which demonstrated diffuse FDG uptake throughout the right pleural space; there is no abnormal FDG uptake elsewhere. A chest MRI showed no evidence of chest wall, diaphragmatic, contralateral, or mediastinal extension. Mediastinoscopy was negative for N2 disease. The patient has been reading on the internet about various treatment options and is curious about your thoughts on who should get chemotherapy and who should undergo a resection."

Treatment/management

Neoadjuvant chemotherapy

Patients with N2 disease, chest wall invasion, and contralateral disease should be referred for neoadjuvant chemotherapy. The preferred regimens for neoadjuvant and adjuvant therapy are platinum-based agents and pemetrexed or platinum-based agents and gemcitabine.

Definitive chemotherapy

Patients who are deemed medically inoperable and those with advanced disease should be referred for definitive chemotherapy.

Cytoreductive surgery

The best chance for cure is complete removal of macroscopic disease (i.e., an R1 resection). Patients with marginal cardiopulmonary function who are unlikely to tolerate an EPP may still be candidates for EPD. The decision to perform EPD or EPP will be based on the patient's physiologic reserve, age, and the extent of disease (minimal versus bulky disease). With either procedure, the goal is a complete macroscopic resection of all tumor.

Adjuvant chemotherapy

Patients who undergo EPD (especially those with node-positive disease) should undergo postoperative chemotherapy. For patients who undergo EPP, those patients with biphasic histology and those with node-positive disease should also undergo postoperative chemotherapy.

Radiation therapy

Radiation therapy can be given to improve local control after EPP (not EPD), to treat and palliate chest wall disease, and to treat a focus of mediastinal disease.

Operative steps

Pleurectomy/decortication

Goals – explore and determine resectability, complete macroscopic removal of all tumor, and mediastinal lymph node dissection. *Note: The incision, exposure, and extrapleural dissection are similar for EPPs and EPDs.*

- Double-lumen endotracheal tube.
- *Tube and lines*: PA catheter on operative side, peripheral IVs, arterial line, Foley catheter, NG tube (to facilitate identification of the esophagus during the extrapleural dissection and to prevent large volume aspiration until resolution of the postoperative ileus).
- Extended posterolateral thoracotomy (divide latissimus dorsi and serratus anterior).
- Excise the 6th rib.
- Begin the extrapleural dissection around the circumference of the thoracotomy, separating the parietal pleura from the endothoracic fascia.
- Continue posterolaterally up to and over the apex of the lung, sweeping the pleura off the subclavian vessels.
- For right-sided tumors, continue along the anterior mediastinum over the SVC to the SVC-azygos recess; avoid injury to the internal mammary vessels.
- Continue extrapleural dissection inferiorly and posteriorly along the azygos for right-sided tumors or along the aorta for left-sided tumors to the retrocrural space and retroperitoneum.
- After completing the extrapleural dissection, the tumor is stripped off the pericardium to the hilar cuff.
- The tumor is incised with a scalpel in-line with the thoracotomy.
- A plane is created between the lung and the visceral pleura. The tumor is bluntly dissected free from the underlying lung to the level of the hilar cuff, where the incision in the tumor is extended down to the hilar reflection. The upper and lower halves of the tumor shell are removed.
- Depending on tumor involvement, the diaphragm and/or the pericardium may need to be resected (and reconstructed).
- Mediastinal lymph node dissection.
- Place chest tubes and close.

Extrapleural pneumonectomy

Goals – explore and determine resectability, complete macroscopic removal of all tumor, and mediastinal lymph node dissection. *Note: The incision, exposure, and extrapleural dissection are similar for EPPs and EPDs.*

- Double-lumen endotracheal tube.
- Tube and Lines: PA catheter on operative side, peripheral IVs, arterial line, Foley catheter, NG tube (to facilitate identification of the esophagus during the extrapleural dissection and to prevent large volume aspiration until resolution of the postoperative ileus).
- Extended posterolateral thoracotomy (divide latissimus dorsi and serratus anterior).
- Excise the 6th rib.
- Begin the extrapleural dissection around the circumference of the thoracotomy, separating the parietal pleura from the endothoracic fascia.
- Continue posterolaterally up to and over the apex of the lung, sweeping the pleura off the subclavian vessels.
- For right-sided tumors, continue along the anterior mediastinum over the SVC to the SVC-azygos recess; avoid injury to the internal mammary vessels.
- Continue extrapleural dissection inferiorly and posteriorly along the azygos for right-sided tumors or along the aorta for left-sided tumors to the retrocrural space and retroperitoneum.
- Palpate the pericardial sac for tumor invasion.
- Avulse the diaphragm from the chest wall, and bluntly dissect the diaphragm off the peritoneum.
- Open the pericardium anteromedially.
- Hilar dissection.
- Dissect and divide the PA (intrapericardial division for right EPP and extrapericardial division for left EPP).
- Intrapericardial division of the pulmonary veins.
- Divide the bronchus under bronchoscopic visualization, leaving a < 1 cm stump.
- Complete the pericardiotomy.
- Complete mediastinal lymph node dissection.
- Mobilize a tongue of greater omentum for bronchial stump coverage.
- Reconstruct the diaphragm with a dynamic patch of 2 pieces of 2 mm PTFE mesh.
- Reconstruct the pericardium with a fenestrated PTFE patch (regardless of side).
- Buttress the bronchial stump with the omental flap.
- Place a 14 Fr red rubber catheter and close.

- Remove air via the red rubber catheter to balance the mediastinum (Right EPP: men 1000 cc and women 750 cc, Left EPP: men 750 cc andwomen 500 cc).

Potential questions/alternative scenarios

"While still in the OR following a right EPP, the patient has a sudden rise in his CVP and PA pressure and a drop in his blood pressure and cardiac output when being turned from lateral to supine."
Turn the patient back in the lateral decubitus position, re-prep and reopen the thoracotomy. The pericardial patch is likely the cause of tamponade and should be replaced with a looser patch.

"On postoperative day number 2 after a right EPP, your patient has a cardiac arrest while in the ICU."
An emergency thoracotomy, removal of the pericardial patch, and open cardiac massage should be performed to address potentially correctable mechanical causes of the arrest (cardiac herniation, a constrictive pericardial patch, kinking of the IVC by the diaphragmatic patch, or a pericardial effusion). Closed chest compressions are ineffective after pneumonectomy. After resuscitation, the patient should be taken back to the OR for a washout and closure.

"A routine CXR on postoperative day number three after a right EPP demonstrates complete filling of the pneumonectomy space and contralateral mediastinal shift."
Place a small drainage catheter in the 2nd intercostal space, midclavicular line to slowly remove fluid to balance the mediastinum. The fluid should be sent for culture and Gram's stain as well as for triglycerides and cell count.

"The culture is negative. The triglyceride level is 900, and the fluid is lymphocyte rich."
These findings are consistent with a chylothorax. (See Chapter 14, Chylothorax for details on management.)

"Five weeks after a left EPP, a patient presents with fevers, malaise, and a drop in his air-fluid level. You are concerned about a possible bronchopleural fistula (BPF) and empyema."
If the patient is acutely toxic, place a chest tube in the pneumonectomy space (above the level of the thoracotomy). The patient ultimately needs a bronchoscopy and open surgical drainage (i.e., a Clagett Window or Eloesser Flap). All synthetic material (i.e., the PTFE patches) should be removed.

"You have a patient booked for a left EPP who you referred for induction therapy. He now returns to the office with a PET-CT for post-treatment staging and he is noted to have uptake along the contralateral costophrenic margin. How would you proceed? What if the patient had only left-sided disease with extensive involvement of the left hemidiaphragm. The read on the PET-CT states that there is questionable extension into the peritoneal cavity. How would you manage this patient?"

Contralateral pleural disease would make this patient unresectable. However this should be confirmed by biopsy, most easily performed with thoracoscopy and biopsy. Peritoneal involvement would also make this patient unresectable. A staging laparoscopy would be prudent in this case to rule out intra-peritoneal disease prior to proceeding with resection.

Pearls/pitfalls

Preoperative evaluation

- Always assure that you have a recent (within the previous 4 weeks) imaging study (i.e., CT, MRI or PET/CT).
- Never biopsy the visceral pleura or nodules on the surface of the lung. Such biopsies often lead to chronic BPFs and impair patients from receiving definitive treatment.

Surgery

- Remove all prior biopsy scars due to the risk for tumor seeding.
- During the extrapleural dissection for a left EPP, it is easy to begin dissecting behind the aorta, thereby injuring the intercostals. To avoid this, begin on the arch and stay in the preaortic plane.
- During diaphragmatic resection for a left EPP, leave a 1-2 cm rim of left crus for suturing during patch reconstruction to prevent gastric herniation.

Postoperative management

- After EPP, extubate in the OR to minimize positive pressure on the bronchial stump.
- After EPD, continue with positive pressure ventilation for the next 24 hours to help tamponade bleeding from the surface of the lung and chest wall.
- PA catheters are essential to optimizing postoperative fluid status and cardiac function.
- For patients with diaphragmatic reconstruction who require long-term postoperative enteric nutritional support, place an open J tube.
- Pneumoperitoneum for laparoscopy can induce a tension pneumothorax. Be cognizant of this potential adverse sequelae.

Suggested readings

- Sugarbaker DJ, RB Bueno, MJ Krasna, SJ Mentzer, L Zellos. *Adult Chest Surgery*. McGraw-Hill. New York, 2009.
- Wolf AS, Daniel J, Sugarbaker DJ. Surgical Techniques for Multimodal Treatment of Malignant Pleural Mesothelioma: Extrapleural Pneumonectomy and Pleurectomy/Decortication. *Semin Thorac Cardiovasc Surg.* 21: 132-148.
- Kaufman AJ and RM Flores. Technique of Pleurectomy and Decortication. *Operative Techniques in Thoracic and Cardiovascular Surgery.* Vol. 15, Issue 4, Pages 294-306.
- DaSilva MC and Sugarbaker DJ. Technique of Extrapleural Pneumonectomy. *Operative Techniques in Thoracic and Cardiovascular Surgery.* Vol. 15, Issue 4, Pages 282-293.

Notes

14. Chylothorax

Ryan A. Macke, MD, and Benny Weksler, MD

Concept

- Presentation and diagnostic workup of chylothorax
- Differences in management of traumatic and neoplastic chylothorax
- Options and justification for medical and surgical management
- Describe the anatomy of the thoracic duct and the steps of thoracic duct ligation
- Pitfalls in management of chylothorax

Chief complaint

"You have successfully completed a redo coarctation repair via left thoracotomy on an otherwise healthy 45 yo man. It is now postoperative day 4. Left chest tube output has been high (> 1 L/day). After starting a regular diet, the chest output changes from serous to milky in appearance."

Differential

Sympathetic effusion, chylothorax, empyema, esophageal perforation

History and physical

Causes of chylothorax can be broadly categorized as congenital, traumatic, and neoplastic. Congenital or primary chylothorax occurs most commonly in neonates and is usually idiopathic in nature. Most cases are treated successfully with conservative management. Traumatic chylothorax is most commonly iatrogenic and can complicate essentially any thoracic operation (most commonly esophagectomy, aortic procedures, left pneumonectomy and resection of posterior mediastinal masses) or lower neck operation (such as radical neck dissection or line placement – particularly in the pediatric population). Blunt trauma resulting in hyperextension of the spine and violent vomiting or coughing can disrupt the thoracic duct at the level of the diaphragm, resulting in a traumatic chylothorax. Neoplastic processes such as lymphoma, primary lung cancer, or metastatic disease from virtually any site can cause obstruction of the thoracic duct, resulting in rupture of lymphatic tributaries and chylothorax. Infection, filariasis, venous obstruction (SVC, subclavian, or jugular veins), cirrhosis, tuberculosis, and pulmonary lymphangioleiomyomatosis (LAM) are less common etiologies of chylothorax. A history of the above procedures, injuries, or conditions and the presence of a pleural effusion, high output serous chest drainage in patients who are not taking oral intake, or milky chest drainage should prompt additional workup to rule out a chylothorax or to confirm the suspected diagnosis. The following chapter focuses primarily on the more common traumatic and neoplastic causes of chylothorax.

Tests

The history of a change in the chest tube output from serous fluid to non-clotting, milky fluid is a classic presentation for chylothorax. Patients who have not begun enteral feedings/oral intake and have high serous chest tube output may be fed high fat content substances, such as heavy cream or olive oil, which will increase output and trigger this characteristic change in appearance. Dyes such as Evan's blue (injected subcutaneously) or methylene blue (added to enteral intake) may also be used. However, oral/enteral intake may not be possible in some patients. Therefore, one should be aware of some of the fluid analyses that may be used to help confirm the diagnosis. Lymph is comprised of fat, proteins, and lymphocytes and even in the fasting state, the concentration of fat is higher than that of serum. The fluid is typically sent for triglycerides first. A concentration of > 110 mg/dL confirms the diagnosis of a chylous leak in 99% of cases, whereas a chylous leak is present in less than 5% of case with a concentration of < 50 mg/dL. In cases where the triglyceride level is equivocal and suspicion remains high, the fluid should be sent for chylomicrons. The presence of any concentration of chylomicrons is diagnostic, as these lipoproteins are not present in serum. Microscopic examination may demonstrate fat globules that stain with Sudan-3 or clear with alkali/ether, with both tests being diagnostic of a chylous leak. Lymphangiography is an invasive test that may be useful in difficult cases, such as failed thoracic duct ligation or left-sided chylothoraces. Lymphangiography may be used to localize the site of leak and plan the approach for additional invasive procedures.

Index scenario (additional information)

"The patient described above is afebrile, hemodynamically stable, and is otherwise doing well on the floor. Chest tube drainage was sent for fluid analysis, showing a triglyceride level of 220 and chylomicrons of 50, confirming your suspicion of chylothorax. Discuss your management going forward."

Treatment/management

Options for management of chylothorax include medical management with lipid-intake restriction or by abolishing all enteral intake and administering total parenteral nutrition (TPN); or invasive procedures such as surgical ligation of the thoracic duct, lymphatic tributary clipping, application of biologic sealant (i.e., fibrin glue), obliteration of the pleural space by surgical or chemical pleurodesis, pleuroperitoneal shunting, or lymphoscintigraphy with thoracic duct embolization or cisterna chyli fenestration.

"Describe the basis for medical management of this patient. How long would you treat medically before deciding to re-operate?"

Medical management has four main components: minimizing chyle production and flow through the thoracic duct, drainage of the chylous effusion to relieve symptoms, replacing fluid losses, and maintaining adequate nutrition. The main role of the thoracic duct is to transport absorbed lipids from the intestine to the venous system. Chyle is composed of lipids (free fatty acids, cholesterol, cholesterol esters, and phospholipids), proteins (such as albumin and fibrinogen), fat-soluble vitamins, enzymes, lymphocytes (mostly T lymphocytes), and antibodies. The thoracic duct also carries extravasated proteins and excess interstitial fluid along with chyle. The composition and volume of chyle depends primarily on the timing, lipid-content, and amount of enteral intake. It takes approximately 90 minutes for ingested lipids to reach the systemic circulation. Long-chain fatty acids are absorbed by the intestine and are transported by chylomicrons in chyle, giving it the characteristic milky appearance. Short and medium chain fatty acids (< 10 carbon atoms) are absorbed directly by the portal system, bypassing the lymphatic circulation. Therefore a diet restricting lipid intake to medium chain fatty acids or complete bowel rest decreases the volume of chyle and increases the chance of spontaneous healing of the duct leak.

An undrained chylothorax will eventually lead to a chylous effusion and compressive atelectasis, resulting in dyspnea in most patients. Drainage is then required, typically by tube thoracostomy. This relieves the acute pulmonary symptoms, however ongoing drainage of a chylous leak leads to loss of important lipids, proteins, vitamins, and lymphocytes, resulting in malnutrition and immunosuppression. Diet restriction helps to minimize these losses. Patients who are maintained on a lipid-restricted diet may be able to maintain adequate nutrition. However, fasting patients should receive nutritional support with total parenteral nutrition (TPN). Commonly used as an adjunct to medical therapy, Somatostatin or its synthetic analog, Octreotide, have been shown to decrease foregut secretions and in turn lymph production.

Spontaneous closure/sealing of thoracic duct leaks are expected in roughly half of patients treated with non-operative/medical therapy. Therefore half of patients will require some form of invasive procedure to prevent ongoing drainage of chyle into the mediastinum and pleural space. Morbidity and mortality increases significantly if the chylothorax has not resolved by one week. High output chylothoraces (> 1 L/day) are less likely to resolve with medical management alone. Cut-offs points for determining failure of medical therapy are controversial. In general, alternative methods to treat the chylothorax should be carried out if the leak fails to seal after 2 weeks of medical therapy or if there is greater than 1 L of output daily. The threshold to abandon non-operative/medical management should be lowered for patients who are immunosuppressed or malnourished.

"You decide to keep treating the patient with bowel rest, octreotide, and TPN. Two weeks have now passed and the patient continues to have ~500 cc/day of chest tube output. Fluid analysis shows a persistently elevated triglyceride level. What would you do next? Describe your approach to thoracic duct ligation."

Persistent chylothorax has been confirmed with the triglyceride level of > 110 mg/dL and the patient has failed to resolve the leak after 2 weeks of non-operative management. Output remains considerable. This leak is unlikely to seal and more invasive measures should be taken.

Suspected location/laterality of the chyle leak plays an important role in surgical approach to thoracic duct ligation. Unilateral chylothoraces can usually be approached on the side of the chylous effusion if direct ligation or tributary clipping is planned. However, the exact location of the thoracic duct injury or leaking lymphatic tributaries may not always be identifiable once in the operating room. In this case, mass ligation of the thoracic duct just above the diaphragm via the right chest is the best approach. Therefore, right-sided chylothorax should always be approached from the right, permitting direct or mass duct ligation. Some planning is needed for left-sided chylothoraces. One approach is to perform lymphangiography preoperatively to localize the leak. Dye (1% Evans blue injected subcutaneously) or high fat containing substances (6 ounces of heavy cream or olive oil enterally) can be administered 2-3 hours preoperatively to assist in identifying the leak once in the chest. A note about methylene blue: this dye may be added to a fat source and given enterally to help confirm a chylothorax; however it widely stains the mediastinum and is not recommended for intraoperative localization. Alternatively, the lymphangiography can be omitted, provocative measures taken preoperatively, and the chest explored by a VATS approach. This avoids redo or second thoracotomy and allows the surgeon to attempt to localize the leak by direct visualization. If the leak cannot be identified with preoperative lymphangiography or by VATS, the safest approach is to perform a mass ligation via the right chest, which will in effect treat the left chylothorax. Some surgeons always recommend a right-sided mass ligation of the thoracic duct, even in left sided chylothoraces. Bilateral chylothoraces should be treated with mass duct ligation via the right chest.

Operative steps

Direct thoracic duct ligation or tributary clipping

- Direct ligation of the thoracic duct or clipping of the duct tributaries may be performed thoracoscopically or via thoracotomy. If an open approach is preferred, the chest can be entered through the previous thoracotomy if one was performed.
- As described above, provocative measures can be taken preoperatively to help identify the leak once in the chest.
- Once adhesions have been lysed and the site located, the duct is ligated proximally and distally with non-absorbable suture.
- If there is no injury to the main duct, but rather leakage is noted from disrupted lymphatic tributaries, the tributaries are clipped.
- The addition of a sealant, such as fibrin glue may be added as a secondary measure following direct ligation or clipping to help seal the leak.
- Drains and chest tubes are positioned near the site of repair to monitor output postoperatively.
- If the site of the chylous fistula cannot easily be identified, dissection in the thoracic duct fat to attempt to find the leak should be avoided, as this may result in additional injury to the duct or disruption of lymphatic tributaries. Failure to identify the leak should prompt one to consider mass ligation of the thoracic duct.

Mass thoracic duct ligation

- Mass duct ligation is performed via the right chest thoracoscopically or open. If a previous thoracotomy is present, the chest may be reentered through the same incision. However, a high thoracotomy may not provide adequate access near the hiatus. A thoracotomy in the 6th or 7th intercostal space is ideal.
- For a VATS approach, a camera port is placed in the 7th or 8th intercostal space in the posterior axillary line. Working ports are placed in the 8th or 9th intercostal space in line with the tip of the scapula and just below the tip of the scapula. A lung retraction port is placed in the 5th intercostal space anterior to the latissimus.
- A retraction stitch may be placed in the tendinous portion of the diaphragm to improve exposure of the hiatus.
- Once the diaphragm is retracted inferiorly, the lung is retracted anteriorly.
- The goal of mass ligation of the thoracic duct is to ligate all tissue in the area limited posteriorly by the azygos vein, anteriorly by the esophagus, and medially by the descending aorta, just above the diaphragm to cease all flow of chyle through the thoracic duct.

- A plane is developed just anterior to the azygos vein and dissection is carried down to the aorta. The esophagus is identified anteriorly and all the tissue between the azygos vein and esophagus is doubly ligated with non-absorbable sutures.
- Large clips may be added proximally and distally for reinforcement.
- Biologic sealant, such as fibrin glue, may be added as well.
- Drains and chest tubes are then placed to monitor postoperative output.
- Pleurectomy or chemical pleurodesis may be performed as an added measure of security to promote pleural symphysis and sealing of leaking tributaries or accessory ducts not addressed by the mass ligation. A fully expanded lung is necessary for this to be effective.

Potential questions/alternative scenarios

"Describe the anatomy of the thoracic duct. What percentage of patients do you suspect have this 'normal anatomy'? What are some common variants seen in thoracic duct anatomy?"

The thoracic duct is the main channel that drains lymph from the entire body to the venous system, with the exception of the heart, dome of the liver, and right upper body (face, neck, arm, chest wall, lung, and diaphragm). The thoracic duct originates at the cisterna chyli, which is located anterior to the spine between vertebral bodies T10 to L3. The duct then passes through the aortic hiatus and ascends to the right of the midline, posterior to the esophagus, between the descending thoracic aorta and azygos vein. The duct then passes behind the aorta, crossing the midline between T5–T6 and ascends through the thoracic inlet along the left aspect of the esophagus. Once in the neck, the duct arches laterally, traveling anterior to the left subclavian and thyrocervical arteries, phrenic nerve, and anterior scalene muscle before passing posterior to the carotid sheath and jugular vein. The thoracic duct then drains into the posterior aspect of the left jugular-subclavian vein confluence.

The right thoracic duct drains the right upper body and typically terminates at the right jugular subclavian vein confluence. This duct is small and rarely seen. It is estimated that this "normal" anatomy is present in only half of patients. Some of the more common variants include multiple terminating trunks draining into the venous system, multiple trunks passing through the mediastinum, variable points of cross-over from right to left, and variable drainage pathways of the accessory ducts draining the right upper body. Less than 40% of patients will drain directly into the jugular-subclavian venous confluence, with the duct commonly terminating at the jugular, subclavian, or both veins.

"You have a patient who is 3 days out from an Ivor Lewis esophagectomy for esophageal cancer. Right chest tube output has been moderate (~500 cc/day). Following initiation of enteral feeds via a jejunostomy tube, you are called because the chest tube has put out 750 cc's of milky fluid so far today. Of note, the patient had a preoperative weight loss of 20 pounds and has a BMI of 21. Discuss how your management may or may not differ from the previous patient and why. Do you perform routine thoracic duct ligation during esophagectomy?"

Post-esophagectomy chylothorax occurs in approximately 1-5% of patients. A more aggressive approach is advocated by many for treatment of this patient population due to higher failure rates with medical therapy alone. Also, many patients who undergo esophagectomy are malnourished and therefore will not tolerate a longer period of medical management due to the nutritional losses that occur. If the chylous leak does not seal after 5 days of medical management, surgical intervention is typically recommended. Drainage of > 1 L/day has been recommended by some to be the cut-off for non-operative treatment failure, while others have shown a lower chance of spontaneous duct closure with > 400 cc's/day. Some even advocate surgical intervention at the time of diagnosis in this patient population. Besides avoiding the malnutrition and immunosuppression that accompanies a high-output chylous fistula, early intervention has the advantage of re-entering the chest at a time where adhesions are soft and minimal. The conduit vascular pedicle is at risk with dissection near the hiatus during mass thoracic duct ligation, making late reoperation a high-risk endeavor.

Although adding a prophylactic mass thoracic ligation to an esophagectomy adds minimal time and risk of morbidity to the procedure, there is not overwhelming evidence to support routine ligation at the time of resection. However, should a ductal injury be identified intraoperatively, direct suture ligation should be performed. It should be noted that identification of a thoracic duct leak intraoperatively is rare since most patients are in a fasting state and without the presence of lipids, the draining chyle will be serous in appearance.

This patient is already severely malnourished and prompt direct thoracic duct ligation (if the injury can easily be identified) or mass ligation of the thoracic duct is warranted.

"Following mass ligation of the thoracic duct, your patient continues to have a refractory right chylothorax. Beside medical management, what are some other options to manage this patient?"

Refractory chylothorax can be problematic. Failure of medical therapy should be treated surgically with direct or mass ligation of the thoracic duct, with success rates upwards of 90% being expected. Reoperation with mass ligation of the duct may be successful in patients who underwent direct ligation or tributary clipping on the first attempt. In patients who have failed surgical ligation or those in which reentrance into the chest is problematic, lymphangiography may be useful to identify the location of the chylous fistula. Once the site is localized, repeat surgical ligation may be attempted after preoperative administration of heavy cream, olive oil, or Evan's blue dye to help locate the leak intraoperatively. Alternatively, thoracic duct embolization or cysterna chyli fenestration may be carried out at the time of lymphangiography. This procedure is invasive, but less so than reoperation. The cysterna chyli is identified by pedal lymphangiography, followed by transperitoneal access of the cysterna chyli using the Seldinger technique. The duct is cannulated and contrast is injected to identify the fistula on delayed imaging. The site or sites of the leak may then be embolized with use of a variety of materials. If the duct cannot be cannulated, the cysterna chyli may be fenestrated under fluoroscopic guidance to promote drainage of lymph into the peritoneal cavity and decrease flow to the thoracic duct, promoting healing of the leak. Chyle is also reabsorbed in the peritoneum, minimizing nutritional losses. Percutaneous embolization or fenestration has reported success rates of roughly 70% with minimal risk of morbidity and mortality, although this procedure is highly operator-dependent. Regardless, this technique is a useful alternative for patients unwilling or unable to undergo reoperation or in refractory cases where mass or direct ligation has failed.

If the refractory chylothorax is low output and the lung is fully expanded with drainage, pleurectomy or chemical pleurodesis may be performed to promote pleural symphysis and sealing of the leak.

"You are re-consulted on a patient you did a mediastinoscopy on 2 weeks ago to confirm the diagnosis of lymphoma. She now complains of dyspnea and has a right pleural effusion. You place a chest tube, confirming the diagnosis of chylothorax. What is the cause of chylothorax in this patient? How would you manage this patient going forward?"

Neoplastic processes may lead to lymphatic duct obstruction by direct invasion, mass effect/compression, or tumor embolism. The obstruction eventually leads to rupture of lymphatic tributaries and accumulation of a chylous effusion. Lymphoma accounts for over half the cases of neoplastic chylothorax. Treatment of the primary lesion with radiation and/or chemotherapy will resolve the chylothorax in many cases, resulting in either shrinkage of the culprit lesion and relief of the obstruction or fibrosis of the lymphatics and closure of the leak. However, the effusion may be symptomatic in some patients, in which case waiting for the systemic therapy to take effect may not be tolerated. Given the abnormal lymphatic drainage in these patients, larger or symptomatic effusions should be drained by tube thoracostomy. Asymptomatic, small chylous effusions may be aspirated or observed, with hopes that initiation of systemic therapy will resolve the leak. It is likely that most duct injuries or leaks do not resolve by healing of the duct itself, but rather are sealed by pleural symphysis. Therefore adequate drainage is necessary for pleural apposition to occur. Some advocate chest tube drainage and chemical pleurodesis via the indwelling tube with such irritants as tetracycline, doxycyline, bleomycin, or talc to promote pleural fusion and sealing of the lymphatic leak. High-output or inadequately drained chylous effusions are unlikely to heal with this technique. Lymphangiography with percutaneous embolization or cysterna chyli fenestration may be a useful alternative in such cases. Surgical intervention, such as pleurectomy and/or duct ligation, is not recommended in patients with non-traumatic chylothorax caused by neoplastic disease in order to avoid delaying initiation of systemic therapy and operating on a typically deconditioned patient. Pleuroperitoneal shunting is one surgical option that has been used in this patient population with some success. These shunts relieve dyspnea by draining the effusion, while nutrients are reabsorbed as the chyle is drained into the peritoneal cavity. Ascites is an absolute contraindication to pleuroperitoneal shunts.

Pearls/pitfalls

- Chylothorax should be in the differential for post-traumatic or postoperative high, serous chest tube
  output. Further workup is needed to confirm the diagnosis.
- Understand the basic principles of medical management for treatment of chylothorax and have a threshold for treatment failure.
- The site of the thoracic duct leak may not be easily identified intraoperatively. Anticipate this scenario "curveball" and have a plan for how to manage it.
- Mass ligation via the right chest can be used to treat right, left, or bilateral chylothorax and is probably the safest answer when describing surgical management of chylothorax.
- Variations in thoracic duct anatomy are nearly as common as "normal" anatomy.
- Thoracic duct ligation and pleurectomy should be avoided when possible for management of neoplastic chylothorax.

Suggested readings

- Johnstone DW. Anatomy of the Thoracic Duct and Chylothorax. In: Shields TW, LoCicero J III, Reed CJ, Feins RH (eds.) *General Thoracic Surgery*. 7th ed. Philadelphia, PA: Lippincott Williams & Wilkins; 2009:827-834.

- Merigliano S, Molena D, Ruol A, Zaninotto G, Cagol M, Scappin S, Ancona E. Chylothorax complicating esophagectomy for cancer: a plea for early thoracic duct ligation. *J Thorac Cardiovasc Surg.* 2000; 199: 453-457.

- Shah R, Luketich JD, Schuchert MJ, Christie NA, Pennathur A, Landreneau RJ, Nason KS. Postesophagectomy chylothorax: incidence, risk factors, and outcomes. *Ann Thorac Surg.* 2012; 93: 897-904.

- Itkin M, Kucharczuk JC, Kwak A, Trerotola SO, Kaiser LR. Nonoperative thoracic duct embolization for traumatic thoracic duct leak: experience in 109 patients. *J Thorac Cardiovasc Surg.* 2010 Mar;139(3):584-589; discussion 589-590.

Notes

115

15. Primary chest wall tumors

Christian C. Shults, MD, and Seth Force, MD

Concept

- Differential for chest wall tumors
- Indicated testing and therapy for the different etiologies
- Techniques for reconstruction
- Adjuvant Therapy

Chief complaint

"A 30 yo man presents with a painless right chest mass that has been slowly growing over the last 5 years."

Differential

Primary chest wall tumor (CWT), adjacent tumors with local invasion, metastatic lesions, or non-neoplastic disease. It is helpful to classify lesions in terms of origin (soft tissue vs. bone/cartilage) and then to sub-classify as benign vs. malignant (** indicates most common with % where available).

- *Benign bony and cartilaginous*: fibrous dysplasia ** (30% of all benign chest wall tumors), osteochondroma ** (50% of all benign rib tumors), chondroma ** (15% of all benign rib tumors), plasmacytoma.
- *Malignant bony and cartilaginous*: chondrosarcoma ** (30% of all primary malignant bone tumors), Ewing sarcoma, osteogenic sarcoma, Askin tumor.
- *Benign soft tissue*: desmoid tumor** (sometimes classified as low grade sarcoma), lipoma, hemangioma, lymphangioma, fibroma, rhabdomyoma, neurofibroma.
- *Malignant soft tissue*: malignant fibrous histiocytoma (MFH) ** (most common primary CWT), rhabdomyosarcoma ** (second most common primary chest wall tumor), liposarcoma, neurofibrosarcoma, leiomyosarcoma.
- *Adjacent tumors (24% of all CWT)*: lung, breast, pleura, mediastinum, skin (including melanoma).
- *Metastatic tumors (32% of all CWT)*: sarcoma and carcinoma.
- *Non-neoplastic conditions*: inflammatory and cystic lesions.

History and physical

The majority of chest wall lesions are the result of metastasis (sarcoma most common) or invasion from adjacent malignancies. Primary chest wall tumors are typically slow-growing masses and 75% are painless. Malignant lesions or lesions arising from bone tend to be painful due to expansion into the cortex or periosteum, destruction of the cortex, or resulting fractures. Important information obtained in the history includes: age (there is an age distribution associated with most masses), symptoms (pain usually indicates malignancy or invasion into bone), history of trauma, and any history of associated disease, weight loss, or previous mass/cancer. The physical exam should focus on whether the mass is soft or firm, fixed or mobile, and tender or painless. A rapid increase in size suggests a malignant lesion. Evidence of previous incisions or trauma should also be assessed.

Tests
- *CXR*: first step, many tumors have a classic radiographic appearance.
- *CT*: highest yield (site, size, bony involvement, screen lungs for metastasis).
- *MRI*: most sensitive, differentiate tumor as well as relationship to critical structures (vascular, neural).
- *PET*: differentiate benign from malignant, delineate tumor grade.
- Diagnosis is ultimately made with biopsy (unless resection planned regardless of diagnosis) and can be performed by core needle biopsy, excisional biopsy (lesions < 5 cm), or incisional biopsy (lesions > 5 cm). It is crucial that the biopsy be performed along the plane of potential surgical resection. Frozen section is usually of little use for diagnostic purposes given frequent bone and cartilage involvement.
- *Labs*: baseline parameters, coags.

Treatment/management
CWTs are a heterogenous group of lesions. However, the general strategy remains the same for most lesions. History and imaging may be enough to make the diagnosis or lead one to have a suspicion of the diagnosis. Tissue should be obtained when the diagnosis remains in questions, although in many circumstances the diagnosis will be made when the lesion is resected. Core needle, incisional, or excisional biopsies are options that must be considered based on the tumor characteristics and suspected diagnosis. Biopsies should not compromise future treatment and care should be take to take biopsies that are oriented within the potential place of resection. Most benign lesions can be observed, unless they are symptomatic. Malignant lesions must be resected. Treatment involves appropriate excisional margins (2-4 cm) for malignant lesions to minimize the chance of local recurrence. Reconstruction may be required and if so, then soft tissue coverage of the reconstruction material may also be required.

"Let's say the lesion in question is slow growing, as mentioned, and the appearance on the CT scan is consistent with lipoma."

Slow growing lesions with benign characteristics on CT scan are likely benign. Treatment includes biopsy to rule out a malignant tumor and confirm the suspected histologic diagnosis. Use of core needle, incisional, or excisional biopsy is based primarily on size. Core needle biopsy is a reasonable first step in larger lesions. However, if a diagnosis cannot be made, then incisional biopsy is needed. Excisional biopsy for smaller lesions (2-4 cm) would also be appropriate.

"Describe your approach to an excisional biopsy (benign or malignant)?"

Excisional biopsy may be appropriate for small lesions or lesions that are thought to be benign, but tissue confirmation is needed. Margins typically only need to be grossly negative in these circumstances. Benign lesions that tend to recur (as noted in other scenarios above and below), chondromas (benign lesion with significant risk of harboring occult areas of malignant sarcoma), or other specific lesions may require "wide" local excision, typically 2-4 cm. Excisional biopsies do not require resection of the overlying skin, however the incisions should be oriented so that if final pathology does demonstrate malignant disease, then the area can be re-resected, including the previous incisions, overlying skin, and surrounding structures. Wide local excision may be accomplished with light monitored sedation versus GETA depending on the size and extent of resection. Oblique incision parallel to the ribs about 2-4 cm on each side of the lesion. Go down through the skin, dermis, and subcutaneous tissue and raise a flap around the tumor leaving fascia on the muscle. Bovie out a circle around the tumor down to the bone with at least 2-4 cm margin of tissue. Ensure that the tumor is freely mobile within the soft tissue and not involving the bone (if the lesion is a primary bone tumor then the rib or bone would be resected with the appropriate margin). Undermine the undersurface of the tumor and hand off the specimen with proper orientation sutures. If the suspicion for malignancy is low, send for permanent, as frozens are not likely to change management. If there is any question about margins, then send the specimen for frozen and/or send a specimen of free margin in the area of concern. Get hemostasis and reapproximate the remaining muscle, subq and dermis. You may need to mobilize the muscle laterally to release tension.

"Let's say instead of a 30 yo man it is a 3 yo boy with what appears to be a hemangioma on the chest wall."

Treatment for hemangiomas in children is non-operative except for cosmetic reasons or complications such as bleeding or ulceration. If there is any question as to the diagnosis, a T2 MRI will show a high signal intensity in the case of hemangioma. Given its benign nature, excision with grossly negative margins is all that is needed.

"What if this lesion were a Lymphangioma?"
Lymphangiomas are benign chest wall lesions that are most commonly found in children. Surgical resection is required to prevent recurrence. OK-432 and acetic acid sclerotherapy may also be used.

"Let's say the patient is a 24 yo woman with a history of trauma to the area and Gardner's Syndrome?"
With a history of Gardner's Syndrome, the desmoid tumor alarm should be going off in your head. 50% of these tumors occur in the abdomen, however the chest wall is the most common extra-abdominal site. They originate from fibroblasts of the deep muscle and connective tissue and most commonly present in the teens – 30's. 62% are painful and are associated with a history of trauma, thoracotomy, and Gardner's Syndrome. They are slow growing and have a very high recurrence rate. Wide local excision with 4 cm margins is optimal. Adjuvant radiation is commonly used to decrease local recurrence rates with both negative and positive margins. There is an 89% 5 year probability of local recurrence with positive margins and 18% if the margins are negative.

"Let's say the patient is a 25 yo man with a CWT on the posterolateral aspect of the 6th rib. The mass is slow growing, asymptomatic, and was incidentally found. The x-ray shows a ground glass appearance of the central area of the rib with thinning of the cortex and irregular calcification in the medulla. How would you manage this patient?"
These are all characteristics of a benign lesion, the most common of which (30%) is fibrous dysplasia. These typically present in the 20-30's on the posterior or lateral aspect of the ribs and are asymptomatic, slow-growing, and are usually found incidentally. They are associated with Albright Syndrome (skin lesions and precocious puberty in girls). Imaging shows the classic ground-glass appearance in the central area of the rib, thinning of the cortex, and irregular calcifications in the medulla. Treatment is local excision for painful lesions. Asymptomatic lesions can be left alone (unless the diagnosis is in doubt). In general biopsies of these lesions are of little yield.

"Let's say the patient is a 20 yo man with growths arising from the cortical bone anteriorly at the costochondral junction along the sternum with caps that feel cartilaginous. X-ray/CT Scan shows a pedunculated protuberance with intact cortex and stippled calcification in the area of the tumor. How would you treat this lesion?"
This is the classic presentation of an osteochondroma. These are cartilage

capped growths that arise from the cortical bone of the sternum anteriorly at the costochondral junction along the sternum. These CWTs most commonly present in the patients 20's with a 3:1 M:F predominance. Imaging findings are as above with a pedunculated protuberance, intact cortex, and stippled calcification in the area of the tumor. Malignant degeneration is rare in these lesions and wide local excision with margins of 2-4 cm is warranted for lesions that are symptomatic, enlarging, or if the diagnosis is in doubt and the patient is an adult.

"You are referred a 30 yo woman with an asymptomatic, slow-growing mass with X-ray/CT findings showing a periosteal lytic mass with a thinning cortex and sclerotic borders. How would you manage this patient?"
This is most likely a chondroma (bening CWT), however it is hard to distinguish chondroma from a malignant, degenerative chondrosarcoma. Therefore treatment is excision with wide margins of 2 cm in all cases. These masses are asymptomatic, slow-growing, most commonly ages 20-40 with M = F. If the lesions proves to be malignant of final pathology (frozen will not help in determining this), then re-resection with 4 cm margins is needed.

"You are seeing another patient, a 60 yo man with pain and no palpable mass in the lateral chest wall. He is also hypercalcemic with a urinalysis positive for Bence-Jones protein. What is the suspected diagnosis and how would you treat this patient?"
Pain with no mass, hypercalcemia, and Bence-Jones proteinuria are key here. This is a plasmacytoma, which is highly associated with multiple myeloma. These CWTs most commonly occur in men, 60-70 yo, and present with pain and no palpable mass. These patients will have Bence-Jones protein in the urine with abnormal protein electrophoresis and hypercalcemia. A bone marrow biopsy will confirm the diagnosis. These patients are treated with surgery for tissue diagnosis only (core needle or incisional biopsy), followed by high-dose radiation. 35% to 55% of patients progress to multiple myelomas, with an overall 5-year survival 25% to 35%.

"You are referred a 60 yo man with a painless slow-growing mass that on CT scan appears to originate from the muscle and grows along the fascial planes between muscle fibers. How would you treat?"
This is a malignant soft tissue Malignant Fibrous Histiocytoma (MFH). This is the most common chest wall sarcoma. It has a male > female predominance and most commonly occurs in the 50's to 70's. These lesions are painless, and slow-growing, originate in the muscle, and grow along the fascial planes between the muscle fibers. Treatment is wide local resection. There is a high local recurrence rate with metastasis 30-

120

50% of the time. 5 year survival is 38%. Adjuvant radiation is given for inadequate margins or high histologic grade. You may also perform re-resection of low-grade tumors.

"A 15 yo boy with a rhabdomyosarcoma is now referred to you. How would you treat this patient?"
Most common in children and adolescents. Treatment is wide local excision and multi-drug chemotherapy. Neoadjuvant therapy followed by surgical excision has a 75% survival rate vs. 25% for surgery alone.

"You are seeing a 50 yo man with a large encapsulated tumor. Previous biopsy of the mass shows a liposarcoma. How would you treat this malignant lesion?"
Liposarcomas occur most commonly in men ages 40-60. They present as large encapsulated tumors. Treatment consists of wide excision to prevent local recurrence. 5 year survival rates are 60%. Other soft tissue malignancies include neurofibrosarcoma and leiomyosarcoma.

"A 40 yo woman presents with a painful, hard, fixed mass at the costochondral angle and with a history of trauma to the region several years ago. The CT scan shows a mixed lytic and sclerotic pattern with an ovulated mass originating from the medulla with cortical lesions as well as some areas of thickened cortex."
This is a chondrosarcoma. This is the most common primary malignancy of the anterior chest wall. It occurs most commonly in 30-60 year olds M = F. It is associated with prior trauma and presents as a painful hard, fixed mass. 80% arise from the costochondral angle and 20% from the sternum. CT scan will show a mixed lytic and sclerotic pattern with a mass originating from the medulla with cortical lytic lesions as well as some areas of thickened cortex. Treatment consists of resection of localized lesions with wide local excision (2-4 cm, or one uninvolved rib above and below). This tumor is radio-resistant and radiation is reserved for positive margins only. Outcome is highly dependent upon the grade of the tumor: Low-grade (mild hypercellularity) – 10 year survival 96% with few metastases. High – grade (marked hypercellularity) have metastases 75% of the time and a 5-year survival of 20-30%. Poor prognostic factors include high tumor grade, large tumor size, incomplete resection, local recurrence, metastasis and patient age over 50 years.

"Walk me through how you would resect this tumor or any primary bone tumor on the anterolateral chest wall."

Operative steps
Chest wall resection for an anterolateral CWT

- Based upon preoperative imaging you would first identify the superior and inferior margins of resection.
- The patient would receive a double lumen tube and an epidural.
- The patient would be positioned in lateral decubitus with the involved side up. (If lateral chest wall lesion.)
- Complete resection is the best chance for cure. Objectives for resection would be a 2-4 cm margin including the rib above and the rib below the tumor as well as involved skin (including biopsy site) and parietal pleura if involved.
- Make an oblique incision parallel to the ribs about 4 cm on each side of the lesion down through the skin.
- Dissect through the dermis and subcutaneous tissue, raise a flap around the tumor leaving fascia on the muscle.
- Get enough exposure to palpate a rib above and a rib below easily.
- Bovie out a circle around the tumor down to the bone with at least 2-4 cm margin of tissue. Score the ribs anteriorly and posteriorly.
- Drop the lung and enter the pleura at the intercostal space below, above, or anterior to the tumor. Note that it is not always necessary to explore the chest at this time if the CT shows no evidence of intrapleural involvement. If there is any doubt, then plan on placing a retractor of choice and exploring the pleural space prior to proceeding.
- Free the intercostal musculature and neurovascular bundles surrounding the upper and the lower ribs. Clear the periosteum 1.5 cm from each border and separate the rib from the underlying pleura. Cut the ribs. An additional 1 cm posterior and anterior margins of the ribs are sent separately and marked appropriately to ensure free margins. Note that in the case of a costochondral tumor, this may require ligation of the mammary artery and resection of the cartilaginous ribs near the sternum. If it abuts the sternum it may require partial resection of the sternum as described below.
- Ligate and divide the neurovascular bundles accompanying the upper and lower ribs that were resected.
- Any soft tissue margin with questionable involvement should be sent for pathologic frozen section to assess whether wider margins are required.

In all patients with a malignant primary chest wall tumor the 5-year freedom from recurrence rate is 56% in patients resected with 4 cm margins and 25% with 2 cm margins.

Potential questions/alternative scenarios

"What if the tumor was not palpable and the patient is obese?"

Multiple options exist. The lesion can be marked by radiology using the CT scanner in an orientation that is perpendicular to the epicenter of the lesion. Alternatively, intraoperative ultrasound could be used to aid with localization. If the lesion involves the rib, a quick VATS can be performed using a camera away from the tumor to identify the boundaries of the tumor and mark with a long spinal needle if needed.

"What if the tumor is adherent to the lung, sternum or the pericardium?"

Tissue adherent to the tumor—including superficial chest wall muscles, lung, thymus, pericardium, or diaphragm—should be resected en bloc. If the sternum is involved, it may require partial or total sternectomy along with excision of the contiguous bilateral costal margins. Try to maintain the circumferential integrity of the chest wall for pulmonary function. If the lower sternum is involved, preserve the manubrium. If the sternal body is involved, a subtotal sternectomy is performed, preserving the upper 2 cm of manubrium and clavicles. If the manubrium is involved, spare the lower half of the sternum. Rigid reconstruction of the sternum is required. Note that advanced primary lung cancers are discussed in chapters 2-3. However, if the lung is adherent to the rib in the setting of a primary lung cancer, then the resection proceeds very much as described above with a few important caveats. It is critical in this scenario to explore the chest before starting your resection. If the tumor is high, then this is easily done through an anterolateral or posterolateral thoracotomy in the 4th or 5th intercostal space. Place your retractor, palpate the lung and assess the degree of chest wall invasion from within the chest. At this point you can either perform the chest wall resection through a separate incision exactly as described above and then perform the lobectomy or perform the lobectomy first followed by the chest wall resection. What if the mass is in the 5th rib in the middle of the thoracotomy exposure that you intended to use for the lobectomy? Enter the intercostal space anterior or posterior to the tumor (depending on location) and proceed as just described. You will obviously not need a separate incision for the chest wall resection in this case as it will be a part your thoracotomy incision. The thoracotomy incision will be closed primarily as usual but the posterior or anterior chest wall defect will require reconstruction as described below.

"How would you reconstruct the defect?"

A subsequent reconstruction may use simple prosthetic placement or more complex tissue transposition techniques. Technique is dependent upon the location and size of the defect.

"Let's say you have a high posterior defect above the 5th rib and < 10 cm?"

All high posterior defects above the 5th rib and < 10 cm do not need reconstruction since the defect will be covered by scapula. Resection that involves the 5th rib can lead to entrapment of the scapula in the defect if it is not reconstructed.

"What if it is an anterior defect?"

All anterior defects < 5 cm do not require reconstruction. Resection of three or more ribs, or removal of two or more ribs with baseline pulmonary compromise needs reconstruction.

"What if you've resected bilateral sternoclavicular joints?"

Resection of bilateral sternoclavicular joints, entire sternum, or upper part of the manubrium needs reconstruction (unilateral sternoclavicular joint not typically reconstructed)

General reconstruction techniques

Materials
- *Rigid reconstruction*: Marlex-methylmethacrylate sandwich, titanium bars, Bio-absorbable bars (biobridge)
- *Non-rigid reconstruction*: Gortex, marlex, bovine pericardium

Technique

Suture prosthetic mesh to the chest wall under tension.

Infected/Irradiated fields: bovine pericardium or processed cellular matrix (Alloderm). A Marlex "sandwich" used when more rigid support is needed: sternal or anterolateral resections. Mesh is measured to 2x the size of the defect. A 2 to 3 mm layer of methyl methacrylate is then poured on one half of the mesh and then the other half of the mesh is folded over. The mesh edges are then sutured to the edge of the wound defect with permanent suture. One technique that is commonly used: drill holes in the exposed rib edges

anteriorly and then posteriorly. Bring in the measured material and use thick non-absorbable sutures (i.e., 1-0 prolene) in an interrupted fashion through the ribs and then the material of choice. Along the top and bottom the suture goes around the staying rib and then through the material. Tie all sutures at the end. Muscle and soft tissue will then be mobilized above this material as needed to achieve complete coverage.

"What if the field is infected?"

Prosthetic reconstruction is contraindicated in infected wounds, in which case skeletal reconstruction should be delayed or biologic material should be used (Biobridge). In these cases, autologous tissue such as muscle and omentum can be used. Soft tissue reconstruction can be used when skeletal stability is not required. Soft tissue options include: split-thickness skin grafts, muscle grafts, or musculocutaneous grafts (Latissimus Dorsi, Pectoralis Major, Serratus, Rectus Abdominus, External oblique).

"A 50 yo man with prior radiation to the chest presents with a rapidly expanding painful mass and elevated alkaline phosphatase levels. The CT scan shows a sunburst pattern and shows the tumor lifting the periosteum. What is the most likely diagnosis based on the imaging findings. How would you manage this patient?"
This is an osteogenic sarcoma. These CWTs are most commonly seen in the long bones. Osteogenic sarcomas represent approximately 6% of all primary chest wall malignancies. These masses are rapidly expanding, painful, and cause elevated alkaline phosphatase levels. CT will show the classic sunburst pattern (sometimes seen on radiograph – representing calcifications at the right angles to the cortex) and Codman's triangle wherein the tumor lifts the periosteum and creates a shadow between the cortex and the raised periosteum. This tumor most commonly occurs in teenagers or adults. It is seen in patients with Paget disease, prior radiation, or prior bone infarction. It is associated with mutations in the RB gene p53. Biopsy can be performed as a core needle, incisional, or excisional. Treatment is neoadjuvant chemotherapy and wide local excision. Outcome is poor with metastasis with a 20% survival rate – lung is the primary site of metastasis. Overall survival is 14-20%.

"A 15 yo boy presents with a rapidly enlarging painful mass. The CT scan shows an onion-peel appearance. What is the most likely diagnosis based on the imaging findings. How would you manage this patient?"
This is a Ewing sarcoma with the classic radiographic appearance of the onion-peel that occurs from the bony destruction and the reactive multiple layers of new periosteal formation. This tumor occurs most commonly in 10-15 yo males (M:F, 2:1). With this presentation you must first get a core biopsy to confirm the diagnosis. This is done with reverse-transcription polymerase chain reaction analysis of the gene locations. Treatment is neoadjuvant chemotherapy followed by wide local excision. Radiation is added for additional cortical control and for positive margins. Survival is 56-65% at 5 years and 43% at 10 years.

"A 17 yo boy presents with a large soft tissue mass that involves the chest wall with pleural thickening. Core biopsy shows small round cells on light microscopy and the cells stained positive for neuron-specific enolase (NSE) and electron microscopy showed dense core granules in the cytoplasm. What is the diagnosis and how would you treat?"
This is an Askin tumor, which is a primitive neuroectodermal tumor

(PNET) from the Ewing sarcoma family of tumors. The radiographic findings will be non-specific. This tumor is difficult to differentiate from other small cell tumors of childhood and young adulthood (Ewing's) especially if only using light microscopy. Positive staining for neuron-specific enolase and dense core granules in the cytoplasm help to differentiate Askin tumors. Workup and treatment are the same as for Ewing's tumor. The presence of a posterior and pleural-based mass in the chest or the presence of a retroperitoneal mass in the abdomen should alert you to the possibility of spread along the sympathetic chain. Presence of these metastatic foci would have significant treatment implications. These tumors are more aggressive than Ewings with a 5 year survival of 16%.

"A 30 yo man presents with a right chest wall soft tissue mass. An incisional biopsy showed plasmacytoma. Do you proceed with resection alone?"
No. Plasmacytoma of the chest wall, even if solitary, should be considered a systemic disease. Resection is reasonable but systemic therapy with radiation and/or chemotherapy is key.

Pearls/pitfalls
- Heterogenous group of tumors (diagnosis is key)
- Needle aspiration not adequate, need tissue for diagnosis, ideally open biopsy
- Plan biopsy to lie within resection margins along the long axis of the tumor
- Most benign lesions can be observed unless symptomatic or otherwise complicated, malignant lesions must be excised
- Complete resection is the most important prognostic factor
- Most CWT are resistant to chemo/radiation
- If there is any doubt as to diagnosis, tissue diagnosis by histologic examination is required
- If suspicion for malignancy you want 4 cm margin, check margins with frozen
- Do not place mesh in an infected field, reconstruct with biologics or native tissue, or plan to return when the infection is cleared for reconstruction
- Must reconstruct
  - Posterior defects below 4th rib
  - All anterior defects > 5 cm
  - Resection of three or more ribs
  - Removal of two or more ribs with baseline pulmonary compromise

- Resection of the manubrium
- Entire sternum

Suggested readings

- Smith MA, Yang SC. Primary tumors of the chest wall. Cameron JL (ed). *Current Surgical Therapy*. Philadelphia: Elsevier 2011:673.
- Allen TC, Cagle PT. Pathology of chest wall tumors. Franco KL, Thourani VH (eds). *Cardiothoracic Surgery Review*. Philadelphia: Lippincott Williams & Wilkins 2012:1169.
- Fabre D, Missenard G, Fadel E, Kolb P, Besse B, Darteville P. Surgical treatment of chest wall tumors. Franco KL, Thourani VH (eds). *Cardiothoracic Surgery Review*. Philadelphia: Lippincott Williams & Wilkins 2012:1178.
- Park BJ, Flores RM. Chest wall tumors. Shields TW, LoCicero J III, Reed CE (eds). *General Thoracic Surgery*. Philadelphia: Lippincott Williams & Wilkins, 2009:669.

Notes

16. Thoracic outlet syndrome

Roman V. Petrov, MD, and Kaj H. Johansen, MD

Concept
- Anatomy of thoracic outlet region
- Variants of thoracic outlet syndrome (TOS): neurogenic, venous, arterial
- Clinical presentation and key physical findings
- Workup of patients with TOS
- Non-operative and operative management of different variants of TOS

Chief complaint
"You are seeing a 29 yo woman who complains of right shoulder and neck pain, occipital headaches, and weakness/numbness of her right arm over the last several months. She is seeking disability benefits and requesting an oxycontin refill."

Differential
Oftentimes patients referred for evaluation of thoracic outlet syndrome (TOS), especially the neurogenic variant, have a long standing history of symptoms and an extensive, fruitless work-up. As such, this diagnosis frequently is a diagnosis of exclusion. Conditions to differentiate: carpal tunnel syndrome, ulnar nerve compression, cervical spine strain, cervical degenerative disk disease/spinal stenosis, brachial plexus injury, fibromyalgia, syringomyelia, polymyalgia rheumatica, structural shoulder injury, compression from tumor (i.e., superior sulcus tumor).

TOS consists of a constellation of symptoms produced by compression of the subclavian vessels and/or the brachial plexus by the musculoskeletal structures of the thoracic outlet. The exact mechanism of compression is not always clear, however the first rib is almost always involved. For this reason, resection of the first rib for decompression is the surgical treatment of choice in most cases. Three variants of thoracic outlet exist – neurogenic (brachial plexus compression, nTOS – 95%), venous (effort thrombosis, Paget-Schroetter syndrome, vTOS - 5%) and arterial (aTOS – 1%).

Understanding the anatomy of the thoracic outlet is critical for treatment of this patient population. A key anatomic region involved in TOS is the scalene triangle, which is bordered by 1) (anterior border) the anterior scalene muscle (ASM) originating from the transverse processes (TP) of C3-C6 and inserting on the first rib 2) (posterior border) middle scalene muscle (MSM) originating from TP of C2-C7 inserting on the superior-lateral surface of the first rib posteriorly 3) (base) superior border of the first rib. The brachial plexus and subclavian artery pass between the anterior and middle scalene muscle, while the subclavian vein passes anteromedial to the triangle.

The brachial plexus consists of 3 trunks traversing the scalene triangle. These include the upper trunk (C5-C6 roots), middle trunk (C7 root) and the lower trunk (C8-T1 roots). Several additional nerves pass through the scalene triangle – the phrenic nerve (C3-C5 roots) travels on the anterior surface of the ASM from lateral to medial before diving under the subclavian vein and down through the mediastinum toward the diaphragm. The long thoracic nerve (C5-C7) passes through the belly of the MSM as it travels distally toward the serratus anterior muscle. The sympathetic chain travels along the posterior inner surface of the ribs and consists of multiple ganglia.

The subclavian artery, after rising from the upper mediastinum, gives off vertebral, internal mammary and thyrocervical branches before entering the scalene triangle. It then arches over the first rib, anterior to the brachial plexus and posterior to ASM. The subclavian vein passes over the first rib anterior to the ASM, but outside of the scalene triangle, and is prone to compression between ASM, first rib, subclavius muscle and the clavicle (costoclavicular space). The thoracic duct can be found on the left side where it enters the junction of the subclavian and internal jugular veins. Compression also may take place between the coracoid process, pectoralis minor (PM) tendon and the chest wall (PM space).

The "classic" anatomy of thoracic outlet is found in less than half of patients and many variations of thoracic outlet region anatomy have been described with additional fibrous bands, muscle structures and bony abnormalities (i.e., cervical ribs). While such anatomic variants are often believed to be predisposing factors, their contribution to symptoms is unclear.

History and physical

A careful review may elicit a history of hyperextension neck trauma (e.g., whiplash). However due to a variable latent period, up to several years between the inciting episode and the appearance of symptoms, a history of trauma can be overlooked. Other conditions predisposing to TOS include repetitive occupational trauma (leads to fibrosis of scalene muscles), bodybuilding (hypertrophy of scalene muscles), poor posture and aging (lead to narrowing of scalene triangle), obesity, pregnancy and others. Clavicular fractures/deformities or a cervical rib can compress thoracic outlet structures and can predispose to TOS as well.

Pain, parenthesis, and weakness are the primary symptoms of nTOS. These symptoms usually affect the arm and hand, most commonly in the ulnar nerve distribution (lower brachial plexus trunk). Extension of the pain to the shoulder, neck, and occipital region is common. Bilateral TOS is not uncommon, although symptoms on one side are usually more prominent. Late, worrisome findings include hand grip weakness and intrinsic hand muscle atrophy.

Physical examination focuses on eliciting symptoms with active and passive range of motion of the arm, neck and head. Degree of disability, such as muscle atrophy and weakness, are assessed as well as sensory abnormalities. Palpation over the scalene triangle may elicit tenderness. Provocative maneuvers include:

- *Elevated arm stress test (EAST)*: arms elevated (surrender positions) repetitive opening and closing of fists elicits typical symptoms.
- *Brachial plexus tension test of Elvey*: arms out, wrists dorsiflexed, tilting of the head produces symptoms on the contralateral side.
- Adson maneuver and Wright test are not useful in diagnosis of nTOS because of their low sensitivity and specificity.

In patients with aTOS, a pulsatile supraclavicular mass or bruit (subclavian aneurysm) and splinter hemorrhages or finger and hand ischemia (signs of distal embolisation) should be sought. Axillo-clavicular venous compression and thrombosis (Paget-Schroetter Syndrome or vTOS) may manifest as upper extremity pain, discoloration and swelling. A prominent net of collateral subcutaneous veins in cases of chronic thrombosis may be present (Urschel's sign).

Tests

nTOS is typically a clinical diagnosis of exclusion and most of the studies are performed to rule out other conditions.

- *Plain radiography, CT, MRI*. Can help identify bony abnormalities, such as spinal stenosis, cervical ribs, disk disease.
- *Electromyography (EMG)*. Usually negative due to the intermittent nature of compression, but may help to exclude other neurogenic conditions.
- *Ulnar nerve conduction velocity (UNCV)*. Has been shown to be useful in nTOS patients and should be obtained in all patients in whom the diagnosis is suspected. Delayed UNCV across the supraclavicular fossa increases the chances that surgical treatment will be needed. Conduction velocities across the median and ulnar nerves are determined at the supraclavicular fossa, mid-upper arm, distal to the elbow, and at the wrist. Normal ulnar nerve velocities at the supraclavicular fossa are > 85 m/s, lower than 55 m/s is considered to be significantly abnormal. Values more distally along

the nerve do not have predictive value in the workup of nTOS, but normally are slower as one moves distally down the nerve.

- *Scalene muscle block.* Relief of symptoms with injection of local anesthetic or botulinum toxin into the belly of ASM is highly sensitive and moderately specific for the diagnosis of nTOS and predicts success of surgical decompression.

Index scenario (additional information)

"The patient admits to having progressive symptoms over several months and now has disabling weakness in her right arm. She is employed as a librarian, but is unable to reach for books on upper shelves and frequently drops objects from her hand. She also admits to frequent tension headaches. On physical examination she has decreased sensation in her medial hand and fingers and internal forearm. Hypothenar atrophy is noted. There is tenderness over the right supraclavicular region. EAST and Elvey tests are positive. Chest and C-spine X-rays do not reveal any abnormalities, MRI is negative. UNCV shows ulnar nerve conduction of 65 m/s and EMG studies were normal."

Treatment/management

Initial management for all patients with a confirmed or suspected diagnosis of nTOS consists of physical therapy. This should focus on stretching the scalene muscles, normalizing posture, and strengthening muscle of the shoulder girdle. NSAIDs, muscle relaxants, and non-narcotic analgesics are adjuncts. Progress is reassessed in 4-6 wks. Two-thirds of the patients with nTOS improve with physical therapy and avoid surgical intervention. Most patients with an UNCV of < 60 m/s will require surgery, but should be treated with physical therapy first. Failure of conservative therapy is an indication for surgical decompression. Indications for surgical decompression without a trial of physical therapy includes nTOS with motor deficits (compared to sensory only), mixed symptoms (both neurologic and vascular symptoms) and vascular symptoms (arterial and venous TOS are always immediate surgical indications, addressed in scenarios below).

Two main surgical approaches currently employed – transaxillary (best for nTOS and vTOS) and supraclavicular (best for aTOS). A posterior transthoracic approach and a VATS approach have also been described.

Transaxillary approach for first rib resection

Pros: cosmetically hidden incision, easy exposure of the first rib, no traction on the brachial plexus.

Cons: poor exposure of scalene muscles, incomplete brachial plexus neurolysis, inadequate vascular exposure.

- Single lumen ETT, supine position with arm elevated above the head with cushion under the shoulder.
- Transverse incision at axillary hairline between pectoralis major and latissimus dorsi, blunt dissection over chest wall to the apex of the axilla. Watch for the intercostobrachial cutaneous nerve.
- Identify first rib, neurovascular bundle beneath the rib, and ASM insertion.
- Divide ASM over a right angle clamp near its insertion on the first rib (protect phrenic).
- Expose the first rib in a subperiosteal plane using a periosteal elevator to strip the intercostal muscle off inferiorly (sweep away pleura to avoid a pneumothorax) and middle scalene muscle off posteriorly-superiorly (watch for long thoracic on its posterior margin).
- A wedge of the first rib is taken out of its mid-portion, including the scalene tubercle (insertion site) to aid with retraction.
- The medial remaining first rib (distal rib) is retracted anteriorly and the subclavian vein is swept off its posterior aspect, the costoclavicular ligament is divided, and the rib is separated from its sternal attachment and removed. Additional bands/adhesions are then removed to completely decompress the vein.
- The posterior remaining first rib (proximal rib) is retracted away from its bed and the subclavian artery and brachial plexus are swept off its posterior aspect. Dissection can be carried in the subperiosteal plane all the way back to its articulation with the transverse process of the first vertebra and the rib disarticulated and removed. Care must be taken to avoid injuring the first thoracic nerve root immediately deep to the rib (avoided by keeping dissection on the rib).
- If the entire rib is not removed, leaving the most distal and proximal extent of the rib in place, the edges of the cut rib should be blunted with a Rongeur forceps. Some advocate removal of the entire rib to prevent future compression by regenerative fibrocartilage.
- Resect any additional fibrous bands crossing the brachial plexus (neurolysis).
- If a cervical rib is present, it should be resected at this time in similar fashion.

- Asses for pneumothorax – consider chest tube.
- Close over JP.

Supraclavicular approach for first rib resection
Pros: wide exposure of all structures, complete scalene resection, complete plexus neurolysis, resection of accessory ribs, obligatory for arterial reconstructions.
Cons: less cosmetic, traction on the plexus during rib resection.

- Single lumen ETT, supine with neck extended or beach-chair position with arm prepped for range of motion during the case.
- Transverse incision two finger breadth above clavicle.
- Divide omohyoid, reflect scalene fat pad laterally, exposing ASM (phrenic).
- Circumferentially dissect ASM (watch for vein anteriorly, artery and trunks posteriorly and phrenic) and divide with scissors from scalene tubercle.
- Reflect ASM superior and resect off TPs at origin (watch for nerve roots).
- Perform complete neurolysis of brachial plexus, consider seprafilm or surgiwrap.
- Retract plexus forward and detach MSM from first rib with periosteal elevator (watch for long thoracic).
- Assess residual compression and need for first rib resection by range of motion of the arm.
- Detach intercostal muscle from inferior aspect of the rib with periosteal elevator and after protecting brachial plexus with the finger divide rib posteriorly (watch for pleura, brachial plexus and long thoracic).
- Depress the rib inferiorly and divide just medial to scalene tubercle, posterior to subclavian vein (watch for the vein).
- Smooth cut edges with a rongeur. The first rib may be removed in its entirety as described above, as well.
- Reapproximate fat pad and close over JP drain.

High posterior thoracoplasty approach for first rib resection
Pros: excellent exposure of nerve roots and brachial plexus, good vascular exposure, good for reoperations.
Cons: larger incision, less cosmetic, uncommon incision/exposure.

- Single lumen ETT, lateral decubitus position.
- Vertical incision between spine and scapula, divide trapezius, rhomboid and posterior serratus.
- Identify and dissect first rib subperiosteally (watch for T1), divide

first rib at the neck, Rongeur out the head.

- Resect cervical rib, fibrous bands, perform neurolysis, consider seprafilm of surgiwrap.
- Perform sympathectomy of T1-3 ganglia (watch for stellate ganglion).

Potential questions/alternative scenarios

"A 48 yo mechanic presents to the ED with pain in his right hand and numbness that began acutely this morning. You notice that he has an absent pulse and petechiae in the first and second digits. His hand appears dusky and motor function is slightly diminished. He notes a similar episode that resolved about a month ago. He does not have a history of arrhythmias (i.e., AF), diabetes, nor peripheral vascular disease. He does complain of symptoms consistent with arm claudication with repetitive maneuvers. How do you proceed?"

This scenario gives an example of aTOS – poststenotic aneurysm with distal embolization. Occasionally acute thrombosis or retrograde thrombosis and cerebral embolization develops. Workup includes vascular lab imaging: CT angiography and/or angiography. In acute arterial thrombosis, endovascular restoration with regional thrombolysis or thrombectomy may be possible and should be attempted first. The patient should be anticoagulated after flow has been reestablished. The primary issue (compression of the subclavian artery) can then be addressed more electively. In elective situations, resection of the aneurysm and bypass or interposition graft is used for reconstruction (proximal and distal control, heparinization prior to clamping) following first rib decompression as described above.

"A 28 yo pitcher presents with acute right arm swelling. He was diagnosed with a subclavian-axillary vein clot on duplex in the ED. How would you manage this patient?"

This is an example of Paget-Schroetter Syndrome, a variant of vTOS. This syndrome typically affects young athletes with excessive/repetitive use of the arm (i.e., pitchers, basketball players, weight lifters). Compression of the subclavian/axillary vein is caused by compression against the first rib by a congenitally, laterally displaced costoclavicular ligament along with a hypertrophied ASM. Diagnose with venous duplex and venogram. Patients should also be worked up for a hypercoagulable state. Initial treatment is with catheter directed thrombolysis (access through basilic vein, cross thrombus with wire and pulse-spray catheter with tPA infusion). After successful thrombolysis, the patient is treated with a heparin bridge and started on Coumadin. Patients with evidence of venous compression should undergo TOS decompression after 3 months of coumadin therapy. Failed thrombolysis is an indication for open thrombectomy and decompression during the same admission versus long-term coumadin therapy if the patient does not wish to have operative intervention.

"Six months after a transaxillary first rib resection, a 55 yo man with nTOS presents with recurrence of symptoms. How would you manage this situation?"

Recurrent TOS – distinguish true recurrence (initial improvement followed by recurrence – due to scarring) vs. false (lack of initial improvement – inadequate surgery – either wrong diagnosis or wrong procedure (i.e., 2nd rib resection). Thorough workup and imaging for assessment of performed procedure. Start with PT. If repeat surgical intervention deemed to be necessary, the preferred approach is a high posterior thoracoplasty.

Pearls/pitfalls
- No confirmatory studies, clinical diagnosis.
- Don't rush to OR. Treat nTOS with PT first.
- Supraclavicular approach offers better decompression, resect a segment of ASM rather than simply detach it.
- Do not overlook aTOS and vTOS—these are game changers and will push you to OR early.
- Not all patients are drug seekers. With appropriate diagnosis and management most get better and return to work.

Suggested readings
- Sanders RJ. Thoracic outlet syndrome: general considerations. Cronenwett JL, Johnston WK, Cambria R, et al. *Rutherford's Vascular Surgery* 7th ed.
- Schanzer A, Messina LM. Thoracic outlet syndrome: venous. Cronenwett JL, Johnston WK, Cambria R, et al. *Rutherford's Vascular Surgery* 7th ed.

Notes

17. Esophageal cancer

Ryan A. Macke, MD, Roman V. Petrov, MD, and Manisha Shende, MD

Concept

- Understand the workup of esophageal cancer, including diagnosis and appropriate staging studies
- Understand the TNM staging system and treatment of early/late stage esophageal cancer
- Understand the indications for surgery, chemotherapy, radiation, and multimodal therapy
- Be aware of the multiple techniques used for esophagectomy, the key steps, and the pros/cons of each
- Understand the treatment of intraoperative and postoperative complications associated with esophagectomy
- Understand the role of the thoracic surgeon in palliation of esophageal cancer

Chief complaint

"You are referred a 63 yo obese, white man with complaints of progressive dysphagia to solids and a 35-pound weight loss over the last 3 months."

Differential

The differential for dysphagia and weight loss is broad and should include a number of esophageal diseases including: esophageal cancer, esophageal motility disorder, GERD/peptic stricture, paraesophageal hernia, esophageal diverticulum, benign obstructing esophageal tumor, and obstruction from external compression (aortic aneurysm, fibrosing mediastinitis).

History and physical

Most patients presenting with symptoms of dysphagia and weight loss due to esophageal cancer will have
locally or systemically advanced disease resulting in obstruction and inadequate oral intake. A complete physical exam should be performed focusing on lymph node basins that would be outside the routine field of resection (cervical, clavicular, and axillary), evidence of other distant disease (pleural or pericardial effusions, ascites, jaundice, headache or other focal neurologic symptoms), and signs of malnutrition. Important information obtained in a thorough history include weight loss, smoking and alcohol use, long-standing GERD, Barrett's esophagus +/- history of dysplasia, hiatal hernia, regurgitation, hematemesis, dysphagia,

odynophagia, and melena. The history and physical will give the surgeon an idea of histology (squamous versus adenocarcinoma) and extent of disease, however most of the pertinent information needed for decision-making will be obtained in the diagnostic workup.

Tests

Workup of patients with suspected esophageal cancer includes a comprehensive constellation of imaging and invasive tests to establish the diagnosis, appropriately stage the disease, and assess for resectability.

- *Barium swallow.* Typically recommended as the initial study for evaluation of any patient with dysphagia. Most importantly, it will identify obstructing lesions (location and extent) that would potentially complicate upper endoscopy or EUS, in addition to assessing for esophageal dysmotility, reflux, hiatal hernias, etc.
- *Upper endoscopy.* Provides direct assessment of the lesion and permits for tissue acquisition to confirm the diagnosis. All suspicious/obstructing lesions should be biopsied to rule out malignancy. Proximal and distal extent of disease should be noted to assist in determining the proximal extent of resection and use of stomach as a conduit. A pediatric endoscope should be available for large, obstructing lesions.
- *PET/CT.* Accuracy in excess of 90% for determining distant disease. CT alone may be used for this purpose, but is less accurate and in the current era is rarely used alone for preoperative staging. May be limited in evaluation of regional nodal disease, as the lymph nodes may be "outshined" by the primary lesion. PET/CT is not sensitive for T staging and is limited in evaluation of brain metastases due to the high FDG-avidity of the brain.
- *EUS.* Serves as an adjunct to upper endoscopy and is the best available clinical tool for T and N staging. FNA of suspicious lymph nodes (short axis > 1 cm, round, hypoechoic) can be performed to confirm nodal disease by cytology. Large, obstructing tumors may not permit passage of the larger EUS scope. Rather than risk perforation, it is probably safest to omit the EUS when the scope cannot be passed easily beyond the lesion.
- *Bronchoscopy.* Should be performed at the time of resection in all patients with respiratory symptoms, upper and mid-esophageal tumors, and squamous cell cancers (more likely to have transmural penetration and invasion into adjacent structures) to rule out airway invasion.
- *CT/MRI brain.* Only used if patient has focal neurologic symptoms to rule out brain metastases.
- *Physiologic testing.* Should include cardiac risk stratification (EKG, stress test), pulmonary function testing, and other tests based on patient comorbidities to assess candidacy for resection.

- *Laparoscopic/thoracoscopic staging.* Although invasive, laparoscopy and/or thoracoscopy allows for direct visual assessment of potential sites of metastasis and lymph node basins, as well as a means to biopsy suspicious lesions or nodes. A combination of PET/CT, endoscopy, and EUS allows for fairly reliable assessment of intrathoracic tumor involvement, making thoracoscopy unnecessary in most cases. Laparoscopy is more accurate at confirming suspected celiac nodal disease than conventional imaging. Enteral access and conduit preconditioning can also be performed at the time of staging laparoscopy for patients who are going to be treated with induction therapy prior to resection.

Index scenario (additional information)

"Barium swallow shows a partially obstructing distal esophageal mass. EGD shows a lesion located at the GEJ 40 cm from the incisors with proximal extension of BE to 38 cm. There is 1 cm of extension onto the cardia. Biopsy proves this to be a moderately differentiated adenocarcinoma. The lesion invades the muscularis propria only on EUS and there is no evidence of suspicious lymph nodes or distant disease on CT, PET/CT, or EUS. The patient is otherwise healthy. What is this patient's clinical stage and how would you manage this patient?"

It is estimated that 30-40% of patients diagnosed with esophageal cancer will be resectable at the time of presentation. Surgery provides the best local control and chance for cure. However, roughly 75% of patients recur distally following resection, suggesting the presence of occult distant disease at the time of diagnosis. As such, treatment of esophageal cancer typically requires a multimodal approach with chemotherapy and radiation therapy playing an important role. Indications for neoadjuvant therapy, the modalities used, and the dosages used for treatment vary considerably between centers. However, most agree that patients with locally advanced disease (T3 or greater) or evidence of nodal disease identified during preoperative staging warrants some form of induction therapy. Concurrent chemoradiation therapy (CRT) is favored by most in the neoadjuvant setting. However, some centers favor chemotherapy alone, omitting radiation to avoid radiation fibrosis and a more complex resection. Adjuvant treatment with CRT or chemotherapy alone is indicated for patients who are found to have node-positive disease or are upstaged on pathologic staging following resection. Postoperative radiation therapy risks damage to conduit blood supply and is discouraged in some, but not all centers. Commonly used first-line chemotherapy regimens include: Cisplatin (or Oxaliplatin) + 5-FU, Epirubicin + Cisplatin + 5-FU, and Paclitaxel + Carboplatin. Trastuzumab may be added in cases with overexpression of Her2-neu mutation. The dose of radiation varies from center to center, however

50 Gy is an accepted dose in the definitive, preoperative, postoperative, or palliative setting with patients receiving approximately 2 Gy/day, 5 days/week, for 5 weeks. It is not uncommon for patients receiving definitive CRT to be treated with higher doses (up to 60 Gy).

Patients with high-grade dysplasia (HGD) or early esophageal cancer (T1a, T1b, T2 and N0) can proceed to resection without delay following thorough staging to rule out evidence of nodal or distant disease. Patients should be assessed for surgical candidacy with a thorough review of comorbidities and physiologic workup. Once the patient has been cleared for surgery, three important decisions need to be made: choice of conduit, route of conduit, and surgical approach.

A gastric conduit based off the right gastroepiploic arcade is the conduit of choice in most centers, providing adequate length for an intrathoracic or cervical anastomosis and requiring only one anastomosis. Selective angiography of the celiac vessels should be performed in patients with prior gastric resection to assess the gastroepiploic arcade. Colon is the next best conduit in cases where the stomach is not usable due to distal tumor extension or the gastroepiploic arcade has been disrupted. The colon blood supply should be assessed with a CTA or mesenteric angiography and colonoscopy should be performed preoperatively to plan for colon interposition. The left colon, based off the ascending branch of the left colic artery, is most commonly used and provides a conduit with good length and matching diameter to the proximal esophagus. Disadvantages include multiple anastomoses (esophagocolic, gastrocolic, and colocolonic) and tendency for conduit dilation in the long-term. The jejunum is a third option, but has limited length. It is the conduit of choice in cases where there is extensive gastric and only distal esophageal involvement, in which case a total gastrectomy and roux-en-y esophagojejunostomy is performed. If the conduit is needed to reach the neck, the jejunum may be used as a free graft, requiring microvascular techniques for the vascular anastomoses to cervical vessels. This technique is used in a few specialized centers and unless one is familiar with these techniques, it is probably unwise to mention during an examination.

Routes for passage of the conduit include posterior mediastinal (native bed), substernal, transpleural, and subcutaneous routes. The posterior mediastinal route is the shortest and preferred path to reach the proximal esophagus for anastomosis and is used for immediate reconstruction. The substernal route is a longer route, but is useful for delayed reconstruction when the native bed has been obliterated, such as occurs following esophageal exclusion. The transpleural and subcutaneous routes are rarely used.

The surgical approach depends on mainly surgical experience and extent/location of disease. Better outcomes are obtained with an approach that the surgeon is most comfortable with, so stick with what you know. Essentially all approaches can be used to resect distal esophageal tumors, however more proximal and mid-esophageal tumors require transection of the esophagus high in the chest to obtain an adequate margin (ideally 5 cm from the primary tumor), necessitating a cervical anastomosis. Remember to note the proximal extent of any Barrett's esophagus, as this should be included in the resection, although a lengthy margin is not required. A *brief* description of some of the more commonly used esophagectomy approaches follows, along with pertinent pros and cons of the approach. Review of the anastomotic techniques commonly used is beyond the scope of this chapter, but it is recommended that the reader become familiar with at least one technique. Studies have failed to show an advantage in survival when comparing these different approaches.

Operative steps

Transhiatal esophagectomy (THE)

Pros: Do not need to reposition, shorter operation, decreased pulmonary complications by omitting a thoracotomy, ease of cervical leak management.
Cons: Decreased LN count, higher blood loss, risk of injuring intrathoracic structures that cannot be clearly visualized (not ideal for proximal and mid-esophageal lesions), higher incidence of anastomotic leaks.

- Supine position, head turned to the right, single lumen ETT

Abdominal phase
- Upper midline laparotomy, stage the abdomen to assure resectability, assess suitability of the stomach as a conduit.
- Divide left triangular ligament and retract left lobe of the liver.
- Divide the short gastric vessels and mobilize the omentum off the greater curvature, preserving the right gastroepiploic arcade.
- Divide the gastrohepatic ligament (watch for replaced L hepatic - preserve if replaced, dividing left gastric distal the replaced take-off, divide if accessory). Divide the left gastric pedicle at its base, sweeping nodal tissue toward the specimen.
- Perform Kocher maneuver so that the pylorus reaches the xyphoid.
- Open pheronoesophageal membrane and dissect out the distal esophagus circumferentially (use narrow Deaver retractor through hiatus).
- Perform pyloromyotomy or pyloroplasty (optional).
- Place feeding jejunostomy (optional).

- Oversew inferior phrenic veins and after opening hiatus anteriorly (optional).
- Perform posterior esophageal mobilization by advancing hand palm up along esophagus to the level above carina. Stay close to the esophageal wall to avulse aortoesophageal vessels after they branch out before entering the wall to minimize blood loss, which can be in excess of 1 liter during this phase (controlled with packing the mediastinum).
- Perform anterior mobilization by advancing hand palm down along esophagus (watch for membranous trachea (injury – blood in ETT, SQE, AL) and left atrium and pulmonary veins (injury – profuse BRB bleeding, hemodynamic instability). Mobilize lateral attachments of the esophagus in a similar fashion.
- Divide stomach along greater curvature (blue or purple GIA), fashioning the conduit. Stomach can be used as a narrow conduit (5 cm) or the whole stomach.

Neck phase
- Left neck incision along anterior border of the left SCM, divide the platysma, omohyoid, reflect straps medially and SCM , IJ, and carotid sheath laterally.
- Expose the prevertebral fascia and mobilize the esophagus circumferentially. After encircling the esophagus with penrose for traction, dissect into superior mediastinum to the level of carina, meeting the dissection plane from below.
- Divide esophagus in the neck with a linear cutting stapler, incorporating one inch penrose drain, secure penrose distally to the specimen and remove specimen retracting it inferiorly through the hiatus and abdomen passing it off the field. Send margins for frozen. Tamponade the mediastinum with sponges for hemostasis.
- Place the conduit into the plastic bag (camera sleeve works), secure to the penrose drain and retract into the neck, maintaining orientation (multiple methods used for passage of conduit, do what you know).
- Perform cervical anastomosis (hand-sewn single or double layer, EEA, side-to-side functional end-to-end, again do what you know).
- Place JP drain into the neck, bilateral chest tubes, pull excess conduit back into the abdomen and secure to the hiatus, place NG tube or pharyngostomy tube and close the abdomen.

Ivor Lewis esophagectomy (ILE)
Pros: increased LN yield, decreased neck morbidity (decreased risk of RLN injury), decreased leak incidence
Cons: lengthier procedure, harder to manage leaks, increased pulmonary morbidity

Abdominal phase
- Supine position, double lumen tube (no lung isolation for abdominal phase).
- All steps of the abdominal phase are performed in the same fashion as the THE approach. However, once the conduit is made, the tip is sewn to the specimen and the specimen is passed through the hiatus for later retrieval in the chest.
- Close the abdomen. Place NG tube Turn the patient in full left lateral position and isolate the lung.

Thoracic phase
- Perform right posterolateral thoracotomy in 6th or 7th intercostal space.
- Mobilize the esophagus anteriorly (off of the pericardium and carina, sweeping all lymphatic tissue with the specimen), divide the R vagus nerve close to the esophagus.
- Mobilize esophagus posteriorly off of the aorta and spine (clip all aortoesophageal and lymphatic branches posteriorly). Make sure to avoid injury to the thoracic duct. If there is any concern of thoracic duct injury – perform prophylactic en mass ligation.
- Divide the azygos vein with vascular stapler (endo-GIA white or gold) and mobilize the esophagus up to the thoracic inlet, staying close to the esophagus to avoid injury to the airway or recurrent laryngeal nerve.
- Transect the esophagus above the azygos vein (performing a high intrathoracic anastomosis minimizes long-term problems of reflux). If there is concern about the proximal margin, an intraoperative endoscopy can be performed for confirmation.
- Pull the remaining specimen and attached conduit up into the chest and cut tacking suture. Pass the specimen off the table and confirm margins by frozen section.
- Pull the NG tube back and perform the anastomosis (hand-sewn single or double layer, EEA, side-to-side, etc) If EEA performed, confirm two rings and send them for frozen as final gastric margin.
- Advance the NG tube into the mid-conduit position and connect to suction.
- Remove any redundancy in the conduit by pushing it back into the abdomen and secure to the hiatus with interrupted sutures.

- Place JP drain posterior to the conduit and bring it out inferiorly. Place one or two (posterior apical and basilar) 28 Fr chest tubes and close the chest.

Three-hole (McKeown) esophagectomy

Pros: Can be used to resect tumors in all locations, increased LN count. Cons: Increased pulmonary complications due to thoracotomy, increased neck morbidity from cervical anastomosis, may need to perform staging laparoscopy first if question of resectability, requires repositioning, longer case.

Thoracic phase

- Double lumen intubation, right lung isolation.
- The chest part of the case is performed first, similar to the fashion described for the ILE, however the esophagus is not divided. The esophagus is mobilized from diaphragm to inlet and chest tubes are placed.

Abdominal and neck phases

- The patient is then repositioned supine, prepping in the neck as well.
- The abdominal and cervical portions of the case are carried out in similar fashion to the THE without the need for intrathoracic mobilization of the esophagus from the abdomen and mobilization of the proximal esophagus distally through the thoracic inlet.

Minimally invasive esophagectomy (MIE)

There exist multiple combinations of laparoscopic and thoracoscopic techniques that have been described to mimic essentially any type of open esophagectomy (ILE – the authors' preferred approach, McKeown, THE). Frequently, these combinations include a mix of open and true minimally invasive steps, better described by the term "hybrid". Regardless of the technique used, the major goal is to minimize morbidity and mortality, blood loss, length of stay, and time to return to activities of daily living. There is now good evidence that has accumulated to support the use of these techniques, however the procedures are complex and describing the details is beyond the scope of this chapter. The basic steps of the operation remain unchanged from the open predecessors of these MIE approaches. If the reader is familiar with one of the forms of MIE, it is recommended that its use for most examination purposes be limited to early stage cancers or high-grade dysplasia.

"Following resection, the path report comes back as T2N1 with 2 of 18 lymph nodes positive. How would you counsel your patient at this point?"

Patients who are found to have lymph node involvement on final pathology have a poorer prognosis. The greater the number of lymph nodes involved, the poorer the prognosis (N1: 1-2 positive nodes, N2: 3-6, N3: > 6). Adjuvant CRT (for those who did not receive induction XRT) or chemotherapy alone should be offered to all patients with evidence of nodal disease, typically 4-6 weeks following resection.

"How would your management change if the preoperative EUS showed invasion beyond the muscularis propria, but without involvement of adjacent structures, and two suspicious periesophageal lymph nodes on EUS? What is this patient's stage? What if the patient had celiac nodal disease rather than periesophageal?"

Both patients have a clinical T stage of uT3 (u for EUS). Patients with T3 disease have an 80% chance of having lymph node involvement, although this may not be detectable on preoperative staging. An attempt should be made to confirm nodal involvement when suspicious nodes are seen on preoperative imaging. Periesophageal lymph nodes can be sampled with EUS-FNA and the aspirates sent for cytologic analysis. Nodes that are 1 cm or greater in the short-axis, round, and hypoechoic on EUS, > 1 cm in short axis on CT or PET, or with FDG-avidity on PET are considered suspicious and should be sampled when possible. Assuming the patient described has positive periesophageal lymph nodes, the clinical stage would be cT3N1. Celiac nodal disease is no longer considered M1 disease, as these nodes can frequently be resected with meticulous dissection. Laparoscopic staging allows for assessment of these nodes. Biopsies should be obtained to confirm metastatic disease within these nodes. Laparoscopy also allows for assessment of resectability. If the celiac nodes appear resectable and the base of the left gastric pedicle appears soft, then the patient may be a candidate for resection after induction therapy. If not, definitive CRT is the best option for the patient. Most centers offer induction therapy to patients with T3/resectable T4 and/or nodal disease. Some centers offer concurrent CRT while others favor chemotherapy alone, as radiation causes inflammation and fibrosis that may complicate resection.

"How would you assess the patient's response to induction therapy? What are the chances of this patient having a complete response to induction CRT? What if the PET/CT scan showed no evidence of disease, would you still resect? What if the histology was squamous cell instead of adenocarcinoma?"

Patients are typically restaged with a PET/CT 4-6 weeks after completion of therapy to allow for completion of treatment effect and resolution of inflammation that may influence the PET scan. The use of EUS for restaging is controversial, as the accuracy is significantly diminished due to treatment effect.The patient should then proceed to resection if there is no evidence of nodal involvement outside the field of resection or distant metastases. Patients treated with definitive CRT who have evidence of persistent disease on post-treatment imaging may be considered for salvage esophagectomy in select cases.

Approximately 25-40% of patients will have a complete response to neoadjuvant therapy. Prognosis is significantly improved in this patient population. Even if restaging PET-CT scan shows no evidence of disease, patients with esophageal adenocarcinomas should be resected. However, there is recent evidence supporting observation in patients with squamous cell carcinomas of the esophagus without evidence of residual disease (by post-treatment imaging and upper endoscopy with biopsy) owing to similar long-term survival in patients with or without surgical resection.

"How would your management change if during preoperative work up you discovered that the patient had an EF of 15%, had an MI 4 months ago, PFTs with a FEV1 of 35% and DLCO of 40%, and that he is wheelchair bound?"

This patient is not a good surgical candidate. Although surgery provides the best chance of cure, the risk of significant morbidity and mortality are too high. Patients who are found to be unresectable or are poor operative candidates should be offered definitive, concurrent chemoradiation therapy. Palliative radiation therapy can be offered for patients who cannot tolerate chemotherapy. Palliative chemotherapy alone does not prolong survival, but can improve quality of life.

"What can you do for this patient's dysphagia? He is not able to eat and continues to lose weight."

A number of options exist to treat this patient's dysphagia and malnutrition. A feeding jejunostomy can be placed to provide enteral access for nutrition. If the patient responds to CRT, swallowing will improve and the tube can be removed. For patients who have dysphagia to saliva and liquids, something should be done to open the esophageal lumen and allow swallowing prior to beginning treatment. Upper endoscopy and gentle dilation (balloon dilation or Savory bougienage) may be enough to provide some palliation, but runs the risk of perforation. Alternatively, the tumor can be debrided/debulked with Nd:YAG laser, photodynamic therapy, or intraluminal radiation (brachytherapy). These methods are also useful for controlling bleeding from friable tumors. Stenting has gained popularity as a palliative treatment for obstructing lesions. Balloon dilation is a good option for cases when the stenting apparatus cannot be passed beyond the lesion. A variety of covered metal (permanent) or plastic (temporary) stents are commercially available. Stents are typically placed with the assistance of fluoroscopy to confirm adequate positioning. Stent migration is a common problem, which is why some discourage the use of stents in patients who are to be treated with radiation therapy, as this local therapy can shrink the tumor and lead to migration. Perforation is less common, but can be a catastrophic event in this ill population. Patients who have stents placed across the GEJ are more prone to reflux and should be treated with carafate and BID PPIs. Stents also provide a good option for palliation of malignant or postoperative tracheoesophageal fistulae (TEF). Stenting of both the esophagus and trachea is discouraged, as the radial force used to expand the stents can cause undue pressure and enlargement of the fistulous tract. Palliative esophagectomy with a substernal gastric pull-up is a reasonable option for patients in good health who have unresectable disease or for patients with TEFs that cannot be controlled with stents.

"You are referred another patient with a biopsy-proven, poorly-differentiated squamous cell carcinoma at 23 cm with invasion into the muscularis propria only and no lymph node involvement. How would you manage this patient?"
Location of the tumor is a primary determinant of surgical approach. All types of esophagectomy can be performed for the treatment of distal esophageal cancers (Ivor-Lewis, McKeown, left thoracoabdominal, transhiatal, MIE). However, tumors extending more proximally than 25 cm require a proximal resection and cervical anastomosis. A transhiatal approach is not ideal for more proximal tumors as tumor clearance and lymphadenectomy cannot be adequately visualized. The McKoewn, or 3-hole, esophagectomy is ideal for more proximal tumors such as the one presented in this scenario. Prior to proceeding with resection, bronchoscopy should be performed to rule out airway involvement, which would make the patient unresectable. Squamous cell carcinomas of the pharynx and very proximal esophagus (within 5 cm of the cricopharyngeus or about 20 cm from the incisors) are treated with definitive chemoradiation therapy, not resection.

"Bronchoscopy is negative for tumor invasion and EUS does not show invasion into adjacent structures. You are now doing a McKeown (3-hole) esophagectomy and as you are mobilizing the esophagus in the chest, you note that the tumor is adherent to the posterior membranous portion of the trachea. How would you proceed?"
Although the appropriate steps were taken prior to resection to rule out unresectable T4 disease, one should still be prepared for unexpected findings once in the operating room (especially on examinations!). Airway involvement makes this patient unresectable and the operation

should be aborted. Addressing the patient's dysphagia and port placement for chemotherapy may be considered before leaving the operating room.

"Returning to the patient with T3N1 adenocarcinoma located in the distal esophagus, following CRT a restaging PET/CT scan shows resolution of FDG avidity in the periesophageal lymph nodes and residual, but decreased avidity in the primary lesion. EUS cannot be done because the tumor is too bulky to pass the scope. You proceed with an ILE and during the abdominal portion you find a suspicious lesion in the left lobe of the liver. How would you proceed? Say there is no liver lesion, but after completing the abdominal portion you are in the chest you find the tumor is adherent to the right inferior pulmonary vein. How would you proceed?"

Every esophagectomy should begin with a thorough search for distant disease or other evidence of unresectability. Laparoscopic staging prior to esophagectomy avoids a laparotomy in cases where distant disease is encountered. Peritoneal and serosal surfaces are carefully examined, with particular attention paid to the liver and omentum. The celiac axis is also assessed to make sure the base of the left gastric is not encased in tumor or there are true celiac axis nodes with tumor involvement that cannot be cleared, which would preclude resection. Suspicious lesions are biopsied and sent for frozen sectioning. If positive, the operation is aborted and the patient is treated with palliative CRT.

The combination of CT and EUS will identify most cases where there is unresectable intrathoracic T4 involvement, but this may not always be the case. In cases where there is concern for tumor invasion into unresectable intrathoracic structures, it may be advisable to perform a staging thoracoscopy to evaluate the area of concern. Airway involvement can usually be ruled out with bronchoscopy. One should be prepared for a situation such as the one presented here, particularly when beginning in the abdomen as is done with an ILE. You are committed at this point, having completed the abdominal portion of the case, so there is no turning back. One option is to leave the involved segment of esophagus adhered to pulmonary vein behind and perform a substernal gastric pull-up, although this might be an overly aggressive approach for some. The remainder of the esophagus is resected, the neck is prepared for a cervical anastomosis, the gastric conduit is brought up through a window created behind the sternum, and the cervical anastomosis completed. A partial upper sternotomy and resection of the left clavicular head is required to avoid compression on the proximal conduit. The patient is then treated with postoperative palliative chemotherapy and radiation (if not given for induction). Another option is to leave the segment of esophagus behind and exclude the patient. The remainder of the esophagus is resected, a cervical esophagostomy is brought out the left neck, the hiatus is closed, and a gastrostomy tube is placed in the tip of the conduit. The patient is then treated with palliative CRT. Finally, the tumor may be shaved off the vein and clips left to mark the area for targeted XRT. Regardless of how this problem is handled, the patient will not receive an R0 resection (it is an R2 resection) and prognosis is extremely poor.

Performing a right lower lobectomy in an effort to obtain an R0 resection may be performed at some high volume centers, however this is probably too radical for examination purposes. T4 involvement that is considered resectable includes invasion of the pleura, pericardium, diaphragm, or adjacent peritoneum.

"You are referred another patient with short-segment BE and a small nodule within the BE at 37 cm that was biopsied and shown to be a moderately-differentiated adenocarcinoma. There was no mass seen on endoscopy. She would like to avoid surgery if possible. What would you offer this patient?"

Nodules or areas of ulceration within a segment of BE should raise the suspicion of HGD or invasive cancer. Endomucosal resection (EMR), which resects a piece of mucosa and submucosa, can be viewed as an extended biopsy. The specimen is then examined and can confirm histologic diagnosis, as well as depth of invasion. Beyond its diagnostic utility, EMR can also be definitive treatment for focal areas of BE with HGD (sometimes referred to as carcinoma in-situ) or intramucosal invasive adenocarcinomas (T1a). Extensive biopsies in the area of BE should be performed to assure that there are no other areas of HGD or invasive cancer. Multifocal disease (HGD or intramucosal cancer) is probably best treated with esophagectomy, although multiple EMRs may be performed. Following EMR, residual areas of BE are typically treated with radiofrequency ablation or other ablative therapies.

The primary early complication of EMR is bleeding, which is almost always treatable endoscopically. Strictures occur later, with a higher prevalence associated with multiple or repeat EMRs. Assuming the margins are negative, this patient will then need to undergo close surveillance with serial endoscopies, initially every 3 months for the first year, then annually.

"You do an EMR and the path returns as invasive adenocarcinoma with a positive deep margin. What is the T stage? What are the chances this patient has nodal involvement? What if the lateral margins are positive, but the tumor does not invade the submucosa?"

A positive deep margin implies that there is *at least* submucosal invasion of the tumor, making the patient *at least* T1b. Once the tumor invades beyond the lamina propria into the submucosa, the incidence of nodal involvement increased from < 3% for intramucosal tumors (T1a) to approximately 25% for tumors that invade into, but not beyond the submucosa (T1b). Patients with T2 lesions have nodal involvement in 25-50% of patients, while positive nodes are present in 75-80% of cases with T3 tumors. The patient should therefore undergo additional work up with CT, PET-CT, and EUS to complete staging. If additional staging reveals T3, resectable T4, or N+ disease, she should be treated with neoadjuvant therapy followed by resection. If she has only T1b or T2 disease, she should be offered resection. If the lateral margins are positive after EMR, but the deep margins are negative, the patient should undergo repeat EMR until lateral margins are negative.

"A patient is now POD 4 from a THE for a pT2N0 esophageal adenocarcinoma of the distal esophagus. He has a low-grade fever and a WBC of 13,000. The cervical wound is erythematous and saliva is seen draining around the penrose drain. How would you manage this patient?"

Cervical anastomotic leaks are more common than intrathoracic leaks, theoretically due to more tension on the anastomosis. Fortunately, these leaks are easily managed with opening of the wound at the bedside. The wound is irrigated, debrided, and dressed with wet-to-dry gauze. The patient is placed on broad spectrum antibiotics and antifungals. A clear liquid diet helps to clear debris intraluminally. Enteral nutrition is maintained with jejunostomy feedings or TPN if no enteral access is in place. Once the fever and leukocytosis have resolved and wound drainage is minimal, a barium swallow can be performed to confirm resolution of the leak. The diet is then advanced and the patient monitored for signs of ongoing leakage. A barium swallow is not needed to confirm the leak if there is enough clinical evidence to suspect a leak. In most case, the wound should be opened without delay.

"The leak has resolved and the patient is now at home, 10 weeks postoperatively, and is tolerating a regular diet. However, she complains of breads and meats 'sticking.' How would you proceed?"

Anastomotic strictures are common after esophagectomy, particularly after a leak. This patient should undergo upper endoscopy and dilation. The scope is advanced distally into the duodenum, a wire passed, the scope is removed and serial dilations performed under fluoroscopic guidance with Savory dilators (the authors' preferred form of dilation, although balloon dilation may also be used). Upper endoscopy is repeated to assess the stricture after every couple of increases in diameter of the dilators or when resistance is met. Blood on the dilator or mucosal tearing at the level of the stricture signifies adequate dilation. Serial dilations every few weeks may be required until maximal dilation has been reached and/or dysphagia resolves. Patients requiring serial dilations may be taught self-dilation with soft-tipped dilators (Maloney), with low risk of perforation with adequate education. Dysphagia that occurs later in the postoperative course should raise suspicion of local recurrence and any abnormalities noted on endoscopy should be biopsied.

"How would you monitor this patient for recurrence of her esophageal cancer?"

Surveillance protocols vary from institution to institution. Having a general idea of how you will follow these patients is necessary. The following is the authors' typical routine surveillance schedule. Postoperatively, patients are seen every 3-4 months for the first year, every 3-6 months for years 1-3, every 6 months for years 3-5, then annually after 5 years. Whole-body PET-CT scans are obtained at least annually for these visits. A CT of the chest, abdomen, and pelvis is obtained for all other visits. Any suspicious findings suggesting locoregional or distal recurrence on CT warrants a PET-CT scan and biopsy if the lesion is FDG-avid or has a suspicious appearance on CT. Suspicion of local recurrence is investigated with upper endoscopy and biopsy. An attempt should be made to confirm all suspected recurrences by biopsy.

Recurrent disease is treated with CRT or chemotherapy alone for palliation. Focal XRT may be considered for patients with painful metastases for palliation, even if treated with radiation previously. Very select cases of local recurrence may be considered for re-resection in good surgical candidates. Patients who were treated with definitive CRT that are found to have a resectable locoregional recurrent or persistent disease may be considered for salvage esophagectomy in select cases if they are deemed to be good surgical candidates.

"You have another patient who is POD 4 from an ILE for a pT3N1 esophageal adenocarcinoma located at 28-35 cm. He remains intubated and has failed weaning trials. He has had marginal blood pressure and poor urine output despite aggressive volume resuscitation. He is febrile to 102.1 this morning. Chest x-ray shows a RLL infiltrate and a right effusion. How would you proceed?"

This patient appears to be septic. There are a number of causes of postoperative infection following esophagectomy and all should be thoroughly investigated. Bronchoscopy should be performed and BAL sent to rule out pneumonia. Urinalysis and urine culture should be sent for possible UTI. Blood cultures should be sent to rule out bacteremia and lines should be changed. The jejunostomy site should be checked for signs of infection. Peritoneal signs should raise suspicion of an enterotomy or leak from the feeding tube site or pyloric emptying procedure. However, first and foremost, one should be concerned about an anastomotic leak or conduit necrosis. A barium swallow cannot be obtained given the patient remains intubated. A CT scan would be helpful to evaluate for pneumonia, empyema, or a leak. However, sending this marginally unstable patient for a scan or swallow (if he was extubated) is unwise. The patient should be promptly brought to the operating room for an upper endoscopy or the endoscopy performed at the bedside to evaluate the anastomosis and conduit.

"The conduit is black."

Gastric conduit necrosis is a rare, but devastating occurrence with a high rate of mortality. However, prompt diagnosis and treatment may be lifesaving for this patient. Any periods of hypotension, evidence of hypoperfusion, fever, leukocytosis, or failure to progress should raise the suspicion of anastomotic leak or conduit necrosis. Imaging only wastes valuable time in these cases, but can be carefully considered in patients who are stable. Prompt upper endoscopy is the gold-standard to rule out conduit necrosis. This patient should be taken to the operating room and the conduit taken down via redo thoracotomy. All necrotic conduit is resected. The remaining stomach is replaced in the abdomen and the proximal esophagus mobilized to the thoracic inlet. The chest is irrigated and drains/chest tubes are placed. The patient is then quickly repositioned supine. The proximal esophagus is brought out the left neck and a cervical esophagostomy (spit fistula) is fashioned. A gastrostomy tube is placed in the tip of the remaining gastric conduit to decompress the stomach and a feeding jejunostomy is placed, if not previously. The hiatus is closed to prevent herniation of intraabdominal contents. If the patient is too unstable, the conduit is resected, the remaining stomach replaced in the abdomen, the hiatus is close from the right chest, and the proximal esophagus is mobilized. The patient is then brought back to the ICU to be resuscitated and the cervical esophagostomy and gastrostomy tube placed at a later time, when the patient is stable. Gastrointestinal continuity can be reestablished with a substernal colonic interposition or gastric pull-up (if there is enough remaining stomach) months down the road once the patient is nutritionally replete.

Pearls/pitfalls
- A thorough preoperative workup is necessary to adequately stage patients with esophageal cancer and to assess resectability.
- Proximal and distal extent of the tumor plays an important role in determining the conduit that should be used and approach taken for resection.

- Chemotherapy and radiation play an important role in the multimodal management of esophageal cancer. Understanding the role of surgery, chemotherapy, and radiation is key to managing this patient population.
- The majority of patients who present with esophageal cancer will be unresectable. It is important to understand the surgeon's role in the palliative treatment of esophageal cancer.
- Morbidity and mortality rates following esophagectomy are significant. Understanding the more common and severe complications (i.e., anastomotic leaks, conduit necrosis, and anastomotic stricture) and having a plan of action is necessary.
- Know how to do at least one type of esophagectomy and be able to describe your preferred anastomotic technique.

Suggested readings
- Schuchert MJ, Luketich JD, Landreneau RJ. Management of esophageal cancer. *Curr Probl Surg.* 2010 Nov; 47(11): 845-946.
- National Comprehensive Cancer Network. Esophageal and Esophagogastric Junction
  Cancers, Version 2.2012. Accessed 10/15/2012.
  http://www.nccn.org/professionals/physician_gls/pdf/esophageal.pdf.

Notes

18. GERD and Barrett's esophagus

Michelle C. Ellis, MD, and Rishindra M. Reddy, MD

Concept
- Work up of gastroesophageal reflux disease (GERD)
- Medical management and surveillance of GERD and Barrett's esophagus (BE)
- Indications for operative intervention
- Options for operative approach
- Endoscopic management of BE

Chief complaint
"A 56 yo man is self-referred to your office with complaints of long-standing heartburn, 'sour mouth', and food sticking. His symptoms have persisted despite trying maximal doses of a number of 'acid-reducer' medications."

Differential
Gastroesophageal reflux disease (GERD), Barrett's esophagus (BE), hiatal hernia, paraesophageal hernia, esophageal motility disorder, esophageal stricture, eosinophilic esophagitis, esophageal cancer

History and physical
Typical symptoms of GERD include heartburn, regurgitation, and dysphagia. Atypical symptoms that have an established association with GERD include cough, laryngitis, and asthma. Additional extra-esophageal symptoms often linked to reflux include dental erosions, laryngitis, laryngeal polyps, and pulmonary fibrosis, though causation has not been clearly established. A history of recurrent pneumonias may be due to aspiration of refluxate, particularly at night. This history is important in elderly, frail patients or those with long-standing interstitial pulmonary disease, as an aspiration event may prove fatal and is a strong indication for surgical rather than medical management of GERD. A thorough review of the patients medications is also prudent. Knowledge of whether H2 blocker or Proton pump inhibitors (PPIs) have been taken and if they provided any relief in symptoms has prognostic value when considering patients for anti-reflux surgery (ARS). It is also important to see how the medications are being taken (PPIs are not as effective if taken PRN, an appropriate course of medical management typically consists of 8 weeks of daily or BID PPI therapy). Any prior history of upper endoscopies and their findings is important as well. Knowledge of a history of BE and whether or not dysplasia was found on previous biopsies is another important piece of information.

- *Endoscopy*: may be normal in up to 70% of patients with GERD, but needed to assess for presence and severity of any esophagitis, BE, stricture, or invasive disease, especially for those patients with alarm symptoms (dysphagia). Approximately 10-20% of patients with GERD seeking care will have a stricture or BE on endoscopy. Any abnormal appearing areas of mucosa should be biopsied.

- *Barium swallow*: provides delineation of anatomy including detection of hiatal hernia, strictures, or esophageal foreshortening. Suspect esophageal shortening in the setting of a large hiatal hernia (> 5 cm) or esophageal stricture. It is recommended that patients with symptoms of dysphagia undergo a Barium swallow prior to endoscopy, which serves as a road map and may key the surgeon in on potential difficulties that may be encountered (i.e., tight stricture that may require a pediatric endoscope to pass, the possible need for dilation, retained food debris from a tight stricture or esophageal motility that may require the patient to be on clear liquids for a few days pre-endoscopy to clear the esophagus).

- *24-hour pH probe (Bravo) testing*: gold standard for diagnosis of GERD. A DeMeester score (abnormal > 14.7) is calculated based on 1) total percent time pH less than 4.0, 2) percent time pH less than 4.0 in the upright position, 3) percent time pH less than 4.0 in the recumbent position, 4) the total number of reflux episodes, 5) the total number of reflux episodes longer than 5 minutes, and 6) the duration of the longest reflux episode. Patients correlate symptoms with a diary of time spent in the upright/supine position as well as meal times. Neither the symptom of heartburn nor the presence of hiatal hernia is necessarily synonymous with GERD. Nocturnal reflux may be associated with a failure of medical therapy, GERD-related strictures, ulcers, or other complications.

- *Esophageal manometry*: provides information on esophageal peristaltic function and lower esophageal sphincter (LES) function during swallowing. Normal LES resting pressure is 15-30 mmHg. LES integrity depends on an adequate overall sphincter length (3-5 cm), as well as the presence of adequate (> 2.5 cm) intra-abdominal length. One must establish the presence of normal peristaltic function prior to surgical treatment, as abnormal peristalsis alone can contribute to symptoms and lead to inadequate symptom relief despite surgery. The amplitude of contractions (< 30 mmHg is considered low in most GI labs), percentage of peristaltic contractions (a normal esophagus will have 100% peristaltic contractions), and whether the esophagus is cleared with the contractions are all important pieces of information that will affect the decision to perform a partial versus a complete wrap during ARS.

- *Impedance monitoring*: useful in patients with non-acid reflux, assesses bolus transit through the esophagus thereby providing additional information on esophageal motility and function.
- *Gastric emptying test*: useful in diabetics or others in which delayed gastric emptying is suspected, also important for reoperations to document whether the vagus nerves are functioning or present (may have been inadvertently divided during a prior ARS).
- *Bernstein acid test*: largely historical, mild hydrochloric acid used to re-create reflux symptoms.

Index scenario (additional information)

"The patient's history and physical reveals long-standing heartburn and occasional dysphagia to meats and breads, especially after large or spicy meals. He has been self-treating with over the counter PPIs intermittently over the past five years with some relief. EGD demonstrates short-segment BE without evidence of dysplasia on biopsy. 24-hour pH study demonstrates an average DeMeester score of 18 over a 2 day period. Manometry shows normal amplitudes throughout the esophagus, 100% peristaltic contractions, and complete bolus clearance. How would you proceed?"

Treatment/management

Symptomatic reflux that persists despite high dose, twice daily proton pump inhibitor therapy is the most common indication for ARS, followed by medication expense, and unwillingness to adhere to lifelong medical therapy. Other indications include endoscopically proven severe esophagitis or mucosal ulceration.These patients should first undergo medical management with BID PPIs for 6-8 weeks without interruption. The upper endoscopy is then repeated to gauge response to therapy. Ongoing or worsening esophagitis is an indication for ARS. Patient with complications of GERD, such as peptic strictures, BE, recurrent aspiration pneumonias, or interstitial lung disease without other known etiologies should be considered for ARS as well. ARS has not been shown to induce regression of BE with or without dysplasia. However by removing the cause of the metaplasia, the risk of esophagitis and more BE should be decreased. Patients with known BE who undergo ARS should undergo surveillance upper endoscopies at the same time intervals as those who are not treated surgically (surveillance discussed below).

Whether a partial (Toupet or Dor) or complete (Nissen) fundoplication is performed, the principal goals of all ARSs remains the same: reduction/repair of any hiatal hernia if present, restoration of at least 2-3 cm of intra-abdominal esophageal length, closure of the widened hiatus, and re-establishment of the esophageal high pressure zone (fundoplication recreates the angle of His). If suspected, BE is identified on preoperative endoscopy (salmon-colored mucosa extending proximally from the squamocolumnar junction, a.k.a Z-line), the patient should undergo biopsy to evaluate for dysplasia or invasive carcinoma. The presence of dysplasia is the greatest risk factor for future development of malignancy. The typical progression to invasive adenocarcinoma induced by GERD is esophagitis without metaplasia, metaplasia (BE) without dysplasia, low grade dysplasia (LGD), high grade dysplasia (HGD), and finally invasive adenocarcinoma. HGD is considered the immediate precursor to invasive cancer, but is also a marker for esophageal cancer. Previous studies have shown that 30-40% of patients with HGD who undergo esophagectomy are found to have synchronous occult areas of invasive cancer elsewhere in the esophagus. The gold standard for endoscopic surveillance is the Seattle protocol, which entails 4-quadrant biopsies taken for every 1 cm of the areas of BE with additional biopsies of suspicious lesions as needed (i.e., areas of nodularity or ulceration). There is high intraobserver and interobserver variation in the histopathologic diagnosis of HGD. Therefore, patients being referred for treatment of BE should have pathology reviewed to confirm the diagnosis. Surveillance should be performed every 3-5 years in those with BE and no dysplasia, every 6-12 months if LGD is present, and every 3 months if HGD is found and has been successfully treated with endoscopic mucosal resection (EMR), or consider surgical intervention. Mucosal directed therapies include radiofrequency ablation and EMR and have become first line therapy for HGD. EMR has the advantage of providing tissue for pathologic examination, aiding in identification of occult invasive cancer. Esophagectomy is now typically reserved for patients with invasive cancers, those requesting surgical intervention, those who fail endoscopic treatment, and those with HGD lesions not amenable to endoscopic mucosal directed therapies.

Operative steps
Open/laparoscopic fundoplication
Indications for minimally invasive approach are the same as open. Caution should be used in the setting of recurrent hernias or large hiatal hernias (> 5 cm), although some centers are approaching large hernias laparoscopically with good long-term results.

- *Port placement.* Varies by surgeon preference, but typically a 10 mm camera port 2/3 the distance from the xiphoid to the umbilicus, 5 mm right anterior axillary line port for a liver retractor, 5 mm right upper abdominal working port, 5 mm left upper abdominal working port, and a 10 mm left lateral subcostal working port. An upper midline laparotomy is made for the open approach.
- Gastrohepatic ligament is incised and a combination of blunt and sharp dissection is used to divide the phrenoesophageal membrane and mobilize the esophagus circumferentially from the crural

attachments. Preservation of the peritoneal lining of the right and left crus is important, as this lining provides strength for closure of the hiatus (bites through the crus muscle alone, i.e., when the lining has been stripped, are more likely to pull through).

- The intrathoracic esophagus is mobilized up into the mediastinum from right to left pleura and pericardium to the pre-aortic plane. This maneuver can provide length to the esophagus to assure that there is at least 2-3 cm of tension-free, intraabdominal esophagus, as GERD can lead to inflammation and scarring that may result in a shortened esophagus with time. If the esophagus is shortened and enough length cannot be obtained with intrathoracic esophageal mobilization, a Collis gastroplasty (wedge gastrectomy) may be performed to add esophageal length.
- Care should be taken to identify and preserve both vagus nerves during mobilization of the esophagus.
- A retro-esophageal window is then made for passage of the stomach in order to create the fundoplication.
- The short gastric vessels are then divided along the upper third of the greater curve of the stomach.
- The posterior hiatus is closed by reapproximating the crura with several interrupted sutures. Anterior sutures may be placed in cases of large hiatal defects due to large hiatal hernias.
- The upper third of the greater curve of the stomach is then passed through the retroesophageal window and a "shoeshine" maneuver of anterior and posterior folds of fundus is performed to ensure there is no resistance and to obtain the desired bulkiness of the wrap.
- The fundoplication is then created over an esophageal bougie (51, 54, and 60 Fr most commonly used) with 3 interrupted sutures to create 2 cm fundoplication, or 4 sutures for a 3 cm fundoplication depending on surgeon preference. It is important to perform the wrap around the segment of intra-abdominal esophagus and not the gastric cardia, as wrapping around the stomach may lead to acid production proximal to the wrap, resulting in ongoing GERD symptoms despite the fundoplication.

Trans-thoracic fundoplication

Esophageal lengthening with a gastroplasty may be more easily performed from the chest, though the transthoracic approach may carry a slightly higher cardiopulmonary risk and postoperative pain issues than a laparoscopic approach. The transthoracic approach may also be useful for patients with prior transabdominal ARS, where a redo approach from the abdomen may be more difficult due to scarring. Some also prefer the transthoracic approach in the setting of a large hiatal hernia.

- The approach is typically via the left chest via thoracotomy through the 6th or 7th intercostal space.
- The inferior pulmonary ligament is divided and the lung is retracted superiorly and anteriorly to expose the esophagus.
- A diaphragm retraction stitch may be helpful to expose the hiatus.
- The esophagus is dissected out from posterior mediastinum and encircled with a Penrose.
- The phrenoesophageal membrane is incised and any herniated stomach is returned to the abdomen after division of the short gastrics.
- A Collis gastroplasty is performed if necessary.
- Posterior crural sutures are placed but not tied; a 360° wrap is performed over an esophageal bougie, as described above, and returned to the abdomen. The crural sutures are then tied.

Potential questions/alternative scenarios

Mortality of both open and laparoscopic antireflux surgery is < 1%. Serious intraoperative complications include splenic injury, and gastric or esophageal perforation. Conversion to the open approach may be needed to aid in visualization or to safely address any of the above complications. Early postoperative complications include gas-bloat syndrome, dysphagia, or stricture due to an excessively tight wrap. Late complications include slippage of the wrap back into the chest, or failure of the fundoplication itself.

"You are doing a Nissen fundoplication and as you are dividing the short gastric vessels (or retracting the stomach), there is bleeding noted to be coming from the left upper quadrant. On further inspection, there is a capsular tear in the spleen. How would you manage this problem?"
Splenic capsular tears can often be managed with application of direct pressure for a period of a few minutes and can be additionally helped with applying one of a variety of topical hemostatic agents available to the area, for example Surgicel (Ethicon, Inc.). Persistent capsular or hilar bleeding may prove to be more difficult to control, necessitating conversion to open and direct control of surgical bleeding. If control cannot be gained with suture ligatures, formal splenectomy may need to be performed.

"You have a patient postoperative day three s/p Nissen fundoplication who is febrile and has peritoneal signs. During division of the short gastric vessels, the vessels were noted to be quite short. Energy was used for division of some of these vessels. How would you proceed? What if the patient had a Collis gastroplasty performed, but presented in the same manner?"

Any patient with peritoneal signs within the early postoperative period should warrant re-exploration to identify the source of either bleeding or perforation. Depending on severity of presentation, a preoperative imaging study such as an upper gastrointestinal contrast study (with water soluble contrast or thin barium) or CT scan can help to localize the areas of concern. Thermal injuries leading to perforation may not be limited to the stomach if care has not been taken during the initial operation to avoid resting the hot blade of the ligating device on nearby bowel. Thermal injuries tend to present a few days postoperatively. It is therefore important to fully evaluate the stomach and surrounding viscous structures for injury. Explorations may be carried out laparoscopically by an experienced minimally invasive surgeon, or by open laparotomy. Given the robust blood supply of the stomach, small perforations or thermal injuries can usually be repaired primarily or close with an endoscopic linear stapler. Drains should be left near the area of injury after the abdomen has been thoroughly washed out. A patient presenting with these symptoms following an esophageal lengthening procedure (Collis) should raise concern for a leak from staple line of the Collis gastroplasty. Most leaks from the staple line can be managed with primary repair and drainage.

"You have a patient who is postoperative day one from a laparoscopic Nissen fundoplication. A Barium swallows is obtained, which shows delayed flow of contrast through a tight wrap. The patient complains of some dysphagia after starting a clear diet. How would you counsel this patient? What if her symptoms persisted beyond a week or two? What if they persisted after dilation?"

If at the initial operation the wrap was performed over an adequate sized esophageal bougie (the authors prefer a 54 Fr bougie), then early dysphagia and tight-appearing wrap on imaging can be attributed to local edema. If no or small sized dilator was used, an early re-exploration to create a looser wrap may be warranted. For those patients who had an adequate sized dilator used can often be managed with continued liquid diet and observation to allow the edema to resolve over time (up to 3 months). If dysphagia persists, endoscopic evaluation and dilation are warranted. The importance of an adequate preoperative work up is highlighted in a patient with prolonged postoperative dysphagia. If a motility disorder was excluded preoperatively in the patient with persistent postoperative dysphagia, then revision may be necessary to relieve an overly tight wrap that has not responded to dilation. Takedown of the wrap with a redo partial fundoplication (Toupet or Dor) should be performed in patients found to have esophageal dysmotility (i.e., low amplitude contractions).

"You have a patient who is two years s/p Nissen fundoplication. She now has recurrent heartburn and regurgitation. How would you work this patient up?"

Workup for recurrent symptoms in a patient that has previously undergone anti-reflux surgery is similar to the initial workup. A barium swallow study may provide useful information regarding whether the wrap remains intact and its location relative to the diaphragm (i.e., slipped Nissen). Manometry is useful as esophageal function may have changed over time. Fundoplications performed on foreshortened esophagi often recur due to the tension pulling the repair up into the chest, putting the crural stitches at risk. It is therefore important to carefully assess esophageal length prior to the initial operation with a barium swallow, as well as intraoperatively following mobilization of the esophagus. A Collis gastroplasty is needed if adequate tension-free length cannot be obtained.

Pearls/pitfalls

- 24 hour pH probe is the gold standard for diagnosis of GERD.
- Patients who fail medical treatment should also undergo a preoperative endoscopy, barium swallow, and manometry prior to any intervention.
- Patients with BE should undergo routine surveillance endoscopy. If HGD is identified, mucosal directed therapy is warranted.
- Gastroplasty in addition to fundoplication should be performed in the setting of foreshortened esophagus to prevent wrap slippage.

Suggested readings

- Krasna MJ (2009). Surgical therapy for gastroesophageal reflux disease. Shields TW et al (eds), *General Thoracic Surgery*. 7th ed. Philadelphia, PA: Lippincott Williams & Wilkins. pp.1913-1923.
- Rice TW, Shay SS, Murthy SC (2010). Surgical treatment of benign esophageal diseases. Sellke FW (ed), *Sabiston and Spencer's surgery of the chest*. 8th ed. Philadelphia, PA: Elsevier. pp. 547-576.
- Rice TW, Goldblum JR. Management of Barrett's esophagus with high-grade dysplasia. *Thorac Surg Clin* 2012 (22) 101-107.

Notes

19. Esophageal motility disorders

Marek Polomsky, MD, and Seth Force, MD

Concept
- Understanding symptoms and presentation of primary esophageal motility disorders
- Manometric characteristics
- Diagnostic work-up and indications for repair of achalasia
- Critical steps for repair of Heller myotomy with partial fundoplication
- Pitfalls and alternative solutions

Chief complaint
"A 48 yo man presents with complaint of progressive dysphagia to both liquids and solids, accompanied by regurgitation."

Differential
The differential for his dysphagia includes motility disorders such as achalasia, nutcracker esophagus, diffuse esophageal spasm (DES), hypertensive lower esophageal sphincter (LES), ineffective esophageal motility (IEM), scleroderma, as well as hiatal hernia, esophageal diverticulum, peptic stricture, eosinophilic esophagitis, and esophageal cancer.

History and physical
A history investigating possible achalasia or other esophageal motility disorders should focus on eliciting classic symptoms of slowly progressive dysphagia for solids and liquids, regurgitation of bland undigested food, and chest pain. Others symptoms suggestive of achalasia include weight loss, aspiration with episodes of recurrent pneumonia or chronic cough, and heartburn. Comorbidities which may affect treatment algorithms include candidal esophagitis, malnutrition, and concomitant cancer, as well as previous thoracic or abdominal surgery. One must be careful to recognize patients that solely have gastroesophageal reflux disease (GERD), where an atypical presentation of reflux can mimic the symptomatology of achalasia. A physical exam focusing on the pulmonary and gastrointestinal exam should be made.

Tests
- *CXR.* A CXR can visualize the presence of a dilated fluid-filled esophagus (typically can see a right sided posterior mediastinal shadow), and the absence of a gastric bubble.

- *EGD.* When performing an EGD, one will often see a dilated esophagus with retention of saliva and undigested food, and a very tight LES making passage of the scope through it very difficult. It is performed to exclude obstruction from tumor or stricture (pseudoachalasia), or infections such as candidal esophagitis. Ringed contractions of the esophagus also suggest abnormal peristalsis that may be seen with other esophageal motility disorders.
- *Barium esophagram.* On a barium esophagram one can visualize a dilated esophagus with the presence of an air-fluid level, a characteristic "bird's beak" at the distal esophagus (from a non-relaxing LES), and aperistalsis. The esophagram can be normal In patients with early achalasia as opposed to patients with late stage achalasia, where a "sigmoid esophagus" may be present. Other motility disorders have characteristic appearances (i.e., corkscrew appearance seen with diffuse esophageal spasm [DES]).
- *Manometry.* Manometric characteristics of achalasia include absence of LES relaxation, elevated LES resting pressure (10-15 mmHg), aperistalsis of the esophageal body, and esophageal body pressurization. There have been variants of achalasia that have been described (i.e., vigorous achalasia) and it is not uncommon for patients with achalasia to have manometric results that do not meet all 4 criteria for the diagnosis. The sine qua non for diagnosis of achalasia is failure of the LES to relax.
- *CT scan.* A CT scan can be useful to assess the integrity of the mediastinum, especially in end-stage achalasia or megaesophagus.

Index scenario (additional information)
"An EGD, barium esophagram, and manometry were performed with findings that were consistent with achalasia. The patient has no history of GERD and no previous surgeries. What is the optimal therapy for this patient?"

Treatment/management
The goal of therapy (both surgical and non-surgical) is to eliminate the outflow obstruction, thus relieving dysphagia, and maintain a barrier against gastroesophageal reflux. Medical therapy includes calcium channel blockers, oral nitrates, and sildenafil. Results of medical therapies are variable and have poor short-term results. Pneumatic balloon dilatation and endoscopic botulinum toxin injections are also alternatives but are rarely effective in the long-term. The most effective and common surgical therapy for achalasia is laparoscopic Heller myotomy with partial fundoplication, which has good long-term outcomes (> 90% relief of dysphagia more than 2 years). While there are

no differences in outcomes, Dor fundoplication (anterior 180° wrap) is typically preferred to Toupet fundoplication (posterior 270° wrap) due to the preservation of posterior crural attachments and being technically easier to perform. Predictors of successful outcomes following Heller myotomy include increased magnitude of preoperative LES resting pressure, minimal degree of preoperative esophageal dilation or tortuosity, and the absence of earlier nonoperative interventions. Infections such as candidal esophagitis, caused by the chronic retained food and secretions in the esophagus, should be treated prior to surgery.

Operative steps
Laparoscopic Heller myotomy with Dor fundoplication
Goals – eliminate outflow obstruction, create a barrier against gastroesophageal reflux.

- Position patient supine in modified lithotomy position, general endotracheal anesthesia (GETA), foley.
- Five working ports to access the upper abdomen, insufflate with CO_2, reverse Trendelenberg positioning.
- The gastrohepatic ligament is divided, making sure to look for a replaced or accessory left hepatic artery. If one is present, the gastrohepatic ligament is opened inferiorly and superiorly to the vessel and a clip is placed on the artery. 15-30 minutes is allowed to pass and the left lobe of the liver is then assessed. If there is discoloration suggesting decreased inflow to the liver, the clip is removed and the artery preserved throughout the dissection, If no ischemia, then the artery is an accessory branch and it can be divided (usually the case).
- Mobilize the esophagus of the right crus by opening the phrenoesophageal membrane. Do the same along the anterior arch of the hiatus, making sure to preserve the anterior vagus nerve. Carry dissection down along left crus to mobilize the esophagus. Division of the short gastrics facilitates dissection along the left crus. The posterior esophagus does not need to be mobilized if a Dor is to be performed, but circumferential mobilization of the esophagus is needed if a posterior Toupet is to be performed, in which case the posterior vagus nerve must also be sought out and preserved.
- Mobilize the intrathoracic esophagus by dissecting in the areolar plane within the mediastinum, dissecting the esophagus from the right and left pleura, as well as the anterior pericardium. Remember the vagus nerves will originate on the right (posterior vagus) and left (anterior vagus) as dissection is carried proximally in the mediastinum.
- Mobilize upper third of the gastric fundus by dividing the short gastric vessels.

- Mobilize the esophagus anteriorly at the hiatus by freeing up the gastric fat pad, going up into the mediastinum and clearing proximally at least 6 to 8 cm of GEJ (in preparation for a full Heller myotomy).

- With a bougie in place (45 or 50 Fr), perform a myotomy starting with blunt dissection using endoscopic Kittners to spread the longitudinal muscle. Then separate the circular muscle fibers from the mucosa, dividing with some type of energy device (hook electrocautery, bipolar, ultrasonic shears, etc.). The myotomy should extend proximally onto the esophagus for 4-5 cm through the GEJ (ensuring division of clasp fibers) and onto the anterior wall of the fundus of the stomach for 2-3 cm. Myotomy edges are carefully separated from the underlying mucosa for 40-50% of esophageal circumference.

- Perform intraoperative EGD to check for completeness of myotomy and to look for an unrecognized mucosal injury prior to proceeding to the fundoplication. Submerging the myotomy under water and insufflating assists with identifying mucosal perforations.

- To create the fundoplication, the mobilized anterior fundus is laid across the myotomy site and the left edge of the fundus is sewn to the left cut edge of the esophageal myotomy with three or four interrupted sutures, taking the highest stitch through the left crural pillar as an anchor. The right side of fundus is sutured similarly to the right edge of the cut esophageal muscle taking the highest suture through the right crural pillar to prevent torsion.

Potential questions/alternative scenarios

"A 59 yo man with severe COPD, ESRD, and a previous laparotomy for gangrenous cholecystitis is diagnosed with achalasia. How would you manage this patient?"

This patient is not a good surgical candidate for surgical treatment of his achalasia, either through a laparoscopic or thoracotomy approach. Depending on the severity of his disease, medical therapy may be tried first. If this were to fail, endoscopic botulinum toxin injection is a reasonable alternative for this patient. Improvement in dysphagia following injection typically lasts 6 months or less and often times requires repeated injections for continued relief. The treatment is also expensive. Botulinum toxin injection should be avoided in patients who are surgical candidates because of the resulting submucosal fibrosis, however prior toxin injection does not rule a patient out for surgical treatment. This fibrosis may make attempts at surgical myotomy more difficult and increases the risk of intraoperative mucosal perforation. As achalasia is a progressive disease, this patient may eventually benefit from a percutaneous endoscopic gastrostomy (PEG) tube for enteral access.

"Your patient develops recurrent dysphagia following myotomy. How would you manage this patient?"

Perform an EGD and a barium esophagram to exclude an obstructing lesion, assess the integrity of the myotomy, and assess for esophageal dilation or tortuosity. Repeat manometry would be beneficial to assess for persistently high LES resting pressure (10-15 mmHg). If an incomplete (not extended proximally or distally enough or bridging muscle fibers are left behind) or a scarred myotomy is suspected, one can perform botulinum toxin injection, pneumatic dilation, redo myotomy, or in certain instances esophagectomy.

"Following completion of your myotomy you perform an intraoperative EGD and notice a small mucosal perforation near the GEJ. How would you proceed?"

Intraoperative mucosal perforation occurs on average 7% of the time and typically is located near the GEJ. If managed appropriately, this complication rarely has any significant clinical consequences. A small defect in the mucosa can be primarily repaired with absorbable suture. Subsequent buttressing with an anterior Dor fundoplication can provide further reinforcement. Endoscopy should always be done at the time of surgery to check for an adequate repair and to assess mucosal integrity. Postoperatively the patient should be kept NPO for 3-5 days, after which a swallow contrast study should be performed to assess for a leak. If there is a leak, the patient should continue to be NPO with NG tube decompression. Further management options include esophageal endoscopic stenting versus reoperation through the left chest or abdomen depending on the size of the leak and the patient's symptoms and clinical status.

"A 67 yo patient presents with long-standing dysphagia and a dilated, tortuous esophagus. Manometry and is consistent with achalasia How would you manage this patient?"

A severely dilated and tortuous sigmoid-shaped esophagus (or megaesophagus) is suspect for end-stage achalasia. Even with esophageal dilation greater than 6 cm and a sigmoid-shaped esophagus, a myotomy can be first-line therapy. But often times the esophagus can be so markedly dilated that standard Heller myotomy can be technically challenging and would not be sufficient to relieve outflow obstruction and permit for adequate esophageal emptying. In such circumstances, a transhiatal or a 3-hole esophagogastrectomy with gastric pull-up and cervical anastomosis can be performed. While patients who have a sigmoid esophagus and a prior failed myotomy are the best candidates for an esophagectomy. Esophagectomy as first-line therapy for achalasia - even in the setting of a sigmoid esophagus - is more controversial.

"A patient presents with severe spasmodic chest pain and dysphagia. You suspect the patient has an esophageal motility disorder. How would you work this patient up?"

After ruling out cardiac and other gastrointestinal sources of chest pain, non-achalasia primary esophageal motility disorders should be suspected. Manometric analysis should be performed. Disorders include nutcracker esophagus (100% peristaltic waves, distal esophageal amplitudes > 180 mmHg), diffuse esophageal spasm (simultaneous pressurizations in 20-90% of the swallows with the remaining swallows having prolonged contractions [> 6 seconds] and the presence of high-pressure amplitudes in the distal segment of the body), and hypertensive LES (resting LES pressure > 40 mmHg, 100% peristaltic contractions). First-line management of most non-achalasia motility disorders is medical therapy. A long myotomy followed by partial fundoplication is associated with good outcomes in these motility disorders when dysphagia and obstructive symptoms are the primary complaints and when the LES resting pressure is elevated with poor relaxation. The proximal extent of the long myotomy should be guided by manometric analysis and should extend past the abnormal and hypertensive contractions until normotensive esophagus is reached. If a myotomy needs to extend above the aortic arch, a right thoracotomy will be necessary.

"A 49 yo woman with dysphagia also has history of Raynaud's phenomena and telangiectasias. What is the suspected diagnosis and how would you confirm this?"

A clinical diagnosis of scleroderma is suspected. Manometric characteristics include a hypomotile esophageal body in 100% of the swallows with a hypotensive LES. In contrast to achalasia, the LES does relax. Also, achalasia affects smooth muscle, therefore contractions in the more proximal esophagus (striated muscle) will be normal. Management is often times supportive therapy with aggressive anti-reflux medical therapy and dilation of strictures if they occur. If antireflux surgery is to be considered, one should perform a partial fundoplication given the impaired esophageal motility associated with scleroderma.

"A patient with long-standing GERD presents with dysphagia."

Diagnostic workup should include EGD, impedance-pH analysis, barium esophagram, and manometric evaluation. Mechanical obstruction may be secondary to peptic stricture, hiatal hernia, or adenocarcinoma. Patients with peptic stricture should be managed first with dilation, followed by anti-reflux surgery once the stricture is adequately dilated. Patients with GERD can also have ineffective esophageal motility (IEM), presumably due to the progressive fibrosis caused by chronic inflammation. IEM is characterized by having at least 30% of the swallows with distal esophageal amplitudes < 30 mmHg, failed contractions that do not transverse the entire esophageal body, simultaneous waves with amplitudes < 30 mmHg, or absent peristalsis. Treatment consists of antireflux therapy or surgery, with reports of improved motility following cessation of the harmful reflux.

"A 72 yo man with a history of GERD is referred to you with a barium esophagram that shows a 'classic' bird's beak appearance of the distal esophagus. He has had progressive dysphagia and a 20-pounds weight loss. He is being referred to you for surgical treatment of achalasia. How would you proceed?"

As stated above, make sure you confirm the diagnosis of achalasia with manometry and upper endoscopy. This patient's history is more suspicious for an obstructing distal esophageal cancer. Upper endoscopy must be performed preoperatively and any suspicious lesions or strictures should be biopsied. Do not fall into the trap of doing a myotomy and fundoplication on a patient with an obstructing esophageal cancer.

"An 81 yo woman with a history of achalasia and a multiple prior pneumatic dilations is referred to you for dysphagia. Manometry appears consistent with achalasia. A barium esophagram shows only a mildly dilated esophagus and question of a filling defect in the mid-esophagus. What is the suspected diagnosis and how would you proceed?"

Remember that long-standing achalasia is associated with squamous cell carcinoma of the esophagus. This patient should undergo upper endoscopy and biopsy of the suspicious lesion. Should this prove to be a malignancy, the patient should undergo esophagectomy following appropriate staging and physiologic testing.

Pearls/pitfalls

- Four manometric characteristics of achalasia are 1) absence of LES relaxation, 2) elevated LES resting pressure, 3) 100% simultaneous pressurizations with aperistalsis of the esophageal body, and 4) esophageal body pressurization. Absence of LES relaxation must be present for the diagnosis of achalasia.
- Perform EGD to look for other associated pathology (pseudoachalasia, infection).
- Surgical therapy for achalasia consists of laparoscopic Heller myotomy with partial fundoplication.
- Length of myotomy should be at least 4 cm on to the esophagus and 2-3 cm on to the stomach.
- Check the completeness of myotomy and for mucosal injury with EGD at completion of myotomy.

Suggested readings

- Heitmiller RF and Buzdon MM. Surgery for Achalasia and Other Motility Disorders. Kaiser LR, Kron IL, and Spray TL.(eds) *Mastery of Cardiothoracic Surgery*.2007; 163-173.
- Hong E and Liptay MJ. Achalasia. Franco KL and Thourani VH. (eds) *Cardiothoracic Surgery Review*. 2012; 1409-1411.
- Herbella et al. Surgical Treatment of Primary Esophageal Motility Disorders. *J GI Surg* 2008; 12: 604–608.

Notes

20. Esophageal perforation

Aaron J. Weiss, MD, and Andrew J. Kaufman, MD

Concept
- Causes of esophageal perforation
- Presentation, diagnosis, and workup
- Operative timing and options
- Pitfalls and alternative solutions

Chief complaint
"A 72 yo woman presents ten hours after undergoing an endoscopy for dilatation of a Schatzki's ring with symptoms of fever, chills, and chest pain."

Differential
Esophageal perforation, acute coronary syndrome, peptic ulcer disease, GERD, gastritis, pneumonia, aortic dissection, tension pneumothorax, pericarditis. The top three most common causes of esophageal trauma include iatrogenic perforation, Boerhaave's syndrome, and external trauma. Iatrogenic injury to the esophagus can occur during flexible or rigid upper endoscopy, esophageal dilatation of strictures or achalasia, sclerotherapy for esophageal varices, transesophageal echocardiography, nasogastric tube placement, endotracheal tube placement, and any endoscopic ultrasound interventions. Boerhaave's syndrome arises from a rapid increase in intraluminal pressure from the patient vomiting with coexisting failure of relaxation of the upper esophageal sphincter. External trauma is exceedingly rare with most cases occurring as a result of high-speed motor vehicle crashes. Perforation from a stab or gunshot wound rarely occurs in the thoracic esophagus due to its location. However, esophageal injury is more likely with neck trauma. Other situations that can lead to esophageal perforation include ingestion of foreign bodies or caustic agents (alkali chemicals worse than acidic chemicals) or injury during another operative procedure such as a thoracic aneurysm repair, mediastinoscopy, or hiatal hernia repair.

History and physical
The physician should have a high index of suspicion based on the clinical situation. Additionally, the presentation may differ based on a number of factors including the cause, location, size, presence of contamination, and length of time elapsed since injury. If stable and alert, the patient should be asked for duration, location, and severity of chest/abdominal/back pain as well as any associated shortness of breath. Elicit history of instrumentation to the esophagus, ingestion of foreign material, trauma, or severe vomiting. A focused physical exam should be performed that

includes vital signs, lung exam, cardiac exam, and abdominal exam. Feel for crepitus and Hammon's sign (systolic crunching sound heard over left sternal border). Mackler's triad consists of subcutaneous emphysema, pain, and vomiting. Focus on signs of sepsis including fever and hemodynamic instability.

Tests

- *Labs.* Acute care panel, complete blood cell count, liver function tests, INR/PT/PTT, type and screen, blood culture x2, troponins.
- *EKG.* To rule out an acute coronary syndrome or an arrhythmia.
- *PA and lateral X-ray, upright abdominal X-ray.* Look for air in the soft tissue surrounding the cervical spine, anterior displacement of the trachea due to air/fluid, widening of the superior mediastinum, "V sign" (emphysema in left lower mediastinum along the aorta and above the left diaphragm), mediastinal widening and pleural effusion +/- a pneumothorax. For cervical esophageal perforations, a lateral neck X-ray may show air in the prevertebral fascia.
- *Esophagogram with water-soluble contrast.* This is the test of choice, but has a 10% false-negative rate. Look for extravasation of contrast into the mediastinum or pleural space. If no leak is seen with water-soluble contrast, the test should be repeated with thin (dilute) barium contrast, which is more sensitive for detecting smaller perforations.
- *Pleural fluid analysis.* Although rarely performed, diagnosis can be made by finding pieces of food, a pH < 6, or elevated amylase levels.
- *CT scan of the chest with IV and PO water-soluble contrast.* A CT should only be done if the patient is stable and if it will either help localize the site of perforation or document the development of any mediastinitis or pleural effusions/empyema.

Index scenario (additional information)
"The patient states that she began having chest/epigastric pain a few hours after undergoing balloon dilatation earlier that morning with rigors setting in shortly thereafter. The patient is tachycardic, normotensive, and febrile to 101.7° F. Besides being tachycardic, the patient's cardiac exam is normal. The lungs are clear to auscultation bilaterally with tachypnea. No crepitus is palpated. Her abdomen is soft, slightly tender in the epigastric region, nondistended, and without rebound or guarding. Esophagram with water-soluble contrast was performed and showed extravasation of contrast from the distal esophagus into the left pleural space. How would you proceed?"

Treatment/management

The basic principles of management include initiation of broad-spectrum antibiotics, copious irrigation and drainage, elimination of any further mediastinal or pleural contamination, and creation of an alternative means of nutrition. Immediate initiation of broad-spectrum antibiotics is paramount. The infection resulting from esophageal perforation is usually polymicrobial and antibiotics should include coverage of MRSA, pseudomonas, and anaerobes in addition to the standard oropharyngeal flora (including yeast). The patient should receive at least two large-bore IV's (possibly a central line) and aggressive isotonic fluid resuscitation. Every attempt should be made to undergo operative repair within the first 24 hours, as the success of operative repair decreases after this time frame. The patient should be counseled on the serious nature of the situation and a discussion should be had covering the various operative interventions that may need to be performed depending on the intraoperative findings. If hemodynamically unstable despite adequate fluid resuscitation, a low dose pressor may be started to maintain a stable blood pressure.

Operative steps

Repair of a distal esophageal perforation

- Large bore IV's, arterial line, general endotracheal anesthesia with placement of a bronchial blocker down the left mainstem bronchus under fiberoptic bronchoscopy or selective-lung ventilation with a double-lumen tube, central line, and urinary catheter.
- An intraoperative EGD is performed first to localize the site of the perforation, determine if there are multiple perforations, and visualize any distal obstructions or mucosal ischemia.
- Position the patient so the left side is up and flexed at the hip to maximize the exposure. Left thoracotomy is performed through the sixth or seventh intercostal space with possible removal of a rib.
- Have the anesthesiologist isolate the lung by inflating the blocker in the left mainstem bronchus. Ensure the patient tolerates one-lung ventilation before proceeding with dissection.
- Retract the lung tissue anteriorly after dividing the inferior pulmonary ligament. The lung may need to be decorticated first if there is extensive pleural contamination. The mediastinal pleura is opened along the entire length of the anterior and posterior esophagus.
- Copiously irrigate and wash out the mediastinum and pleural space. Debride any necrotic tissue.
- Localize the site and extent of perforation. A longitudinal myotomy may need to be performed to fully expose the mucosal defect. Assess the degree of contamination and quality of tissue at the site of injury.

- If primary repair is possible, approximate the full thickness of the mucosa and submucosa over a 40-46 Fr bougie using an interrupted absorbable suture. It is important to make sure the repair is free of tension. The muscular layer is also reapproximated with a running absorbable suture. Have the anesthesiologist pass an NG tube through the esophagus and into the stomach under tactile guidance by the surgeon to ensure no disruption of the repair.
- Buttress the repair with a pedicled flap, as this will increase the rate of successful repair.
- Continue drainage by irrigating and washing out the mediastinum and pleural space again. Place as many large bore chest tubes as needed to ensure adequate postoperative drainage.
- Close in an anatomic fashion and transport the patient to the intensive care unit for monitoring.

Potential questions/alternative scenarios

"What flaps can be used to buttress a primary repair of an esophageal perforation?"

Multiple options exist for buttressing the repair and include an intercostal flap (remember to plan for this when performing the thoracotomy and mention to a potential examiner), pleural flap, pericardial fat pad, diaphragmatic pedicle graft, omentum on-lay graft, rhomboid flap, or latissimus dorsi flap.

"Due to the patient initially refusing surgery, operative intervention is not performed until 48 hours later. Should primary repair be performed, and if not, then what should be done?"

If greater than 24 hours has passed from the time of esophageal injury, there is an increased rate of failure for primary repair of a perforation. This is typically due to worsening mediastinitis, poor tissue quality, and hemodynamic instability. However, the decision to primarily repair or not must be assessed on a case by case basis. Don't jump to esophagectomy and bipolar exclusion in a stable patient who may still be a candidate for repair based on time from injury alone. One must take into account the physiologic status of the patient and assess the area of injury in the operating room. Perforations caused by iatrogenic injury from endoscopy may be relatively clean and have minimal contamination if the patient remains in a fasting state. If this type of patient is stable and the tissue appears viable, attempting primary repair is reasonable, even after the 24 hour window. In contrast, a patient with Boerhaave's syndrome who has gross contamination of food debris, saliva, etc. will likely have rapid progression of mediastinitis and tissues unsuitable for primary repair. This may even occur earlier than the 24 hour mark (so don't jump to primary repair just because the patient is 12 hours out from injury either).

If primary repair is not thought to be feasible, a number of options exist. If the area of perforation is relatively small, the mediastinum should be debrided, the area of injury exposed, and a T-tube may be placed through the site of injury and brought out through the chest wall. This creates a controlled esophagocutaneous fistula that allows for adequate drainage of the esophagus and gives the tissues around the site of perforation time to heal. Additional chest tubes are placed after complete decortication has been performed to ensure adequate drainage of the pleural space. Enteral access in the form of a feeding jejunostomy and possible gastrostomy tube placement for gastric decompression are also helpful. If there is extensive mediastinal contamination or a large injury, bipolar esophageal exclusion should be considered. The manner in which this is carried out depends on the stability of the patient. In a relatively stable patient, the lung is decorticated, the mediastinum is debrided, and the site of injury is located. The esophagus is then divided proximal and distal to injury and the perforated segment of the esophagus is resected, drains are left in the esophageal bed, and wide drainage of the pleural space with multiple chest tubes is carried out prior to closure. If the patient remains stable, they are repositioned supine and a jejunostomy tube is placed for enteral access, a gastrostomy tube is placed for gastric decompression, and a proximal cervical esophagostomy is brought out the left neck for proximal diversion. If the patient is unstable, decorticating the lung, washing out the chest, debriding the mediastinum, and resecting the perforated segment of esophagus is all that should be done. Drains are placed, including placement of a NG tube in the proximal esophageal stump, and the patient is closed. The remaining steps of the bipolar (meaning proximal and distal) exclusion are carried out when the patient is more stable. Delayed reconstruction can then take place at a later time with completion esophagectomy followed by a substernal gastric pull-up. If the stomach is not usable as a conduit, a substernal colon interposition would be the next best option. The posterior mediastinal space will be obliterated, so do not attempt to pass the conduit through the native bed in cases of delayed reconstruction.

"What should be done if there is an obstruction distal to the site of the perforation during a primary repair?"

Studies have shown that if primary repair was performed without treatment of a distal obstruction to the site of the perforation, mortality approaches 100%. However, with treatment of the distal obstruction and the perforation, survival increases significantly. Attempts should be made to do an intraoperative dilatation for a distal stricture prior to repair. An esophagomyotomy opposite the site of perforation should be performed in cases of achalasia prior to attempting repair. In cases of a malignant obstructing lesion with a more proximal perforation, the patient should undergo esophagectomy and bipolar exclusion as described above. A substernal gastric pull-up may then be performed at a later date if appropriate (depending on stage on cancer, if they need adjuvant therapy, etc). Patients that have undergone multiple prior dilations for tight peptic strictures, achalasia, or other anatomical obstruction, consideration should be given to performing a formal esophagectomy at the time of perforation. Since these perforations are identified at the time of dilatation or shortly after and patients are usually in a fasting state prior to dilatation, there is minimal contamination. Performing a formal esophagectomy with immediate reconstruction can be considered in these cases. If there is extensive contamination due to a delay in diagnosis of the perforation, then esophageal exclusion may be the safest treatment plan.

"If the perforation occurred in the cervical esophagus, what surgical approach should be taken? What about if the perforation were in the mid-esophagus?"

For cervical perforations of the esophagus, the incision should be made anterior to the left sternocleidomastoid (SCM) from the sternal notch to the level of the cricoid cartilage. After lateral retraction of the SCM and carotid sheath and medial retraction of the trachea and thyroid, use blunt finger dissection to expose the prevertebral space. Often adequate irrigation and drainage will allow for the esophageal injury to heal on its own without any repair. If there is evidence of leakage into the mediastinum, then drainage of the pleural space is required as well. For injuries to the mid-esophagus, the approach is through a right thoracotomy. Distal esophageal perforations can be approached from the right or left chest. If a pleural effusion is seen or there is extravasation of contrast into the pleural space, the approach should be on the side of the effusion.

"Are there any minimally invasive options in this setting?"

Various minimally invasive options exist including video-assisted thoracoscopic surgery that utilizes three to four trocars to perform the same procedure as the open approach. Most of the experience with this approach has been done in the setting of an iatrogenic esophageal perforation that was picked up early before extensive mediastinitis could set in. Insertion of an endoscopic esophageal stent or prosthesis is another option for patients who are too sick to tolerate open surgery with the hope that more definitive repair can be performed once the patient's status improves. Endoscopic clipping of the perforation is another option but is only applicable to a small subset of stable patients with little signs of frank infection. Despite the existence of these minimally invasive options, operative intervention is still considered the standard of care.

- Early diagnosis and treatment are of the utmost value to optimize outcome following an esophageal perforation.
- A variety of tests and imaging are useful in diagnosing an esophageal perforation with the standard being an esophagogram with water-soluble contrast followed by thin barium if the initial study is negative and suspicion of perforation is high.
- Operative intervention within 24 hours maximizes the surgeon's chance of doing a primary repair. Buttressing of the repair should be performed and the surgeon can choose from many options.
- The etiology of perforation, clinical status of the patient, time from injury, extent of mediastinitis, and quality of tissue surrounding the injury should all be taken into account when determining whether primary repair is appropriate.
- Cervical perforations can typically be treated with drainage alone, assuming there is no leakage into the pleural space.
- Intrathoracic perforation should be approached on the side of extravasation of contrast or pleural effusion. If neither are present, distal perforations can be approached from the left or right, whereas mid- and proximal esophageal perforations are best approached from the right chest.

Suggested readings

- Wu JT, Mattox KL, and Wall MJ Jr. Esophageal Perforations: New Perspectives and Treatment Paradigms. *J Trauma*. 2007. Nov;63(5):1173-84.
- Wiener DC. Esophageal injury. Mery CM and Turek JW. *TSRA Review of Cardiothoracic Surgery*. 2011. 212-217.

Notes

21. Esophageal diverticula

Carlos J. Anciano, MD, and Manisha Shende, MD

Concept

- Pulsion vs. traction diverticula (false vs. true)
- Anatomical level guides differential and intervention (Zenker's, mid-esophagus, epiphrenic)
- Minimally invasive and open approaches are valid
- Concomitant underlying disorders
- Treatment aims to relieve distal obstruction, treat associated disorder, and avoid leakage at site of diverticulectomy and myotomy

Chief complaint

" A 72 yo man arrives to your clinic with complaints of difficulty swallowing, sensation of food getting stuck in his throat, and occasional choking and regurgitation of food when eating. "

Differential

Esophageal motility disorders (i.e., achalasia), neuromotor degenerative disorders, esophageal diverticulum, esophageal stricture/ring, GERD, hiatal hernia, cancer.

History and physical

Focus on evaluating dysphagia: patterns, progressiveness, saliva vs. liquid vs. solids. Look for regurgitation of digested or undigested meals, aspiration history, halitosis, and cervical bruits on swallowing. Changes in tone of voice and globus sensation suggest more proximal pathology. Respiratory issues such as new onset asthma, pneumonia, or pulmonary abscesses are commonly related. Up to 50% of proximal diverticula are associated with GERD. Progressive dysphagia or changes in symptom pattern may suggest progression of an underlying dysmotility disorder, hiatal hernia, or stricture. Chest pressure or spasm-like pain suggest more distal esophageal pathology and associated motor disorders. Loss of weight and old age should increase the suspicion of malignant disease.

Tests

- *Contrast esophagram.* Typically the first step in the workup of dysphagia. Imaging should include views of the cervical esophagus to the stomach, as well as video cine recordings. Contrast pooling on post-swallow images will help to identify important characteristics of diverticula. Evaluate size, base/neck of diverticula, location and number of diverticula. Tertiary contractions, spasms, and esophageal quivering may suggest a motility disorder, but this is best confirmed with manometry. Evidence of reflux, rings, strictures, or filling defects should prompt further work up as well.

- *Manometry/pH studies.* Obtained selectively to determine etiology of diverticulum. A hypertensive upper esophageal sphincter and GERD are associated with Zenker's diverticula, while a number of motility abnormalities are commonly associated with epiphrenic diverticula.
- *CT scans.* Most useful for workup of mid-esophageal traction diverticula to evaluate for pulmonary or mediastinal inflammatory processes, such as granulomatous disease (i.e., TB, histoplasmosis). May also be helpful in planning operative approach (i.e., laterality).
- *EGD.* Perform carefully to avoid perforation. Can confirm presence and location of diverticulum, as well as evaluate for mucosal lesions. Therapeutically allows for dilation of strictures and allows for clearance of retained debris.
- *Labs.* Blood counts pointing to acute or chronic respiratory infections, blood losses, as well as nutritional status chemistries are useful.

Index scenario (additional information)

"The patient's breath is foul as he speaks and states he sometimes regurgitates chewed up lunch when he goes to bed at night. Contrast esophagram shows a 4 cm posterior cervical outpouching with retained contrast on post-swallow scout. Where do you go from here?"

Treatment/management

This patient has a Zenker's diverticulum (a false, pulsion diverticulum). Given his symptoms, operative repair should be recommended. Patients with Zenker's are typically older (50% are > 70 yo and 20% are > 80 yo at presentation), therefore it is important to assess cardiopulmonary reserve and nutritional status preoperatively. Once the patient has been deemed an adequate surgical candidate, one must then decide between endoscopic or open surgical treatment. Ankylosis of the jaw, cervical kyphosis, a prominent orbital arch, and a diverticulum < 3 cm (cannot fit stapler) or > 8-9 cm (creates a cloaca when stapled transorally) should prompt one to opt for an open approach. A narrow diverticulum neck with a larger pouch is an ideal candidate for endoscopic treatment with transoral stapling. Hiatal hernias and GERD are not uncommon in patients with Zenker's diverticula, with some proposing that there is compensatory tightening of the cricopharyngeus to protect from aspiration of refluxate, which then leads to the pulsion diverticulum. One must determine which pathology is more symptomatic (GERD/hiatal hernia vs. Zenker's), in which case the more symptomatic of the two is treated first. Treating both in the same setting significantly increases operative risk in a typically older patient population and should be avoided.

Operative steps

Diverticulectomy/diverticulopexy

Goals – relieve obstruction/high-pressure area/dysfunctional sphincter by cricopharyngeal myotomy, prevent collection of food debris within the diverticulum by pexy vs. resection.

- Supine patient with head slightly to right, ETT to prevent aspiration of retained debris. Left cervical oblique incision from hyoid to 1 cm above clavicle, retract sternocleidomastoid and carotid sheath laterally, larynx and thyroid medially.
- The omohyoid and middle thyroid vein may be divided for improved exposure.
- Avoid positioning retractors medially and dissect directly on the esophagus to minimize the risk of injury to the recurrent laryngeal nerve in the tracheoesophageal groove.
- Dissect out the diverticulum circumferentially to the base, which can be facilitated by placement of a 36-44 Fr bougie (probably safest to place over a guidewire to avoid perforation of the diverticulum).
- Cricopharyngeal myotomy is performed approximately 135° laterally, extending inferiorly at least 4 cm and proximally at least 2 cm on to striated muscle. The edges of the myotomy are separated approximately 90°.
- For diverticula < 2 cm, myotomy alone is sufficient treatment. Larger diverticula can be resected, most commonly done with a linear cutting stapler placed parallel to the long axis of the esophagus. The diverticulum may also be resected followed by hand-sewn reapproximation of the mucosa with 4-0 absorbable suture. Remnant omohyoid or strap muscle may be used to cover the repair. Salivary fistulae have been reported in up to 25% of patients undergoing diverticulectomy. Alternatively, pexy of larger diverticula to the more proximal prevertebral fascia prevents collection of debris within the lumen and has a significantly lower risk of fistulization.
- Retropharyngeal drain and layered, interrupted closure.

Transoral stapling

Goals – relieve obstruction with myotomy while creating a common channel between diverticulum and esophageal lumen to prevent collection of food debris.

- Supine patient, ETT to prevent aspiration of retained debris, shoulder roll, head slightly extended.
- Flexible esophagoscopy is performed first and a guide wire is placed in the true esophageal lumen for orientation.
- Rigid esophagoscopy is then performed with Weerda retractor. The top blade is positioned in the esophageal lumen while the lower blade is positioned in the diverticulum.
- The common wall between the true lumen and the diverticulum (which contains the cricopharyngeus) is centered in the view. A long stitch placed in the apex of the common wall aids with retraction during stapling.
- A linear cutting stapler with a dulled anvil tip is passed through the rigid esophagoscope. The stapler is positioned with the blunted end in the diverticulum and the cartridge in the true lumen. Serial firings may be needed for larger diverticuli.

Potential questions/alternative scenarios

"Now you are seeing a 54 yo man complaining of crushing chest pain, dysphagia, heartburn, and regurgitation. After ruling out cardiac reasons for his chest pain, you obtain a Barium swallow, which shows a 7-8 cm outpouching in the distal esophagus. How would you manage this patient?"

This patient has an epiphrenic diverticulum (false, pulsion diverticulum). His symptoms of heartburn and spasm-like pain suggest a concurrent motility disorder, which are common in patients with epiphrenic diverticula. Epiphrenic diverticula, particularly small ones, will likely be asymptomatic or present with mild symptoms. Some surgeons argue that all epiphrenic diverticula should be treated surgically, while other believe that patients who are asymptomatic or with mild symptoms can be treated conservatively. Conservative, or medical management, consists simply of chewing food well and intake of adequate liquids with meals. Patients who are symptomatic should unquestionably be treated surgically. Common associated symptoms include dysphagia, chest pain, food retention, aspiration, and regurgitation. Since many patients with epiphrenic diverticula have an underlying functional or mechanical distal obstruction that contributes to the formation of the diverticulum, it may be unclear if the symptoms are due to the diverticulum itself or the accompanying esophageal pathology. For this reason, epiphrenic diverticula should always be addressed when other esophageal pathology is being treated surgically. Manometry will uncover underlying esophageal spasm, achalasia, or a nonspecific motility disorder that may affect the surgical plan. pH studies will identify GERD, which may have lead to strictures or rings. EGD can visualize rings, strictures, areas of narrowing (external or internal compression), and allows for preoperative dilation. CT may assist with determining the best operative approach (chest or abdomen, left or right chest). A clear liquid diet may be required for a few days preoperatively to clear the esophageal lumen and diverticulum of debris. Treatment remains a myotomy extending proximal to the most cephalad diverticulum and distally past the area of incomplete relaxation (manometry guides). The myotomy is typically performed 90-180° away from the neck of the diverticulum. If further than 1 cm onto stomach (especially if non-relaxing lower esophageal sphincter), consider an antireflux procedure in the form of a partial fundoplication. When high amplitude contractions and spasm-like motility is present, it is best to perform a long proximal myotomy. Right-sided pouches, need for long myotomy (proximal to the aortic arch), and higher epiphrenic diverticula should be approached from the right chest. Distal, smaller, or left-sided pouches may be approached from the left chest or abdomen. Favor an open, posterolateral thoracotomy approach unless extremely comfortable with VATS techniques. If the base is wide and the pouch small, myotomy alone suffices in most cases. For large diverticula, those with narrow necks, or diverticula in which the endoscope passes preferentially into the pouch, perform a diverticulectomy over a 50-54 Fr bougie with a linear stapling device. The esophageal muscle and/or pleura can be reapproximated to buttress the staple line. The myotomy should then be performed at least 90° away from the staple line. Be compulsive about elevating the muscle layer away from mucosa with right angle clamps or the energy device of choice before division to avoid injury to the underlying mucosa. If the mucosa is perforated, primarily repair with absorbable suture, buttress the repair, and rotate the site of myotomy. Local drainage (i.e., Jackson-Pratt) near the staple line in addition to chest tube drainage of the pleural space is recommended. Contrast esophagram is routinely obtained in the early postoperative period before starting a diet. Save abdominal laparoscopic approaches for very small, distal diverticula, with distal manometry-guided targets (i.e., LES in achalasia). Approaching diverticula through the chest and performing abdominal fundoplication if symptoms of reflux in a second stage is perfectly valid treatment plan. Aim to prevent recurrence, protect your suture line, and treat dysmotility. Injury to one vagus nerve is of little clinical significance while bilateral injury may require a gastric emptying procedure require a gastric emptying procedure.

"You walk in the office to meet a 43 yo spelunker complaining of solid food dysphagia, stating that occasionally food 'won't go down' (while pointing to sternum). He reports occasional regurgitation of undigested food, as well as occasional blood-streaked emesis. How would you manage this patient?"

Contrast esophagram is the first test of choice for dysphagia, which in this case shows a 6 cm outpouching in the mid-esophagus. There seems to be contrast outside of esophagus, for which a non-contrast CT scan will help to clarify. The CT shows that the extraluminal densities are actually calcifications in the mediastinum. This mid-esophageal (true, traction) diverticulum, demographics, hematemesis, and mediastinal findings should prompt the further imaging (CT scan). Granulomatous disease (i.e., histoplasmosis, TB) should be suspected. Treatment of symptomatic mid-esophageal diverticula remains myotomy and diverticulectomy with certain considerations. Hematemesis or hemoptysis raises concerns for erosions, airway-esophageal fistulae, vascular-esophageal fistulae, granulation tissue bleeding, ulceration and esophagitis. CT angiography is appropriate in surgical planning that may require vascular control as part of the plan. Chronic cough, changes in imaging such as bronchiectasis or airway to esophageal fistula should lead to anticipated pulmonary resection. All mid-esophageal diverticula should be approached from the chest via thoracotomy or a VATS approach if uncomplicated and the surgeons possesses the skill set needed. The level of the thoracotomy will depend on the exact location of the diverticulum, however most can be approached through the right chest in the 5th or 6th intercostal space. Careful entry into the chest and consideration for intercostal muscle harvesting is needed. The myotomy should be carried at least 1 cm proximal and distal to neck of the diverticulum, 90-180° away from the neck. Pulmonary function testing preoperatively is also appropriate. Airway repair follows classic principles with interposition of live pedicle tissue (see Chapter 23, Tracheal strictures and fistulae). Treatment of his primary pulmonary disease (histoplasmosis or TB) is also needed.

Pearls/pitfalls
- Pulsion diverticula (i.e., Zenker's, epiphrenic) are protrusions of the mucosa through a weak area in the muscle layers (false), potentiated by some anatomic or functional distal obstruction. Traction diverticula arise from inflammation of surrounding tissue that leads to pulling of all layers of the esophagus (true).
- Diverticula < 2 cm, myotomy suffices, resect large and narrow neck diverticula.
- Cancer in Zenker's diverticula is rare; most are squamous cell carcinomas resulting from neglect of the condition. When limited to the diverticulum, diverticulectomy suffices for long-term survival. Not having muscularis, further involvement requires a case-by-case, more aggressive approach.
- If a Zenker's patient is hoarse, document vocal cord exam before surgery and anticipate management in case of recurrent nerve injury.

- Diagnose motility disorders before treating the diverticula. If LES is normal on manometry, limit to < 1 cm gastric extent of myotomy. If compromised, extend > 2 cm and perform a partial fundoplication.
- If motility is normal, myotomy to 1 cm above level of most proximal diverticulum suffices.
- Ask Zenker's patient to open mouth and extend neck in clinic to see if they are candidates for transoral stapling.
- Suppurative lung disease with mid-esophageal diverticula require conscientious planning with PFTs, CTAs, esophagrams, cardiac clearance, etc.

Suggested readings

- Esophageal Diverticula. Shields TW, LoCicero J, Reed CE, and Feins RH (eds). *General Thoracic Surgery.* Lippincott Williams & Wilkins. 7th edition. 2009.
- Peracchia A, Bonavina L, Narne S, et al: Minimally invasive surgery for Zenker's diverticulum: Analysis of results in 95 consecutive patients. *Arch Surg* 1998; 133:695-700.

Notes

22. Paraesophageal and diaphragmatic hernias

Philip W. Carrott, MD, and Benjamin D. Kozower, MD, MPH, FACS

Concept
- Management of acute and chronic presentations of paraesophageal hiatal hernias
- Preoperative work-up
- Open and laparoscopic repairs
- Assessment of esophageal length
- Fundoplication options

Chief complaint
"You are asked to see a 70 yo woman who was admitted overnight to the gastroenterology service for anemia and upper gastrointestinal bleeding. They performed an upper and lower endoscopy this morning and saw evidence of a large hiatal hernia with over half of her stomach above the diaphragm. Linear erosions were seen on the stomach mucosa at the hiatal narrowing, but there were no signs of ischemia."

Differential
Paraesophageal hiatal hernia (likely Type III by the classification of hiatal hernias), peptic ulcer disease, large epiphrenic diverticulum, esophagitis, tumor (GIST or gastric cancer)

History and physical
A thorough history usually uncovers multiple issues related to the hernia that have been evolving for some time. Hiatal hernias are long in evolution unless there is a congenital component to their origin (i.e., Bochdalek (posterior) or Morgagni (anterior) diaphragmatic hernias). The typical paraesophageal hernia patient will describe a spectrum of gastrointestinal and gustatory complaints including dysphagia, reflux, chest or abdominal pain, early satiety, decreasing meal size, regurgitation, and avoidance of late meals. In addition, patients with larger hernias will frequently complain of increasing shortness of breath that is often inaccurately attributed to aging rather than the dysfunction in respiration caused by mass effect of the hernia. Also, patients with paraesophageal hiatal hernias are often found to have occult anemia and GI bleeding from ulcerations/erosions caused by constriction of the stomach at the hiatus and movement in and out of the chest with respiration (Cameron lesions). As described in this patient, Cameron lesions are linear ulcers or erosions seen within the herniated portion of the stomach in patients with large paraesophageal hernias.

In the acute presentation, initial symptoms will more often be significant chest or abdominal pain due to ischemia. Patients may also present with nausea and inability to vomit due to complete or partial esophageal obstruction. Urgent NG tube decompression with or without endoscopy should be performed to relieve the intragastric pressure when possible. Signs of sepsis, unrelenting pain, or inability to pass a NG tube suggest complete esophageal/gastric obstruction, typically from a volvulized intrathoracic stomach. This may lead to gastric ischemia or frank necrosis. Therefore these signs should prompt emergency surgical intervention without any further delay for diagnostic studies. Patients who present acutely but are stable and without signs of ischemia, are handled differently. Fluid resuscitation, electrolyte replacement, and appropriate diagnostic studies are carried out prior to proceeding to the operating room, typically during the same hospitalization. Chronic paraesophageal hernias that do not present with acute symptoms can be handled on an elective basis. Results of repair are significantly worse for patients who undergo repair in the setting of acute symptoms, therefore elective repair of chronic paraesophageal hernias should not be delayed beyond a few weeks.

Tests

- *Imaging.* A contrast esophagram (a.k.a Barium swallow or UGI contrast study) is the cornerstone of diagnosis for paraesophageal hernias and should be obtained in most cases for diagnosis and definition of anatomy. Paraesophageal hernias are routinely imaged incidentally on CT scans and chest plain films, but these exams provide little additional information regarding the hernia not provided by the UGI. The one exception would be gastric wall perfusion seen on a contrast CT scan performed for abdominal pain, although this is not a necessary part of the work-up and is better assessed endoscopically. The UGI should be omitted in patients who present with signs of obstruction.
- *Labs.* Routine preoperative labs including CBC, BMP, and coags are typically all that are needed. Patients who present acutely frequently have electrolyte disturbances due to diminished oral intake and vomiting.
- *Endoscopy.* Routine endoscopy should be performed prior to any paraesophageal hernia repair to rule out other problems, such as esophagitis, Barrett's esophagus, malignancy, or ischemia. The timing of endoscopy either at diagnosis or prior to operative repair is not important. Upper endoscopy is particularly important for patients who present acutely, as signs of ischemia or necrosis will alter the operative plan.

- *Manometry/pH/impedance studies*. These esophageal function tests may be helpful in patients with a long history of reflux or regurgitation who may have esophageal dysmotility. The abnormal configuration of the esophagus likely produces some dysmotility and poor peristalsis. Therefore, some surgeons opt to forego these studies, assuming there is some degree of motor dysfunction. Large hernias may complicate the placement of probes needed to carry out these studies, in addition to making interpretation of the results more difficult.

Index scenario (additional information)

"The patient reports a 3-year history of anemia, the cause of which was not previously determined. She also reports that she feels full quickly and has occasional epigastric abdominal pain after meals. She was told that she had a hiatal hernia some years ago and was prescribed a proton pump inhibitor for reflux symptoms, although she no longer has regular reflux. The patient undergoes an UGI swallow study revealing a Type III giant paraesophageal hiatal hernia. How would you advise this patient?"

Treatment/management

Most patients who present with a paraesophageal hernia are symptomatic at the time of presentation. Indeed, in fit patients, if symptoms related to the hernia are affecting their daily life, such as early satiety, breathlessness, anemia, dysphagia, or significant reflux symptoms, the hernia should be repaired. The usual preoperative work-up for the patient's age and comorbidities should be undertaken as appropriate. Paraesophageal hernias may be classified as "giant" if over 50% of the stomach is herniated into the chest on preoperative imaging. The classification is well-known and relates to what is herniated, along with the location of the gastroesophageal junction (GEJ), (Type I – sliding hernia of the GEJ, Type II – herniation of the fundus with the GEJ in the abdomen, Type III – both the GEJ and stomach are herniated into the chest, and Type IV – Type III with other organs herniated into the chest). Type III is the most common "giant" paraesophageal hernia, and there is some debate as to the existence of Type II, since the GEJ is almost always herniated with the stomach. The most common method of primary repair for giant paraesophageal hernias is via laparoscopy, although key steps are the same for all approaches. Redo surgeries are possible via laparoscopy, but thoracic surgeons should be aware of the Belsey Mark IV (thoracic) repair, another useful approach for redo operations. The key steps include reduction of the hernia by dissection and removal of the hernia sac, establishment of adequate intra-abdominal esophageal length, hiatal closure, and a fundoplication of some sort to minimize reflux.

Laparoscopic repair

- Dissection begins at the hiatus, dividing the gastrohepatic ligament (pars flaccida). The sac is incised on the right crus, leaving the peritoneal covering on the crus, which provides strength for the hiatal closure.

- The sac is everted and blunt/sharp (with energy) dissection is carried out to divide the attachments of the sac to the mediastinum and mobilize the intrathoracic esophagus. The vagus nerves must be identified and preserved.

- Entry into the pleural space should be avoided when possible to avoid development of a tension pneumothorax due to insufflation. If the pleura is violated and a tension pneumothorax does develop, a pigtail pleural catheter or chest tube should be placed. A sustained positive pressure breath at the end of the procedure is usually sufficient to expel most of the insufflation and the chest tube is removed the following day.

- The short gastric vessels are divided along the upper third of the greater curve of the stomach in preparation for the fundoplication.

- The sac is completely removed from the mediastinum, typically from right to left, and excised. It is frequently easier to dissect the sac from the left crus after dividing the short gastric vessels.

- A bougie is then passed to assess the hiatus (54 or 56 Fr works for most patients). The right and left crus are then re-approximated with interrupted sutures beginning posteriorly (with the bougie pulled back in the upper esophagus). The authors use 0 Ethibond with or without pledgets, depending on the state of the crus. If the peritoneal lining of crus is stripped, the sutures are more likely to pull through the muscle and pledgets should then be considered.

- The bougie is replaced to assess the completeness of the closure. Occasionally anterior sutures are required for large hiatuses. Tight reapproximation of the crus should be avoided, as this will lead to postoperative dysphagia and possible obstruction.

- Esophageal length is then assessed. If there is less than 2 cm of intra-abdominal esophagus, Collis gastroplasty is undertaken with a thick tissue stapler to add the needed length.

- We typically perform a fundoplication with the neo-fundus by wrapping the esophagus anteriorly (180° - Dor). A 270° posterior wrap (Toupet) is also an option for patients with severe reflux. Some surgeons also perform a complete wrap (Nissen) but it is essential that it is truly a "floppy" wrap and that the patient has normal esophageal motility preoperatively. The stomach may also be secured to the diaphragm to help reduce the risk of recurrence.

Thoracic repair (Belsey Mark IV)

- Left anterior thoracotomy via the 6th or 7th intercostal space (should be based on preoperative imaging). If a re-do surgery, Chest CT scan should be obtained.
- Mobilize the sac anteriorly and posteriorly off the posterior pericardium and aorta/spine. It is frequently helpful to enter the sac if the anatomy is unclear.
- Excise the sac from the crus and stomach.
- Mobilize some fundus into the chest, usually dividing a few short gastric vessels.
- The right crus can be challenging to find as this is the deepest extent of the dissection. However, dissection of the hernia sac posteriorly will lead one to the right crus. The crus are grasped with a Babcock clamp and pledgeted 0 Ethibond sutures are placed in a horizontal mattress configuration to reapproximate the crus. These are left loose until the stomach is reduced to the abdomen.
- The fundoplication is performed by rolling the fundus up to the GEJ and securing it to the esophagus and itself. The needles are left on the second row of sutures so that they can be placed through the diaphragm anteriorly. The Belsey spoon may be used for retraction.

Open abdominal repair

- The basics of an open repair are the same for the above described laparoscopic approach.
- The Hill repair is used principally in the Pacific Northwest and is performed similarly to the laparoscopic method, but the fundoplication is performed with 5 silk sutures which are used to bring a small amount of fundus lateral to the vagus nerves around the esophagus, and then the sutures are passed through the crural repair posteriorly, anchoring the GEJ to the crural repair. A lengthening procedure is not typically needed as the repair can place some tension on the esophagus.
- Other fundoplications may be utilized in an open abdominal operation, as described above.

Potential questions/alternative scenarios

"Following mobilization of the esophagus, you determine that the esophagus should be lengthened. How is this determination made? Also, during laparoscopic repair you find that you and are having trouble closing the hiatus. How would you close a hiatus that won't come together?

At least 2 cm of tension-free, intraabdominal esophagus is recommended to decrease the risk of recurrence. Extensive mobilization of the intrathoracic esophagus as proximal as the inferior pulmonary veins aids significantly in obtaining this length. However, the esophagus may be significantly shortened from a chronic paraesophageal hernia and/or from chronic reflux that leads to fibrosis and presbyesophagus. If full esophageal mobilization does not obtain enough length, a stapled wedge fundectomy (Collis gastroplasty) is most commonly used to lengthen the esophagus. The wedge should be performed with a bougie in place (typically a 54 or 56 Fr.) to avoid inadvertent narrowing of the esophagus. In order to determine if there is enough intraabdominal esophagus, the GEJ must be clearly seen, which is most easily done by mobilizing the esophageal fat pad off the GEJ anteriorly.

The difficult hiatus is a problem without an easy solution. Polypropylene mesh has been used with some success, but there have been a number of reports of erosion into the esophagus. If there is too much tension on the crural repair, a biologic mesh such as acellular dermis or absorbable mesh should be used. In addition, it may help to start closing the hiatus anteriorly where there is a little less tension. During laparoscopic cases, a pneumothorax may be induced with insufflation to create a "floppy" diaphragm, which may permit adequate reapproximation of the hiatus. Adhesions to the liver and spleen should also be taken down to ensure the the crus are not tethered laterally. Decreasing the insufflation pressure may also help to take tension off the hiatus.

"How would you treat Barrett's esophagus if found on preoperative endoscopy?"

Barrett's esophagus should be assessed with biopsy and histologic analysis. Biopsy-proven Barrett's should be followed with repeat endoscopies and biopsies. The recommended biopsies of 4 quadrants every centimeter of Barrett's should be performed yearly to look for dysplasia or cancer. Guidelines recommend surveillance every 1-3 years for uncomplicated Barrett's, with recommendations of either maximal PPI therapy or anti-reflux surgery for these patients. Patients with low-grade dysplasia should be followed every 6-12 months and high-grade dysplasia every 3 months if no eradication therapy (EMR, RF ablation, or esophagectomy) is carried out. Repair of a paraesophageal hernia and creation of a fundoplication does not alter the surveillance protocol.

"At laparoscopy, you see the stomach seems to enter the abdomen with the GEJ located intraabdominally, but then herniate posteriorly through a separate diaphragmatic defect. How would you manage this?"

Other defects in the diaphragm are rarely seen, but are possible in adults. Bochdalek (posterior paraspinal) and Morgagni (anterior parasternal) hernias can be closed primarily or repaired with Gore-tex mesh. The dissection can be disorienting since these defects have presumably been present since birth. Bochdalek hernias are more likely to involve the stomach. Much less is known about the natural history of these hernias, as they are most commonly found incidentally. Most surgeons recommend treatment for those that are symptomatic or those that appear to have incarcerated bowel or other abdominal viscera.

"The patient now has had 3 previous repairs, and has recurrence of her paraesophageal hernia with the wrap from the previous surgery in the chest. How would you approach this hernia?"
Once a patient fails multiple redo antireflux surgeries/hernia repairs, the chance of a successful repair is less likely as the risk of recurrence increases with each redo operation. If this patient was unable to eat, unable to maintain their weight, or had other severe symptoms (significant abdominal pain or anemia from the hernia), many surgeons would offer the patient an esophagectomy. A roux-en-y "near" esophagojejunostomy may be another alternative if the patient has not lost a significant amount of weight already. If an esophagectomy is to be performed, there should he consideration for an intrathoracic anastomosis (Ivor Lewis or left thoracoabdominal approach) since the stomach may not be a suitable conduit due to the multiple reoperations. One should also be prepared to use an alternative conduit, such as colon, in these circumstances.

"A 45 yo patient without previous surgery has a symptomatic hernia and a BMI of 39 with insulin-dependent diabetes and sleep apnea. How would you approach this patient?"
A patient that has significant reflux, a paraesophageal hernia, and morbid obesity qualifies for bariatric surgery and should be evaluated by a bariatric surgeon prior to consideration of paraesophageal hernia repair. The paraesophageal hernia would be repaired as usual, but a roux-en-y gastric bypass would benefit this patient more in the long-run. Most patients will actually gain weight following paraesophageal hernia repair since the repair restores normal function to their stomach. Some surgeons advocate a "near" esophagojejunostomy, which leaves only a small gastric pouch, thus removing all acid producing cells and preventing ongoing reflux.

"How would you follow these patients over time?"
Recurrence rates for paraesophageal hernia repairs range from 15-50%. Some surgeons do not offer routine postoperative follow-up of these patients, only seeing patients back in the office if symptoms recur. Due to the high recurrence rates, others chose to follow these patients annually or even more frequently with a barium swallow.

"A 76 yo man presents with chest pain, nausea, and inability to vomit. The ED is unable to pass a NG tube, which can be seen coiled in the chest. The patient has a history of a long-standing paraesophageal hernia. He has a low grade fever, is tachycardic, and with marginal blood pressure. Upper endoscopy reveals patchy areas of ischemia in the stomach and an area suspicious for necrosis. How would you manage this patient?"

This is a life threatening complication of paraesophageal hernias and the patient must be operated on urgently. The most likely cause is gastric volvulus with resulting ischemia and progression to frank necrosis due to obstruction, distension, and decreased perfusion. If no frank necrosis is present, quickly reducing the hernia and performing a gastropexy (tacking the greater curve to the anterior diaphragm/anterior abdominal wall) may get the patient off the table quickly and to the ICU for resuscitation. The stomach can then be reassessed later endoscopically. Cases where there is gastric necrosis are more complicated. In these cases, the hernia may be reduced and the area of necrosis is resected. Depending on the degree of resection, a gastrojejunostomy (Billroth II or Roux-en-Y) may be needed. This can be performed in a staged fashion if the patient is too unstable. In cases where the majority of the stomach is necrotic, a Roux-en-Y is needed. If there is distal esophageal necrosis, the patient must undergo bipolar exclusion with resection of the necrotic stomach and esophagus. The esophageal stump must be drained, either with a pharyngostomy tube or by placing a drain in the stump and bringing it out through the abdominal wall. If time permits, a feeding jejunostomy is placed. Reconstruction with a substernal colon interposition can then be carried out in a delayed fashion once the patient has recovered.

Pearls/pitfalls

- Preoperative work-up should be thorough and include, at a minimum, UGI and upper endoscopy.
- Presentation with pain should have NG tube placement or endoscopy to relieve possible obstruction.
- Urgent/emergency surgery for unrelenting pain or signs of ischemia.
- Must resect the hernia sac.
- Secure the stomach to diaphragm or anterior abdominal wall to prevent recurrence.
- Mesh is rarely indicated, but when truly necessary a biologic mesh is preferred.

Suggested readings

- Carrott PW, Hong J, Kuppusamy MK, et al. Clinical ramifications of giant paraesophageal hernias are under appreciated: making the case for routine surgical repair. *Ann of Thoracic Surgery* 2012; 94:421-8.
- Oelschlager BK, Pellegrini CA, Hunter JG, et al. Biologic prosthesis to prevent recurrence after laparoscopic paraesophageal hernia repair: long-term follow-up from a multicenter, prospective, randomized trial. *J Am Coll Surg* 2011; 213:461–468.
- Whitson BA, Hoang CD, Boettcher AK, et al. Wedge gastroplasty and reinforced crural repair: Important components of laparoscopic giant or recurrent hiatal hernia repair. *J Thorac Cardiovasc Surg* 2006; 132:1196-1202.

Notes

23. Tracheal strictures and fistulae

Michael P. Robich, MD, and Daniel Raymond, MD

Concept
- Diagnosis and workup of tracheal strictures and fistulae
- Management
- Conduct of the operations and pitfalls
- Managing complications

Chief complaint
"You are consulted by the MICU to see a 77 yo woman with diabetes, respiratory failure due to pneumonia, and newly discovered bilious secretions from the tracheostomy. You are familiar with the patient as you placed the tracheostomy one month ago."

Differential
Gastroesophageal reflux disease, aspiration, tracheoesophageal fistula

History and physical
Patients at risk of developing a benign tracheoesphageal fistula (TEF) usually have risk factors including diabetes, corticosteroid use, immunodeficiency, infection, hypotension, prolonged intubation, neck trauma, caustic ingestion, foreign body ingestion, iatrogenic injury during tracheal or esophageal surgery, and granulomatous infections. High cuff pressures (30 cm of water (22 mmHg)) can impair mucosal blood flow and the concurrent presence of a nasogastric tube can contribute to development of a TEF. In ventilated patients, bilious secretions or tube feeds in the endotracheal tube or tracheostomy, gastric dilatation, and loss of tidal volumes are signs that may suggest a TEF. In non-ventilated patients, signs of TEF include persistent cough, fever, and dyspnea. Recurrent pneumonias are common in both groups of patients.

Tests
- CXR may demonstrate the endotracheal tube outside of the trachea and gastric dilatation.
- Contrast esophagography can identify the fistula. Water-soluble contrast should be avoided when TEF is suspected (iso-osmolar contrast is recommended if communication with the airway is suspected).
- CT scan may show a defect between the trachea and esophagus, as well as extra-luminal fluid collections.

- Direct visualization is the mainstay of diagnosis. Bronchoscopy will often reveal the defect. In ventilated patients the endotracheal tube must be withdrawn to examine the trachea at the point of contact with the balloon. Esophagoscopy can also be utilized to visualize the tracheal cuff protruding into the esophageal lumen.

Index scenario (additional information)

"The patient has bilious secretions and is noted to have volume loss on the ventilator. CXR shows a moderate-sized gastric bubble, but is otherwise unrevealing. How will you manage this patient?"

Treatment/management

This is the classic picture for TEF. A bronchoscopy from above the tracheostomy (either transnasally or transorally) should be performed to examine the trachea with focus on the area where the balloon sits. Once the diagnosis is confirmed, a plan for management can be made. Esophagoscopy should be available as well for a thorough examination.

Spontaneous healing is rare in this situation and surgical intervention is usually needed. If non-operative treatment is to be attempted, the first step is to minimize further soiling of the airway. Keep the head of the bed elevated > 30°. The tracheostomy cuff should be repositioned distal to the TEF, but above the carina, with minimal cuff pressures. An adjustable flange tracheostomy tube or distal XLT (longer distal limb of tracheostomy) may be helpful in these situations. Endotracheal intubation with a single lumen tube may be required in cases where a tracheostomy cannot be adequately positioned. Efforts should be made to wean the patient from the ventilator, as the positive pressure provided by the ventilator keeps the tract open and minimizes the chance of closure. The patient's nutritional status needs to be aggressively optimized. Removal of the NG tube is important. Placement of a gastrostomy tube will allow continued enteral feeding and venting of the stomach.

If the patient cannot tolerate a period of non-operative management, covered tracheal or esophageal stents can be utilized as a temporizing measure to allow time for the patient to be optimized for surgical treatment, or in some rare cases may facilitate spontaneous closure. Stenting can cause extension of the TEF, particularly when both a tracheal and esophageal stent are used as the radial forces place unwanted pressure on the area of communication. Stenting should only be used with caution and by those with experience.

Once the patient has been optimized, an operative plan can be made. Preoperatively, a strategy to ventilate the patient needs to be made. If the fistula is small and will not require tracheal resection, the tube can be placed distally to allow repair. If tracheal resection is needed, proximal low tidal ventilation, distal high-frequency jet ventilation, double lung ventilation with distal airway isolation, or cardiopulmonary bypass can be utilized. In cases where primary repair or simple resection is not possible, esophageal exclusion (described in Chapter 20, Esophageal perforation) may be need to be performed as a last resort.

Operative steps

Takedown of TEF and primary tracheal repair

- *Incision*: a low collar incision with extension to the left. Subplatysmal flaps are raised.
- Dissect down to the tracheoesophageal groove, divide the left inferior thyroid artery to improve exposure. Dissection between the trachea and esophagus in the groove should be on the esophageal wall to avoid disrupting the anterolateral blood supply of the trachea and avoid injury to the recurrent laryngeal nerves.
- The fistula is identified circumferentially, sharply resected, and sent for pathologic analysis.
- The defects are debrided back to healthy tissue.
- The membranous tracheal defect is closed with interrupted 3-0 or 4-0 vicryl with the knots on the outside.
- The esophageal defect is closed in two layers (Mucosa- 4-0 vicryl interrupted, muscularis and adventitia- imbricating 3-0 vicryl interrupted).
- A sternocleidomastoid (SCM) flap is created by dividing the SCM distally and mobilizing an adequate length to cover the repair. The tracheal and esophageal repairs should be separated by the flap. The rotational flap is then sewn onto the esophagus with interrupted 4-0 vicryl.

Takedown of TEF and repair with tracheal resection

- *Incision*: collar incision for anterior approach to the trachea.
- The pretracheal plane is developed above and below the fistula and the trachea is dissected circumferentially at the level of the defect. Dissect bluntly on the trachea to avoid damage to the recurrent laryngeal nerves.
- A transverse tracheal incision is made below the fistula. The endotracheal tube is removed, a sterile tube is placed in the distal trachea, and cross-field ventilation initiated.
- The trachea is divided proximally and the fistula is resected from the esophagus.
- The esophagus is repaired in two layers and a muscle flap placed.
- The trachea is then reapproximated end-to-end with interrupted 4-0 vicryl.

- A new endotracheal tube is placed distal to the repair.
- Postoperatively efforts should be made to extubate the patient as soon as possible.

"The TEF is large and won't be amenable to simple closure or resection. How will you manage?"

If the fistula is too large for the management strategies mentioned above, the defect can be dissected with a rim of esophageal wall. The rim of esophagus can then be approximated to re-create the membranous trachea with interrupted 4-0 vicryl. The esophagus is closed in two layers and a muscle flap placed. Reports have also described use of biologic prostheses, autologous pericardium, or aortic homograft to reconstruct the back wall of the trachea.

"A patient is found to have a left broncho-esophageal fistula. What is the appropriate surgical approach once the patient is deemed appropriate for surgery?"

The distal trachea, carina, and both mainstem bronchi can be approached via right thoracotomy or sternotomy. The defect should be resected and repaired as previously described. If extra length is needed to obtain a tension-free repair, the inferior pulmonary ligament can be taken down and a hilar release performed (opening the pericardium in a U-shape anterior to the hilum, curved under the inferior pulmonary vein, and posterior to the hilum). Neck flexion will also take tension of the anastomosis in the case of a tracheal resection. A sleeve resection with reconstruction can also be performed for bronchial fistulae. A muscle, pericardial, or pleural flap is placed to buttress the repair.

"A 67 yo man presents one year after esophagectomy for esophageal adenocarcinoma with complaints of persistent cough, increased secretions, fevers, and chest pain. Bronchoscopy shows a TEF at the anastomosis and biopsy reveals cancer recurrence. How will you manage this patient?"

Malignant TEF is associated with esophageal, pulmonary and tracheal cancers. Make sure to do an endoscopy and take biopsies to determine if there is recurrent cancer present. Malignant TEFs are often a sign of advanced disease with a poor prognosis and survival rates of less than 10% at 12 months. As such, management is geared toward palliation and avoiding significant morbidity. Covered tracheal and/or esophageal stents offer a reasonable management strategy. Esophageal exclusion with end cervical esophagostomy, gastrostomy tube for distal decompression, a feeding jejunostomy may be the only option in some cases to prevent ongoing soilage of the airway. Esophageal exclusion and bypass is often associated with significant morbidity and is generally not a good

195

palliative option if other options exist. Chemotherapy and radiation may be of some benefit.

"The ER consults you to see a patient that was transferred from a rehab center with blood in the tracheostomy tube. The tracheostomy was placed 4 weeks prior to presentation. As you are examining the patient, massive bleeding from the tracheostomy begins. How will you manage this?"

The differential in this case scenario includes: mucosal irritation from suctioning, tracheitis, bleeding tracheal granulation tissue, alveolar hemorrhage, and tracheoinnominate fistula (TIF). Given the history, and since it is a potentially fatal complication, one must presume that TIF is the diagnosis until proven otherwise. TIF is caused by erosion of an endotracheal tube balloon eroding into the innominate artery. It is usually caused by pressure necrosis by the tube. With the advent of lower pressure tracheostomy tube balloons, the incidence of TIF has decreased over time. However when it does occur, the mortality is near 100%. Factors that predispose to formation of TIF include: prolonged intubation, high cuff pressures to prevent air leak, poorly positioned tracheostomy, tracheostomy placed below the 4th tracheal ring, high-riding innominate artery, hypotension, sepsis, medical comorbidities (diabetes, infection, steroid use, malnutrition), and prior radiation. The peak time frame is 2-4 weeks after tracheostomy, with 75% occurring in the first month. Most patients, similar to the above example, will present with a small sentinel bleed hours to days prior to massive bleeding.

In the case of TIF, over-inflation of the cuff balloon may *temporarily* tamponade the bleeding. This has been reported to be successful in 85% of cases. If this does not work, the tube can be slowly withdrawn while applying anterior pressure. If this maneuver fails, an oral endotracheal tube can be placed and the tracheostomy tube removed. With the tracheostomy removed, digital pressure through the stoma can be applied to compress the innominate artery against the sternum as the patient is transported to the OR for immediate operative intervention.

Concurrent to the efforts to stop the bleeding, the operating room should be alerted and volume/blood resuscitation initiated. The distal airway should be cleared and diagnosis confirmed with bronchoscopy.

The choices for repair include: simple ligation, resection of affected innominate artery, direct repair of the defect, and bypass of the fistula with a graft. Endovascular stenting has also been described. Because of the emergency and contaminated nature of the operation and the associated high mortality, ligation of the innominate artery is generally recommended. In cases where bleeding has ceased from the above mentioned measures (i.e., this was a herald bleed), consideration can be given to CTA of the neck and chest to further delineate the anatomy prior to proceeding to the operating room, however this should be done with caution.

Repair of tracheo-innominate fistula
- *Incision*: median sternotomy or partial upper sternotomy
- Innominate artery is exposed by dissecting the thymus and retracting the brachiocephalic vein
- Achieve proximal and distal control
- Ligate the artery

Tracheal stenosis
Index scenario (additional information)
"A patient presents following a complex postoperative course including tracheostomy after a major abdominal surgery. The patient was discharged ultimately to a rehabilitation unit and was decannulated in the unit over two months ago. The patient currently complains of progressively worsening dyspnea on exertion and stridor over last few weeks. How will you evaluate and treat?"

Differential
Postintubation airway pathology includes benign strictures, granulomas, and tracheomalacia. Benign and malignant neoplasms, vocal cord dysfunction, prior airway trauma, and infection should also be considered.

Tests
- *CXR*: a high posteroanterior and lateral CXR can delineate some tracheal pathology, but CT scan shows more detailed information.
- *Dynamic airway CT*: can show highly detailed 3D reconstructions to demonstrate functional tracheal problems (i.e., tracheomalacia).
- *Laryngoscopy*: can be performed in the office setting on an awake patient for an initial assessment of the hypopharynx, vocal cords, and proximal trachea.
- *Bronchoscopy*: essential to make the diagnosis, plan treatment, and intervene as a definitive treatment or a bridge to definitive treatment.
- *Pulmonary function tests*: may see early flattening of the expiratory portion of the flow-volume loop (obstructive pattern).

"On bronchoscopic examination the patient has an anteriorly pointed, arrow-shaped stenosis that occurs at the level of the prior tracheotomy. How will you manage?"

Any patient with a history of endotracheal intubation developing symptoms of airway obstruction (wheezing, stridor, or exertional dyspnea) should be investigated for an obstructing tracheal lesion. Stomal stenosis is caused by enlargement of the tracheotomy and eventual healing with granulation tissue. As the granulation tissue contracts it narrows the tracheal lumen. The stoma can be enlarged due to leverage forces from equipment attached to the tracheostomy, a large tracheotomy at the time of insertion, or infection. Patients may present late, as they may not regain enough functional activity to manifest airway obstruction for some time. For a patient to be symptomatic at rest, the tracheal diameter is typically less than 30% of normal. Having the patient extend the neck or inspire rapidly may illicit stridor. Diagnosis can be made on laryngoscopy, which should be carried out prior to more invasive procedures requiring anesthesia.

Bronchoscopic evaluation of tracheal stenosis should be undertaken in the operating room with careful planning preoperatively by the surgical and anesthesia teams. The patient should initially be evaluated awake with local anesthesia and the anatomy should be confirmed. Intravenous anesthetic is provided without muscle relaxant until the airway is controlled, which may require suspension laryngoscopy and rigid bronchoscopy. The glottis and vocal cord function should be assessed in addition to the stenosis. If the tracheal lumen is less than 5 mm in diameter, dilation can be performed with graduated Jackson dilators. This will often provide only temporary relief, which can allow delay of the operation until the tracheal mucosa is healed and the patient is medically fit for surgery. If the stenosis is greater than 5 mm the bronchoscope should cross and will provide dilation. Gentle insertion of the tip of the bronchoscope into the stenosis with a rotatory motion and light pressure, typically allows it to advance past the stenosis. Other interventional pulmonary techniques such as balloon dilation, stenting, bouginage, or Nd:YAG laser debridement can be used (if you discuss this option remember to lower FiO2 to ≤ 30% prior to using an energy source in the trachea). However, because the ischemic injury is full thickness, endoluminal therapies are not usually curative. Definitive treatment is resection of the affected area after careful assessment of the location and length of the stenosis. An anesthetic plan involving cross table ventilation, preservation of blood supply and achieving a tension free repair are keys to success of the operation.

For patients who cannot tolerate tracheal resection or who have long strictures not amenable to resection, a redo tracheostomy may be needed. Care must be taken to make sure the distal end of the tracheostomy is distal to the stricture. The tracheostomy can eventually be exchanged for a tracheal T-tube. The soft, silicone T-tube is passed through the tracheostomy stoma and has three limbs: a shorter proximal limb that is directed toward the vocal cords; a longer distal limb that is directed toward the carina and should pass the stricture, and a short limb that passes externally through the tracheal stoma. When the external limb is uncapped, the patient can inhale/exhale through the T-tube. When the T-tube is capped, it acts as a stent, covering the stricture and allowing the patient to breathe and speak normally. It is important to measure the distance from the vocal cords to the stricture and from the carina to the stricture (done with flexible bronchoscopy). T-tubes with varying limb lengths are available or custom T-tubes can be ordered from the manufacturer. It is important to make sure the limbs are not too long, as uncontrollable coughing will be caused by irritation of the vocal cords or carina (depending on which limb is too long). T-tubes provide a good long-term option for inoperable patients, as they are better tolerated than tracheostomies, rarely cause stricturing, and allow the patient to speak and breathe normally. It is important to note that patients with T-tubes cannot be placed on mechanical ventilation, as a significant amount of the tidal volume will escape proximally out the nose and mouth (if necessary, the nose and mouth are sealed to prevent loss of volume, which is obviously not an option when the patient is awake). The T-tube is instead pulled out the stoma (easily done at the bedside) and a cuffed tracheostomy is placed (making sure the distal tip passed distal to the stricture) through the stoma. Bronchoscopy and tracheal suctioning can be performed easily through T-tubes and there is little risk of migration.

Operative steps

- Low collar incision +/- upper hemisternotomy.
- Dissection is carried out immediately adjacent to the trachea to avoid damage to the recurrent laryngeal nerves. Circumferential dissection of the trachea is carried out only at the level of stenosis and not more than 1-1.5 cm of normal trachea. This will help preserve the lateral blood supply to the airway.
- Anterior and posterior mobilization of the trachea to the level of the carina is important to limit tension on the anastomosis.
- The stenotic segment can be identified by external abnormality or via transillumination during intraoperative bronchoscopy.
- The airway is divided sharply with care not to injure the esophagus posteriorly.
- The distal airway can be intubated with a sterile endotracheal tube and ventilator circuit.

- Ensure a tension-free anastomosis. The anastomosis is most commonly created with 4-0 vicryl or PDS in a running, interrupted, or combined fashion.
- The patient should be extubated in the OR.

Potential questions/alternative scenarios

"During a mid-tracheal resection the anastomosis is under undue tension. How will you remedy this?"

Cervical flexion will provide enough tracheal length for most repairs. A stitch can be placed from the chin to the chest ("Grillo stitch") to maintain flexion postoperatively. Dissection on the anterior and posterior surfaces will preserve the blood supply and provide length. Suprahyoid laryngeal release will provide 1-1.5 cm of length, but postoperative dysphagia is a common sequelae.

"Six weeks after tracheal resection a patient develops massive hemoptysis and dies. How could this be prevented?"

A tracheoinnominate fistula can occur when the innominate artery is mobilized and subsequently erodes into the airway. An interposition muscle flap at the time of initial operation can be used to decrease the risk of this rapidly fatal complication.

"A 69 yo patient with a tracheal stenosis presents in acute respiratory distress. Critical care is unable to intubate the patient. You are called for an emergency airway."

Patients with critical tracheal stenosis are at increased risk of obstruction from minimal amounts of secretions. Furthermore, a high grade stenosis will prevent effective positive pressure ventilation. Thus the patient must be kept spontaneously ventilating while be transported to the operating room. Use of paralytics prior to control of the airway will likely be lethal. During transport, preparations should be made for fiberoptic intubation, rigid bronchoscopy, jet ventilation, and emergency surgical airway placement. Start with mask ventilation first. Fiberoptic bronchoscopy can be performed, although in an emergency rigid bronchoscopy is often necessary to quickly dilate the stricture and establish an airway. Once the stenosis is dilated, place a tube exchanger (can ventilate through tube exchanger with jet as you pull out rigid), and a small ETT (pediatric). Once the patient is stabilized, further plans can be made for more definitive management. (redo tracheostomy, resection, T-tube placement, etc).

"You are asked to see a patient with multiple severe medical problems and a tracheostomy for 3-4 months. On bronchoscopy you note a circumferential distal stricture 3.5 cm proximal to carina, but distal to the tip of the tracheostomy. The patient is improving, but has required increasing vent support and has higher airway pressures. How will you manage?"

The most common post-intubation lesion is cuff stenosis, which occurs at the level of the sealing cuff (balloon). The radial pressure exerted from the cuff causes circumferential pressure necrosis, which can cause cicatricial scarring and stenosis. Large volume, low pressure balloons have helped decreased the incidence, however over-inflation can lead to damage of the trachea. This typically occurs within 3-4 cm of the cricoid cartilage and is a circumferential stenosis. Definitive management is resection with primary anastomosis. However, in patients that are poor surgical candidates or need mechanical ventilator support other options exist. A tracheostomy with a longer flange may be able to cross the narrowing as a temporary solution. Endotracheal stenting can also provide relief in the patient not fit for surgery. However, these stents tend to cause granulation tissue and the proximal and distal ends of the stent, essentially converting a single stricture into two. Focal circumferential stenoses of the trachea can be balloon dilated. The technique involves incremental inflation with frequent deflations to assess progress and check for injury to the airway. Topical application of mitomycin-C can retard restenosis. In stenosis involving only the cartilaginous rings of the trachea, balloon dilation should not be used as the risk of perforating the membranous airway is high. In the case where a stent in placed and the ends become obstructed by granulation tissue, options include serial debridement (YAG-Nd laser), serial dilations, or removal of the stent and placement of a T-tube to cover all the strictures segments.

Pearls/pitfalls

- A period of non-operative optimization of the patient's pulmonary and nutritional status should
  be instituted prior to repair of TEFs whenever possible.
- Try to extubate the patient as soon as possible after repair of TEFs or tracheal resections.
- Avoid injury to recurrent laryngeal nerve and have a low index of suspicion for nerve injury, which should be investigated with laryngoscopy.
- TIFs are life-threatening complications. Therefore significant hemoptysis in a patient with a prior tracheostomy must be thoroughly investigated. Ligation of the innominate artery may be the fastest and safest way to save the patient's life.
- Patients presenting with tracheal strictures must be handled with caution, particularly when presenting acutely. Rigid bronchoscopy

and the ability to jet ventilate is crucial. A plan is needed to do whatever is needed to obtain access beyond the stricture to ventilate. Once this is accomplished, planning for more definitive surgical treatment can take place.
- Options to treat tracheal strictures in the long-term include resection for focal strictures, while dilation, debridement, tracheostomy, and tracheal t-tube are options for more complex strictures (long, multiple) or inoperable patients.

Suggested readings

- Cooper JD, Grillo HC. The evolution of tracheal injury due to ventilatory assistance through cuffed tubes: a pathologic study. *Annals of Surgery*. Mar 1969;169(3):334-348.

- Wright CD. Management of tracheoinnominate artery fistula. *Chest Surg Clin N Am* 6 (1996), pp. 865–873.

- Wain JC Jr. Postintubation tracheal stenosis. *Semin Thorac Cardiovasc Surg*. 2009 Fall;21(3):284-9.

Notes

24. Malignant lesions of the trachea
Timothy J. Pirolli, MD, and William D. Ogden, MD

Concept
- Presentation and workup of tracheal tumors
- Differential diagnosis
- Principles of surgical resection
- Airway management during resection
- Postoperative care and adjuvant therapy

Chief complaint
"You are referred a patient with complaints of a cough and wheezing that's been getting worse for the last few months. The patient's pulmonologist told him he had a mass in his airway."

Differential
Primary malignant tumor of the trachea, metastatic tumor to trachea, benign tracheal mass, tracheal strictures, external compression of trachea by mediastinal mass, aspirated foreign body, adult-onset asthma

History and physical
A detailed H&P focusing on duration and progression of symptoms (hoarseness, cough, wheeze, stridor, dyspnea, hemoptysis, dysphagia) should be made. Other key components include examining the patient's functional status, a thorough review of systems, evaluation of comorbidities, medications and smoking/substance abuse history. A complete physical exam (focusing on the airway/lungs/lymph nodes/oropharynx) must be performed.

Tests
- *CXR.* Airway narrowing, mediastinal widening or evidence of metastatic disease.
- *CT scan of neck and chest.* May help delineate invasion of surrounding structures, metastatic disease. Critical for defining the length of the tumor.
- *Bronchoscopy (rigid or flexible) +/- biopsy.* Direct examination of tumor with tissue sampling if feasible. Length of the tumor is assessed, as well as distance from the vocal cords and carina.
- *Endobronchial ultrasonography (EBUS).* May assist in distinguishing primary tracheal tumor from external compression/infiltration of extrinsic tumor; may clarify extent of invasion.

- *Pulmonary function tests.* Evaluate for upper airway obstruction, flattening of expiratory and inspiratory phases, normal preoperative assessment.
- *Basic labs:* CBC, BMP, INR/PTT.
- *PET scan/MRI brain/abdomen CT.* Examination for extra-tracheal sites of possible primary tumor or metastatic disease.
- *Upper endoscopy, esophageal ultrasound.* If concern for invasion into esophagus.
- *EKG/stress echo.* As part of preoperative cardiac workup if warranted.

Index scenario (additional information)

"A 61 yo man with an 80 pack-year smoking history has been referred to you by his pulmonologist after increasing wheezing and coughing that was not responsive to bronchodilators prompted a workup that revealed a mid- tracheal mass. He has no other comorbidities except for hypertension. CT scan shows a tracheal mass measuring 2.0 cm long in the mid-trachea. PET scan reveals no metastatic disease. What further workup would you perform and what are his options?"

Treatment/management

The patient has confirmed radiographic findings of a tracheal mass without evidence of distal metastases. The next step in the workup should be bronchoscopy (flexible +/- rigid) to examine the tumor, assess its length and resectability, and to biopsy the mass. Once a tissue diagnosis has been made, the decision on management must be addressed. Most tumors present as locally advanced disease at time of presentation. The majority of primary tracheal malignancies are either squamous cell carcinoma (SCC) or adenoid cystic carcinoma (ACC). Histology has prognostic importance for survival, with ACC and mucoepidermoid tumor having the best outcomes. SCC is more likely to present with hemoptysis, whereas ACC is more likely to present with obstructive airway disease. Survival in surgically resected patients is superior to non-resected patients in both major histologies. Lymph node involvement has been shown to result in decreased survival but does not preclude surgical resection. A standardized oncologic staging system has not yet been developed.

Surgical resection of the tracheal tumor should be considered for any patient who has a resectable tumor without metastatic disease and who would tolerate the surgery. Resectable tumors are typically less than 4.5 cm in length (MGH data), have minimal invasion into the mediastinum, are amenable to negative margins (although in ACC resections, positive margins may be accepted and respond to radiation therapy). No preoperative chemotherapy or radiation is warranted prior to resection of a tracheal tumor. Involvement of the larynx/subglottic tumors should portend a laryngotracheal resection and be performed at an experienced high-volume center or in conjunction with an otolaryngologist.

Tumors that are a direct extension or metastasis from other primary sites to the trachea are rarely resectable. Certain cancers such as some T4 NSCLCs and thyroid cancers that involve the airway may be amenable to resection only after a full metastatic workup is otherwise negative and the patient is an ideal surgical candidate. These surgeries are undertaken only if en-bloc resection of the tumor is curative.

Operative steps
Tracheal resection for a mid-tracheal tumor
Goals – resect the tracheal mass with negative margins with minimal disruption to tracheal blood supply and create a tension-free anastomosis.

- Adequate PIVs/central venous access is critical. Radial arterial line.
- Total intravenous anesthesia or slow induction of inhaled anesthetic agents is optimal to minimize risk of airway collapse. No muscle relaxants are given until the airway is secured. A rigid bronchoscope and jet ventilation equipment should be ready if collapse occurs prior to intubation. For intrathoracic tumors, cardiopulmonary bypass on stand-by may be warranted.
- Pre-incision bronchoscopy. Placing a 25-gauge needle percutaneously into the airway to define the upper/lower limits of the tumor under direct visualization may be helpful.
- Collar incision for upper/mid tracheal lesions (R thoracotomy or median sternotomy for lower tumors). Skin flaps are raised, strap muscles split, and the trachea is exposed with a pretracheal release from cricoid to sternal notch. The thyroid isthmus is divided and dissected off the trachea. The manubrium may need to be partially divided and retracted laterally.
- Define upper and lower borders of resection and dissect circumferentially around the trachea, staying close to trachea to minimize disrupting the main blood supply to the remaining trachea. Recurrent laryngeal nerves travel laterally in tracheoesophageal groove on each side. Avoid them. Pass a tape around the trachea. Remove any lymph nodes.
- Prior to excision of the trachea, a separate corrugated tubing setup should be passed off to anesthesia in preparation for cross-table ventilation. Tubing is connected to a flexible endotracheal tube (Tovell tube) and managed by the surgeon (assistant) on the field.

- Traction sutures are placed laterally on the trachea 1 cm below level of transection, incorporating 1-2 tracheal rings. Transect the trachea anteriorly between rings just distal to the tumor. Healthy cartilage should be present at the cut margin.continuous suctioning of the airway is needed to prevent secretions and blood from passing into the distal airway.
- Communicate with the anesthesiologist as the ETT is withdrawn and Tovell tube is advanced into the distal airway through the tracheal incision by the surgeon. Jet ventilation may be used during this period.
- Circumferential dissection is carried out proximally and distally for a maximum of 1 cm dissection of the remaining trachea to maintain blood supply. Traction sutures are placed proximally. The trachea is then divided proximal to the tumor and the resected trachea/tumor is removed: maximum ~4.5 cm length (~8 tracheal rings). Send the specimen for frozen section of margins. Positive margins for ACC are accepted.
- The neck is flexed to assess tension on the airway and the traction sutures a retracted to bring the proximal and distal trachea together. Interrupted 4-0 coated Vicryl sutures (some surgeons use prolene) are placed starting at the midline posteriorly with the knots placed to lie outside of the trachea. Sequentially, sutures are placed on either side of the 1st suture 4 mm apart and 4 mm from the cut edge of trachea through cartilage. The sutures are clipped to the drape and continued around circumferentially without tying the knots until all sutures are placed. The anterior sutures are then placed in a similar fashion and the Tovell tube is removed as the endotracheal tube is advanced beyond the anastomosis. An alternative method is to advance the ETT beyond the area of resection into the distal trachea and place the sutures circumferentially without placing a Tovell tube.
- Neck is kept fully flexed and the anterior sutures are tied. If there is tension evident on the anastomosis, release maneuvers should be performed. The first maneuver should be the Montgomery suprahyoid release performed by dividing the hyoid muscles through a small horizontal incision and dividing the hyoid bone laterally, giving 1-2 cm more mobility. Other release maneuvers include a suprathyroid laryngeal, hilar (pericardial release for intrathoracic tumors), and inferior pulmonary ligament releases.
- Once the anterior sutures are tied and the tails cut, the posterior sutures are tied, working from lateral to the posterior midline on one side and then the other.
- A "guardian stitch" fashioned at the end of the case secures the underside of the chin to the chest at the level of the manubrium, keeps the patient's neck flexed and reminds them not to extend.

- Bronchoscopy after completion. Extubate immediately if possible, ICU care.
- Bronchoscopy of patient 1 week after surgery prior to discharge.
- Adjuvant therapy with 54-60 Gy of radiation 2 months postoperatively for most patients.

"What is the blood supply to the trachea?"
Lateral arcade of arteries arising from superior and inferior thyroid arteries (main supply of cervical trachea), internal thoracic arteries and bronchial arteries (main supply of lower trachea).

"A patient presents with a life-threatening airway obstruction. She was previously diagnosed with a large, mid-tracheal lesion that you recently biopsied. The lesion is suspicious for malignancy and you are still awaiting the results. In the meantime she presents in extremis. How would you manage this patient?"
If you do not have an airway, you cannot ventilate this patient. Therefore emergency measures need to be carried out to obtain a patent airway. The patient should be transported to the OR immediately. IV sedation should be administered rather than general anesthesia. A rigid bronchoscope provides the best chance of establishing an airway in patients with an acute obstruction due to intraluminal or extraluminal disease. If the tumor is not circumferential, the beveled tip of the rigid scope is advanced along the free area of tracheal wall, distal to the tumor. Jet ventilation may then be instituted to "catch up." Of note, it is useful to have a number of rigid scopes available, including pediatric rigid scopes, to facilitate passage (pediatric - 3.5, 4.0, 5.0, and 6.0 mm and adult - 7.0, 8.0, 9.0, 11.0, 14.0 mm sizes). Once the patient is stabilized, the rigid scope can be used to core out the tumor and to enlarge the lumen. Bleeding can be tamponaded with the rigid scope or with energy sources such as electrocautery, Nd:YAG laser, or argon plasma beam. These energy sources can also be used to perform additional tumor debridement (which may have been helpful at the time of biopsy in this patient), however, their use in the acute setting is unlikely to be tolerated as a low FiO_2 is required to prevent combustion within the airway. A tube exchanger can then be passed through the rigid scope and an appropriately sized endotracheal tube passed over the tube exchanger after the rigid scope has been removed. If the tumor is circumferential and almost completely obstructive, the rigid scope is used to core out the lesion until a lumen is present and the scope can be advanced beyond the obstruction.

A note about acute airway obstruction from extrinsic compression/ lesions—the rigid scope is still useful in this situation to obtain a patent airway, stenting the airway open and allowing ventilation distally. An airway stent may then be used in the acute setting to maintain airway patency (but should not be used in the acute setting for intraluminal lesions). Although measures such as tracheostomy and radiation can be useful tactics to provide airway patency, they should not be used in the acute setting. Elective resection may be carried out in the patient once airway patency is secured and workup is completed for surgical resection, should the tumor be resectable and the patient is an operative candidate.

"Which major histology has a better survival following resection? Which responds better to radiation therapy?"
Adenoid cystic carcinoid (as opposed to squamous cell) for both.

"You are referred a 79 yo man with a 2 cm mid-tracheal tumor who presents with increasing dyspnea and hoarseness. He has ESRD, poorly controlled DM and ischemic cardiomyopathy with EF 30% and has PET-positive masses in RUL."
This patient is a poor operative candidate and surgical resection would not be curative (and would be very high risk). Tissue diagnosis is needed to confirm cell type of the tumor. Assuming this is a squamous cell carcinoma, he should only be offered radiation therapy (dosing of at least 60 Gy in daily fractions of 1.8-2.0 Gy). Measures may be needed to debride the tumor if his symptoms do not improve with radiation therapy. There have been no trials that define the role of chemotherapy as a treatment for unresectable disease.

"You are referred a patient with a biopsy proven SCC of the trachea measuring 2 cm and located in the distal trachea 2 cm proximal to the carina. What would your approach be to resection? What if it involves the carina?"
A median sternotomy provides good exposure to the distal trachea and gives access to the neck if release maneuvers are required. The sternum is opened, as is the anterior pericardium. The tracheobronchial bifurcation can then be accessed between the SVC and ascending aorta by opening the posterior pericardium. Distal tracheal tumors can also be approached via a right posterolateral thoracotomy, which is particularly useful if parenchymal resection is required in conjunction with a carinal resection. Carinal tumors have higher perioperative morbidity and mortality, but can be undertaken by experienced surgeons.

"You are referred a patient with a long tracheal tumor measuring 6 cm in length? What are contraindications for resection?"
The trachea is approximately 11 cm long. Long tumors have been shown to be the most common reason why resection was not feasible. Some

report resection of lesions up to 6 cm, but the risk of significant tension on the anastomosis is greater if greater than 4.5 cm is resected. Absolute contraindications for surgery include over 50% of tracheal length, multiple positive lymph nodes, mediastinal invasion of unresectable organs, a mediastinum that has been irradiated with > 60 Gy, and distant metastases for SCC. Distant metastases or mediastinal lymph node involvement requires tissue diagnosis, by mediastinoscopy, EBUS, percutaneous biopsy, etc.

"When is airway stenting appropriate?"
Airway stenting may be used to maintain airway patency in patients with aggressive, unresectable tumors that recur and obstruct the airway. Airway stenting is also a good option for the treatment of airway obstruction caused by external compression. However, stents constitute palliative therapy only and must be used in conjunction with tumor debulking (rigid bronch, mechanical coring, Nd:Yag laser, cryotherapy, argon beam, etc.). Montgomery T-tubes or metallic stents are used for symptom-relief and life expectancy is minimal.

"Following tracheal resection, your patient has significant laryngeal edema and is not able to extubated. How would you manage this patient?"
Leave a small ETT and keep the patient intubated for 48 hours to allow for the edema to subside. Adjunctive measures include corticosteroids for 24-48 hours, fluid restriction, elevation of the head of the bed, and close monitoring in an ICU setting. The patient should be brought back to the OR 48 hours later and extubated with the help of anesthesia. If extubation is unsuccessful or the patient does not meet criteria for extubation, placing a tracheostomy tube two rings below anastomosis may be warranted. Consideration should be given to covering the anastomosis with a pedicled strap muscle flap for reinforcement.

"Another patient now 6 days after tracheal resection of a 3 cm lesion develops fever, crepitus over the neck and chest, and stridor. How would you manage this patient?"
Dehiscence of the tracheal anastomosis is of primary concern in this scenario. This suspicion should be immediately confirmed with flexible bronchoscopy. An endotracheal tube should be placed over the bronchoscope to avoid additional separation of the anastomosis and to assure adequate ventilation. A definitive airway is then established in the operating room with a tracheostomy distal to the anastomosis. The area surrounding the dehiscence is then debrided and drained. Finally, the defect is controlled with a muscle flap (i.e., strap muscles or sternocleidomastoid). Delayed re-operation may be attempted to revise the anastomosis once the patient has been stabilized and the infection is

resolved. An alternative treatment in the short-term may be a covered stent for those patients who are not stable enough to undergo extensive reoperation early on. In this case, tracheostomy and drainage must be established prior to stenting. Esophageal injury should also be ruled out in this scenario (Contrast esophagram, EGD) should the bronchoscopy fail to show a dehisced anastomosis.

Pearls/pitfalls

- Tracheal tumors are uncommon, usually present as locally advanced disease, and appropriate patient selection for surgery is key to successful outcomes.
- Full evaluation of extent of disease including bronchoscopy and tissue diagnosis is essential for preoperative workup.
- IV induction of anesthesia, immediate intubation, and excellent communication with anesthesiologist is vital.
- Release maneuvers are critical to mobilizing trachea to avoid tension on the anastomosis.
- Minimal circumferential dissection is critical in order to maintain the tracheal blood supply; if needed, compromise oncologic principles of clear margins to favor a tension-free anastomosis.
- Avoid the recurrent laryngeal nerves! Never sacrifice both nerves if tumor is involved.
- Patients with unresectable tumors should receive radiation therapy or tumor debulking/stenting for palliation.
- Adjuvant radiation therapy is warranted for most tumors, especially with positive margins. ACC responds especially well.

Suggested readings

- Gaissert, HA et al. Treatment of tracheal tumors. *Seminars in Thoracic and Cardiovascular Surgery.* 2009; 21(3): 290-295.
- Gaissert HA and DJ Mathiesen. Primary Tumors of the Trachea. *Pearson's Thoracic & Esophageal Surgery.* 3rd Edition. Philadelphia: Churchill Livingstone, 2008. 312-320.
- Honings J et al. Clinical aspects and treatment of primary tracheal malignancies. *Acta Oto-Larynggoligca.* 2010; 130: 763-772.
- Macchiarini P. Primary tracheal tumors. *Lancet Onc.* 2006; 7: 83-91.
- Merritt RE and Mathieson DJ. Tracheal Resection. *Pearson's Thoracic & Esophageal Surgery.* 3rd Edition. Philadelphia: Churchill Livingstone, 2008:376-382.
- Wigle DA and S Keshavjee. Upper Airway Tumors: Seconday Tumors. *Pearson's Thoracic & Esophageal Surgery.* 3rd Edition. Philadelphia: Churchill Livingstone, 2008. 321-325.

Notes

25. Mediastinal masses

Gabriel Loor, MD, and Daniel Raymond, MD

Concept
- Differential for an anterior mediastinal mass
- Diagnostic options
- Management options pertinent to each possible etiology
- Staging the tumor
- Conduct of the operation and pitfalls

Chief complaint
"You're second clinic appointment has arrived. She is a 52 yo woman who presented to her primary care physician with complaints of generalized weakness and vague chest discomfort. She eventually had a chest CT scan that identified a 2.5 by 3 cm anterior mediastinal mass."

Differential
Thymoma, germ cell tumor (GCT), lymphoma, thyroid or parathyroid masses.

History and physical
Focus on symptoms and exam findings associated with Myasthenia Gravis (MG) including ocular muscle weakness (diplopia, blurred vision), dysphonia, dysphagia, or progressive generalized weakness. Note that 15-30% of MG patients have a thymoma. Ask for any history of fevers, night sweats, chills or malaise consistent with lymphoma or GCT. Listen for stridor (indicative of airway compression) and decreased breath sounds or pericardial rub (indicative of pleural effusion or pericardial involvement). Obtain a detailed past medical history including prior malignancies, smoking history, prior chest surgery or radiation, history of cardiopulmonary disease, and details of significant comorbidities. Be aware of other autoimmune disorders associated with thymoma including systemic lupus erythematosus, pure red cell aplasia, pure white cell aplasia, and hypogammaglobulinemia.

Tests
- *Imaging*: chest CT is required and this patient already had one done. Review the quality of the scan, the location of the mass and its relationship to neighboring structures (vessels, pericardium, phrenic nerve). Note whether it appears encapsulated or invasive. Review the scan for evidence of metastatic disease including pleural effusion, pleural nodularity and mediastinal adenopathy. Thymomas classically present as a solid mass with lobulations. GCT are

rounded without lobulations. They may be calcified or have thick walls.

- *Labs*: prior to any thought of an invasive procedure, serum markers should be ordered. Beta human chorionic gonadotropin (B-HCG), alpha-fetoprotein (AFP) and lactate dehydrogenase (LDH) are elevated with non-seminomatous GCTs, but often normal with most seminomatous GCTs as well as thymomas or lymphomas. Notably, one-third of seminomas produce B-HCG but none make AFP.

- *CT-guided core needle biopsy*: this allows definitive tissue diagnosis and helps identify tumors that are not primarily treated with surgery (lymphoma and malignant germ cell tumors). In cases where the diagnosis is still indeterminate you should consider additional measures including anterior mediastinotomy (Chamberlain procedure), video assisted thoracoscopic surgery (VATS), or mediastinoscopy for biopsy. If the clinical setting and characteristics of the mass point to an obvious etiology, then you might be justified in foregoing the biopsy if it is potentially hazardous. An example of this would be a patient with symptomatic MG and a lobulated thymic mass very typical of thymoma who already had an indeterminate biopsy.

Index scenario (additional information)

"The patient's history and physical reveal ocular weakness and dyspnea that worsens throughout the day. She has no other comorbidities. The mass on CT appears lobulated without calcification and is centered on the right superior pole of the thymus. B-HCG and AFP are normal. How would you proceed with diagnosis and treatment of her mediastinal mass?"

Treatment/management

Note that no mention has been made of a positive tissue diagnosis. The clinical suspicion for MG is high in this patient. Neurology consultation should be obtained and testing to confirm the diagnosis should be undertaken including serologic studies, repetitive nerve stimulation, and single fiber electromyography. The CT characteristics are typical of a thymoma. Her neurologic evaluation reveals seropositive myasthenia gravis and her tumor markers are negative for a germ cell tumor. Given the diagnosis of myasthenia gravis, you forego the needle biopsy and make an operative plan.

Ask about any cardiac symptoms or comorbidities which might necessitate an echo or stress test. An older patient with an isolated mass, who is diabetic with a history of angina should clearly undergo an echo, stress test, and EKG. At least an EKG should be ordered otherwise. PFTs are helpful in predicting postoperative respiratory issues, although they would not be helpful in the presence of an active MG flare. Define the stage for this patient – CT scan suggests a localized tumor without metastatic disease. This patient is clinical stage I. There is no evidence of advanced regional invasion into neighboring structures. [Masaoka staging system]

- *Stage I*: no evidence of microscopic extracapsular invasion.
- *Stage II*: microscopic or macroscopic invasion through the capsule into the surrounding fat or pleura.
- *Stage III*: Invasion of adjacent structures (pericardium, great vessels, lungs).
- *Stage IVa*: pleural or pericardial metastasis.
- *Stage IVb*: lymphogenous or hematogenous metastasis.

MG patients must be medically stabilized prior to surgery, the surgeon needs to work closely with the neurologist regarding appropriate timing of surgery. Medical treatment options include:

- Oral anticholinesterases (pyridostigmine)
- Plasmapheresis (any patient with active disease or "MG crisis")
- IVIG is another possibility in lieu of plasmapheresis
- Corticosteroids, Mycophenolate mofetil, cyclosporine and azathioprine

Operative steps

Trans-sternal thymectomy

Goals – explore, stage, total thymectomy with surrounding fat, identify and preserve phrenic nerves.

- Single lumen ETT, central venous catheter, arterial line, foley.
- Full median sternotomy, expose and explore the thymus, identify extent of disease.
- Open pleura bilaterally to assess for lung metastases and to identify the location of both phrenic nerves.
- Free up the right inferior horn of the thymus.
- Free up the right superior horn (resect the thymic-thyroid ligament).
- Ligate the lateral vessels coming from the mammary.
- Make a 1 cm incision above the right phrenic nerve on the mediastinal pleura, remove this superficial pleura and fat with the thymus.
- Repeat these steps on the left side.
- Divide the venous branches draining into the innominate vein.
- Carefully dissect both superior horns of the gland into the neck and divide small arterial branches from the inferior thyroid arteries.

"Postoperatively, the patient is extubated and doing well. 5 hours later you are called to evaluate the patient for generalized weakness and respiratory distress."

Daily spirometry may be used to track the patient's strength and identify exacerbation of the myasthenia gravis. This patient will require reintubation for respiratory compromise. Postoperatively most thymectomy patients are extubated within 6 hours. This includes MG patients. Plasmapheresis may be required for MG patients exhibiting ocular weakness or respiratory weakness, although patients in acute distress warrant immediate re-intubation and plasmapheresis can then be initiated.

"Preop – 65 yo woman with no symptoms of muscle weakness, fevers or malaise. She has a history of diabetes and occasional angina. She had a recent stress test that was negative for coronary disease. Serum markers were all negative."

In this patient the diagnosis is less clear. A CT-guided needle biopsy should be performed.

"The pathology comes back indeterminate cells."

This patient requires an anterior mediastinotomy for tissue diagnosis. She already had a recent stress test but otherwise would require one. She will eventually require an echo and PFTs prior to any definitive resection. Know the steps and pitfalls of an anterior mediastinotomy (see Chapter 6, Mediastinal staging).

"The tissue biopsy reveals largely lymphoid cells mixed with occasional epithelial cells."

This pathology is typical of a thymoma and the patient should proceed with a thymectomy as described.

"The patient's CT scan is suggestive of an invasive carcinoma involving the innominate vein. Intraoperatively, you find evidence of fibrotic tissue along the inferior aspect of the vein."

In general, all tissue that is safe to resect should be removed en bloc with the thymus. This includes the not uncommon scenario involving invasion of major venous structures. If the tissue is fibrotic and you are not ready to commit to a venous resection, then send a shaving for frozen section. If it comes back positive then proceed with resection. If negative, then leave clips along the area for postoperative XRT if warranted. Venous resections come in several variaties. If a limited resection of the inferior portion of the innominate or less than 50% of the superior vena cava (SVC) diameter is required, then resection with primary reconstruction can be performed. Larger areas or any resection where a primary closure appears to reduce flow may be approached with a saphenous vein patch. Thus, the legs should have been prepped circumferentially if there was any suspicion based on the CT. Alternatively bovine pericardium can be used as a patch. Obtain proximal and distal control. For an isolated segment of innominate vein, clamping proximally and distally for a short period of time is well tolerated (30-45 min). For involvement of the SVC, options include clamping the SVC for 20-30 min or cardiopulmonary bypass with additional venous drainage of the right innominate vein. When clamping the SVC, watch for hemodynamic instability. Usually this responds to volume loading and careful anesthetic management. SVC reconstruction options range from primary repair to patch reconstruction or reconstruction with a PTFE tube graft 18-20 mm in diameter. Patients with PTFE reconstructions should be on coumadin postoperatively. These venous resections can be challenging and it may be a good idea to have a senior partner available for assistance.

"The thymic tumor invades the right upper lobe of the lung and pericardium."
Studies show superior survival for patients who undergo debulking followed by adjuvant chemoradiation therapy (50 Gy + platinum-based chemotherapy) compared with patients who only undergo surgical biopsy followed by definitive CRT. Tissue that is reasonable to resect should be removed en bloc. In this case, the involved portion of the lung should be wedged with a surgical stapler, which can be done via sternotomy by opening the right pleura. The pericardium should additionally be resected to a negative margin. If the tumor invades the heart or great vessels, the tumor should be debulked and a rim of tissue left surrounding the involved structure. Clips should be placed to guide XRT postoperatively. Note that a clamshell incision is another alternative approach if preoperatively it is clear that the tumor involves the right or left pulmonary hilum. Be prepared for the possibility of a pneumonectomy or sleeve resection and perform the appropriate preoperative evaluation (see Chapter 4, Pneumonectomy and sleeve resection).

"You are referred a 50 yo man with intermittent fevers and chest pain who is found to have a large mediastinal mass. Serum markers are negative. The initial CT-guided tissue biopsy is consistent with lymphoma."
Patients with a diagnosis of lymphoma in the anterior mediastinum rarely require an operation. However, after a dialogue with the pathologists and oncologists, there may be a need for more tissue. This can be achieved via VATS, mediastinoscopy or anterior mediastinotomy. The treatment for these patients is CRT with a variety of regimens (MOPP – mustargen, procarbazine, prednisone, vincristine; ABVD – doxorubicin, bleomycin, vinblastine, and dacarbazine). Avoid doing an endobronchial ultrasound

and fine needle aspiration (EBUS-FNA) in this situation, as it is unlikely enough tissue will be obtained to perform the needed flow cytometry for lymphoma.

"The initial tissue biopsy is consistent with a GCT."
This patient should be evaluated for a primary gonadal tumor although in some instances no primary gonadal site may be found. The management and prognosis for GCT depends on the type of GCT (benign teratoma, seminoma, and non-seminomatous). Thus, in the absence of obvious clinical characteristics and serum markers indicative of seminomatous GCT, a tissue diagnosis is required. A benign teratoma is the only GCT for which surgery alone is indicated. No adjuvant chemotherapy or XRT is needed. Seminomas have an excellent prognosis. They are very chemo- and radiosensitive and do not require surgery. Non-seminomatous mediastinal GCT include choriocarcinoma, embryonal carcinoma, teratocarcinoma and mixed cellular types. Klinefelter syndrome is associated with non-seminomatous GCT. Non-seminomatous GCT have a poor prognosis and an aggressive multimodality approach has been advocated by several groups. This treatment involves a cisplatin-based combination chemotherapy regimen followed by surgery for residual disease in certain circumstances.

"A 58 yo woman presents with a history of recurrent cough. A CT scan shows a 4 by 6 cm cystic appearing mass adjacent to the right mainstem bronchi. What is your approach to this patient?"
The CT characteristics are typical for a bronchogenic cyst. The majority of these lesions are benign. If diagnosis is uncertain, further information can be obtained with a T2 weighted MRI, which will have a characteristic appearance, or endoscopic ultrasound with biopsy/aspiration of cyst fluid. With characteristic findings on CT, biopsy is not necessary. The treatment of choice for symptomatic bronchogenic cysts is complete surgical resection. The approach is dictated by the location and in this scenario a right VATS or posterolateral thoracotomy would be best. Care is taken to identify and avoid injury to the venous or arterial branches. The cyst is dissected free from surrounding tissue and sent to pathology for definitive diagnosis.

"What if the lesion were asymptomatic?"
This remains an area of debate. Generally speaking, resection is recommended for children and young adults with any cyst impacting anatomy. For adults with small, asymptomatic, classic-appearing cysts, conservative monitoring with serial CT scans/MRI is justifiable. If there is evidence of change in the cyst or the patient develops symptoms, then resection is indicated. Additionally, patients should be educated about the challenges of cyst resection if it becomes infected.

"A 50 yo man presents to your clinic with vague left lower back pain. An MRI was ordered by his primary physician which showed a 6 by 6 cm mass at T5 near the left costovertebral junction. What is the approach to this lesion?"

The most common posterior mediastinal neoplasms are nerve sheath tumors such as a schwannoma or neurofibroma. Malignant tumors of nerve sheath origin are in the differential, but far less common. Ganglionic and paraganglionic tumors are also in the differential. Functioning paragangliomas or pheochromocytomas may have a characteristic constellation of symptoms that includes hypertension, sweating, and palpitations. This should prompt a workup that includes urine catecholamines and metaiodobenzylguanidine (MIBG) scanning. The patient should be evaluated for any evidence of neurologic involvement. An MRI is the imaging modality of choice and is useful for determining extension into the spinal canal. Schwannomas may be positive by PET and high uptake does not necessarily indicate a malignant process. Complete resection is advocated for any symptomatic tumor and encouraged for asymptomatic tumors unless the patient has a high surgical risk. Small tumors (< 3 cm) are the least likely to grow and be malignant. If the patient is asymptomatic and not an ideal candidate or apprehensive, serial imaging is reasonable. VATS and open resection are options. VATS may be appropriate for smaller non-invasive tumors < 3 cm in size if the operator has experience with this modality. Otherwise the open technique involves a left posterolateral thoracotomy. The pleura is opened around the tumor with a margin of 1-2 cm. The neurovascular bundle is clipped or ligated and the tumor is removed. One important variant is the "dumbbell" tumor, which involves the spinal cord. For these tumors neurosurgery should be involved for a single or staged approach including a hemi-laminectomy or foraminectomy for complete resection.

Pearls/pitfalls

- Involved structures are resected en bloc with the thymic mass.
- Always spare one phrenic nerve .
- *If total resection is not possible*: debulk as much as possible and leave clips along the perimeter.
- *Extension into the lung hilum*: clamshell incision.
- *GCT*: evaluate for primary gonadal tumor.
- *Elevated serum markers = non-seminomatous*: platinum-based chemotherapy followed by surgery.
- *Lymphoma*: chemotherapy, surgery only for tissue diagnosis.
- *MG*: stabilize medically prior to OR

Suggested readings

- Mornex F, Resbeut M, Richaud P, et al. Radiotherapy and chemotherapy for invasive thymomas: A multicentric retrospective review of 90 cases. The FNCLCC trialists. Federation Nationale des Centres de Lutte Contre le Cancer. Int J Radiat Oncol Biol Phys 1995;32(3):651-659.
- Venuta F, Rendina EA and Coloni GF. Surgery of the superior vena cava: resection and reconstruction. CTSnet. Thoracic techniques. 2009.
- Nichols FC and Trastek VF. Thymectomy (Sternotomy). Kaiser LR, Kron, IL, Spray TL (eds). Mastery of Cardiothoracic Surgery. 2007.
- Attia P. Mediastinal disease. Yuh DD, Vricella LA, and Baumgartner WA (eds). Johns Hopkins Manual of Cardiothoracic Surgery. 2007.

Notes

II. Adult Cardiac Surgery

26. Management of the porcelain aorta

Mark Joseph, MD, and Andy C. Kiser, MD

Concept
- Management of the Porcelain Aorta in relation to Coronary Artery Bypass Grafting (CABG) and Aortic Valve Replacement (AVR)
- Preoperative considerations
- Revascularization options
- Operative strategies and myocardial protection
- Pitfalls and alternative solutions

Chief complaint
"A 70 yo man with previous h/o Hodgkin's lymphoma presents to his primary care physician with intermittent chest pain on exertion. CXR shows calcification of the aorta and is otherwise is unremarkable."

Differential
Angina, aortic stenosis w/aortic calcification, PE, dissection, mediastinal mass

History and physical
Clarify the duration and character of the chest pain to distinguish between possible etiologies. The calcium on the CXR raises concerns for a porcelain aorta although the CT scan is needed before establishing the diagnosis. Look for risk factors associated with this disease including atherosclerotic risk factors (diabetes, smoking, HTN, family history), radiation for Hodgkin's, renal failure/hemodialysis and aortic stenosis. Physical exam should focus on peripheral pulses, and cardiopulmonary exam.

Tests
- *EKG*: evidence of arrhythmias and previous or ongoing ischemia.
- *Echocardiography*: valve function and EF.
- Cardiac catheterization.
- *CXR*: look for other lung pathology.
- *CT scan*: CT scan is warranted in patients with strong risk factors for ascending aortic atherosclerosis or if there is evidence of aortic calcification on ECHO or CXR. Look for concomitant disease such as dissection or aneurysms.

"Angiogram reveals significant 3 vessel disease: Left main (80%) and ostial LAD (80%), circumflex (75%) and mid RCA lesions (70%). Echo reveals AVA of 0.4 mm, peak gradient of 80 mmHg and mean gradient of 40 mmHg with a jet velocity of 4 m/s2. Diffuse circumferential ascending aortic calcification is noted on the CT scan. EF is 55%."

Treatment/management
There is a spectrum of ascending aortic calcification from multifocal patchy disease to diffuse involvement. The CT scan is helpful for preoperative planning although the final decision is made in the OR with careful palpation and the use of an epiaortic ultrasound. This patient meets criteria for CABG - AVR but is not likely to have a safe place to clamp and cannulate. In addition, he likely needs a LIMA-LAD, S-PDA and S-OM and thus needs room for proximals. If you can find a place to clamp and cannulate then that is a reasonable but unusual opportunity. Axillary artery cannulation affords you more real estate on the aorta for placement of the clamp. If you did find a safe place to clamp you may still have considerable difficulty finding a place for proximals. The safest and most reliable alternative is axillary artery cannulation, circulatory arrest, replacement of the ascending aorta, AVR, and CABG.

Operative steps
Goals – bypass coronary lesions, replace the aortic valve, protect the heart, and minimize manipulation of the aorta using a "no touch" technique.

- Central line +/- Swan, large peripheral IV's, arterial line, general endotracheal anesthesia (GETA), foley with temperature monitoring.
- Check the intraoperative TEE for evidence of AI or other unexpected pathology and to evaluate ventricular function.
- Median sternotomy, gentle palpation of aorta to determine extent of calcifications, and epiaortic ultrasound.
- Decide whether you can clamp or if you need circulatory arrest.
- Harvest the appropriate conduit depending on revascularization scheme (arterial and/or venous conduit).
- Heparinize (400 mg/kg), right axillary cannulation with a side graft, bicaval cannulation, retrograde coronary sinus catheter, once ACT is above 480, initiate cardiopulmonary bypass (CPB), (cool to 20°), place LV vent through right superior pulmonary vein (RSPV).
- While cooling you can perform the distal anastomoses with a stabilizer or simply wait.

- Once cool and EEG is silent, circ arrest, myocardial arrest, distal ascending graft anastomosis (may need limited endarterectomy to ensure a healthy aortic wall, consider felt reinforcement), deair the graft, clamp the graft, rewarm, hemostasis, inspect, resect and debride the aortic valve, complete any remaining distals, AVR, proximal ascending graft anastomosis and complete the proximal vein anastomoses from the new ascending graft.
- Root vent, deair, unclamp, wean from CPB.

Potential questions/alternative scenarios

"You begin cooling and the patient fibrillates."

If you do have AI you will almost certainly fibrillate and over distend during cooling and you will have no place to clamp. Have an LV vent in place to protect you from over distending. You can attempt to defibrillate but it is often not helpful. IV lidocaine load can be tried as well. The key is to prevent overdistention until you are ready to circ arrest.

"Same patient but no need for AVR."

The most common approach in this setting is a beating heart CABG with or without axillary artery cannulation and CPB support. The decision to use support depends on how well the patient is expected to tolerate manipulating the heart and which vessels need to be grafted. An off pump LIMA-LAD is a safe operation to describe. It involves harvesting the mammary, traction sutures on left side of the posterior pericardium, full heparinization, a commercially available immobilizer to stabilize the heart at the region of the LAD target, silastic vessel loops proximally and distally, and a shunt if needed. The patient has to be adequately fluid resuscitated and potentially on pressors to tolerate the manipulation.

"The LIMA-LAD is completed off pump. How do you revascularize the Cx territory and the PDA with a porcelain aorta?"

An arterial graft (radial or free RIMA) fashioned as a Y off the LIMA or a RIMA in situ through the transverse sinus are options for a high OM. Options for the PDA include a RIMA in situ (may have issues with length here, usually reaches the RCA well), a SVG with proximal anastomosis to the innominate, carotid, subclavian, right axillary, or internal mammary arteries or the descending aorta; alternatively, if no SVG due to a prior CABG then consider an *in-situ* gastroepiploic artery (become familiar with this prior to suggesting it as an option).

"The circumflex and PDA disease is quite distal, the EF is 40% and you do not expect the heart to tolerate excessive manipulation for a completely off pump CABG. What are your options?"

Use right axillary and venous cannulation, go on pump to empty the heart while you use the stabilizers to graft your targets. You still have issues with needing long conduits to the lateral OM and PDA. Assuming no place on the aorta for a proximal, the best option may be a long RIMA in situ to the PDA and long radial from the LIMA to the lateral OM. Options for Y grafts include sizing and fashioning the end to side Y anastomosis first then completing the two distals or doing the distals first and then the end to side. Make sure the heart is full when sizing these arterial grafts. If you anticipate using the right axillary as inflow for a vein graft to the PDA in the not so uncommon event that the RIMA does not reach then plan your axillary cannulation on the left. Other alternatives for the PDA or lateral OM include the in-situ gastroepiploic or a proximal vein off the descending aorta. The descending aorta can be accessed with an incision in the retropericardium. With the heart decompressed, elevate the heart out of the pericardial well and open the leftward pericardium behind the left phrenic nerve. Using a side biting clamp, the descending aorta can serve as an alternative for conduit inflow. Another alternative is to use the HeartString III (MAQUET, Wayne, NJ, USA) proximal anastomosis device if a small area of soft ascending aorta is available. Yet another option is a hybrid procedure with LIMA-LAD and stents to the PDA and/or circumflex. Always remember the significance of the lesion you wish to graft, the run off and the distal target. A non significant lesion on a nondominant right with excessive scar tissue , poor target and poor runoff is not worth the risk of "creative" coronary grafting strategies. Also remember that a sent is a reasonable option when appropriate.

Pearls/pitfalls
- Look for signs or risk factors for a calcified ascending aorta and get a CT scan if concerned.
- Need to replace the ascending with a graft if performing an AVR in the setting of a porcelain aorta.
- Beating heart CABG with or without CPB assist is an option for patients with a porcelain aorta in need of a CABG.
- For beating heart CABG where there is no space on the aorta for proximals anticipate alternative grafting strategies especially for the distal PDA and lateral circumflex. Hybrid procedures with LIMA-LAD and stents to the PDA and/or circumflex may be an option if the anatomy is favorable. Also consider the HeartString III device if you are comfortable and familiar.
- Axillary cannulation is preferred over femoral for same reason retrograde cardioplegia is preferred to avoid the "sandblasting" effect from the aorta towards the coronary ostia.
- If the ascending aorta cannot be safely replaced consider a hybrid approach with LIMA to LAD and PCI +/-TAVR if both valvular and coronary disease are present.

Suggested readings
- Leyh R.G., et al. Management of porcelain aorta during coronary artery bypass grafting. *Ann Thorac Surg* 1999; 67(4):986-988.
- Mills N.L., Everson C.T.: Atherosclerosis of the ascending aorta and coronary artery bypass. Pathology, clinical correlates, and operative management. *J Thorac Cardiovasc Surg* 1991; 102(4):546-553.
- Sabik J.F., et al: Axillary artery: an alternative site of arterial cannulation for patients with extensive aortic and peripheral vascular disease. *J Thorac Cardiovasc Surg* 1995; 109(5):885-890.discussion 890-1.
- Sundt T.M., Barner H.B., Camillo C.J., et al: Total arterial revascularization with an internal thoracic artery and radial artery T graft. *Ann Thorac Surg* 1999; 68:399-405.

Notes

27. Cardiopulmonary bypass pitfalls

Juan G. Penaranda, MD, and Harold M. Burkhart, MD

Concept
- Establishing access for CPB
- Initiating CPB
- Maintaining CPB
- Separating from CPB
- Pitfalls that arise in each of the above steps

Chief complaint
"A 77 yo diabetic man is undergoing a CABG AVR. Describe any preoperative workup relevant to CPB."

Differential
Non applicable

History and physical
Any patient requiring CPB needs to have a comprehensive systems based history and physical to identify history of stroke, renal disease, coronary lesions, intestinal angina, respiratory problems, bleeding disorders, or peripheral vascular disease.

Tests
- Comprehensive labs (CBC, BMP, Coags, LFTs)
- Head CT if recent stroke
- Carotid duplex if stroke or bruits
- Mesenteric duplex if evidence of intestinal ischemia
- ABIs for evidence of peripheral vascular disease
- Coronary angio to identify critical lesions
- PFTs for history of respiratory problems
- Chest CT scan for any patient with calcification on CXR

These tests allow risk stratification, identification of lesions that require preoperative intervention and identification of lesions that modify the lowest acceptable MAP on CPB.

Index scenario (additional information)
"The patient has a creatinine of 1.7, and a carotid duplex showing a 60% asymptomatic left carotid lesion. Chest CT shows a normal appearing aorta without calcification."

Treatment/management

This patient will require CPB in order to perform the combined CABG AVR. His MAP should be kept at the upper range of normal to ensure adequate renal and brain perfusion. A useful rule of thumb is MAPs = decade of age (i.e., 77 = 70-80 mmHg). Mild hypothermia (32-34° C) can be considered to decrease the tissue oxygen demand.

Operative steps

Cannulation

- Median sternotomy.
- Palpate the aorta for calcification.
- Ensure you are high enough to complete all your proximal procedures.
- Give Heparin (400 Units/kg).
- Place purstrings.
- Check your systemic pressure (ideally < 70 mmHg).
- Cannulate the aorta with a 21-24 F arterial cannula and secure the cannula.
- Check your line (assess the swing and line pressure with a test transfusion). Visualize the proximal aorta with the test transfusion.
- Cannulate the RA with a dual stage cannula that drains both the RA and IVC.
- Alternative venous cannulas include right angled IVC/SVC cannulas, 3 stage SVC cannula, or long femoral vein cannulation.
- ABC's - A: anticoagulate, B: be sure you are high enough, C: calcification.

Initiation

- Check your ACT and make sure you are > 480.
- Go on CPB - forward flow is initiated to ensure there is no obstruction.
- Empty out - drain the heart once forward flow is confirmed.
- Hold ventilation.
- Flush cardioplegia, specify your desired temperature, and complete any required dissection prior to cross clamp and arrest.
- Specify your temperature.
- ABC's - A: ACT, B: breathing - hold ventilation, C: circulation (forward flow and drainage, PAPs, CVP should be low).

Maintenance

- Check for asystole (clamp, antegrade/retrograde).
- Aortic vent on.
- Check for optimal MAPs (usually 50-80 mmHg) - higher age or greater atherosclerotic burden may require higher MAPs.

- Flow is usually 2.1-2.5 L/min.
- Assess perfusion via lactate, venous saturation, urine output.
- Cooling to mild hypothermia (32-34°C) may allow a decrease of flow and MAPs when needed.
- Check drainage - heart should be empty, CVP and PAP should be low.
- Check sats, ABG, oxygenation, visual inspection of arterial blood - should be bright red).
- ABC's - A: asystole B: breathing (oxygenation) C: circulation (forward flow, drainage).

Releasing the cross clamp
- Deair the left atrium and root.
- Administer hot shot cardioplegia (institution specific).
- Drop your flows, vent on, head down, release the clamp, resume your flows.

Weaning from CPB
In general you need to be warm, have rhythm and be ventilating in order to come off.
A more detailed but useful mnemonic follows:
A - Anastomosis
B - Beat of the heart (fibrillation, pacing wires), Breathing - ventilation
C - Circulation (fill up the heart and eject), assess Contractiliy
D - Degrees (36° C)
E - Echo (function, valves, air), Electrolytes
F - Flows (gradually reduce while observing function and hemodynamics)
G - Gases (ABG)
H - Hypertension (vasodilate)
I - Inotropes
J - Juices (urine output throughout the case)

Potential questions/alternative scenarios
"5 minutes after the cross clamp is released the heart begins to over distend. You notice a lack of spontaneous contraction. What do you do?"
There are 2 considerations - one is that the valve has a leak of some degree and the second is that the heart is not ejecting to overcome any regurgitant volume. Usually the first maneuver will be to squeeze the heart to get it to decompress from the apex up towards the LVOT. Check your PAP which will give you a clue as to how effectively you are decompressing. Try to pace or tap the heart to encourage ejection but ultimately the solution may be to cross clamp.

"You attempt to pace but have no capture despite well placed leads. Anesthesia tells you there is 1+ central AI. Perfusion tells you that the potassium has been 7 meq/L and they have struggled to bring it down. The patient has not made urine during the case. You cross clamp the aorta, turn up the root vent and empty out the heart. After 10 minutes the potassium starts to decrease and the heart contracts."

Now you know the etiology. There is some leak but it is hard to truly estimate it without contractility. Knowing the electrolytes is an important component of the weaning process as is the production of urine output. If the potassium does not decrease options include hemoconcentration, IV insulin and glucose, lasix, or bicarb. Usually the perfusionist is able to get the potassium down but it may take some time. Another option would be to vent the heart while you wait for the K to resolve. While you wait it would not be unreasonable to open the aortotomy and explore the aortic valve for any major defects especially if you were told that the AI was moderate-severe. But in the absence of something obvious and only 1+ AI, wait until you are ejecting to analyze the valve and decide on replacing or not. Once you are ready, release the cross clamp, pace prn, ventilate, fill up the heart, eject, wean your flows and check the echo carefully.

"A 60 yo male patient has just undergone a mitral valve repair. You release the cross clamp. The heart begins to fibrillate. The echo does not demonstrate anything more than a trace to 1+ central aortic jet. You try to defibrillate but are unable to cardiovert. Describe your approach to defibrillating the patient."

Internal paddles are set at 10-20 Joules and gradually increased. If you cannot cardiovert give IV lidocaine and or amiodarone (150 mg IV) and try again. There are several issues that can make it hard to cardiovert: distention, air, low systemic pressures, electrolyte abnormality, poor oxygenation, and hypothermia. In addition, consider coronary ischemia or valvular incompetence. If the heart appears distended and or the PAPs are elevated, the initial step is to manually squeeze the heart while emptying out with CPB. If the heart continues to over distend then place a PA vent or LV vent. After placing the vent and decompressing the heart you should be able to cardiovert to sinus rhythm. Make sure the root vent is on to evacuate any air. Increase your perfusion pressures to > 75 mmHg both for improved coronary perfusion and to flush out any air that may have embolized. Give lidocaine and or amiodarone. Optimize your oxygenation, electrolytes and temperature. Check the echo to ensure that you do not have AI. Anything greater than 1+ warrants consideration for replacement (see previous scenario). On the differential, is damage to the non-coronary leaflet with placement of the mitral stitches. If this appears to be the problem by echo, arrest the heart and explore the aortic valve. If there is evidence of coronary ischemia as evidenced by ST changes or new regional wall motion abnormalities then bypass with a vein graft. If you cannot defibrillate even after venting and reversing all of the above then clamp, arrest and try again.

"Describe the components of the CPB machine."
Blood drains into the venous reservoir by gravity or vacuum assist. It is then pushed by centripetal or centrifugal pumps into the oxygenator/heat exchanger. It then continues on to the arterial air filter and back to the patient.

"You are starting a mitral valve repair and ask the anesthesiologist to give the heparin. After the cannulas are in you ask your perfusionist if the ACT is adequate for bypass. He is having trouble and tells you a standard dose of heparin has been given and the ACT is only 200 seconds and is not going up. How do you deal with this issue?"
Antithrombin III deficiency is the most common reason for an inadequate ACT despite appropriate heparin dosing. An additional dose of heparin solves the problem in most cases. If the ACT does not respond appropriately to a second dose of heparin, one should consider administering either fresh frozen plasma or recombinant antithrombin III.

"You end up giving a dose of AT III and the ACT is now adequate for bypass. Soon after going on CPB, the perfusionist alerts you of a high aortic line pressure. What is your checklist for this situation?"
- Obstruction on the arterial circuit (kink in or clamp on line)
- Malposition of the aortic cannula
- Cannula too small for full CPB
- Evidence of aortic dissection: systemic pressure will be low and the ascending aorta will be abnormal

"You checked the systemic pressure and it is normal. You inspect the ascending aorta and it looks normal without evidence of swelling or discoloration. You trace out the arterial line and there are no kinks in the circuit. Upon inspection of the cannulation site you notice there is an excessive angulation of the cannula suggesting that the tip is against the lateral aspect of the innominate artery. You reposition the cannula and the line pressure comes down."

"Your perfusionist now tells you there is poor venous return and a drop in venous reservoir volume after snaring the caval tapes. The right atrium is not distended and the PAP is low. The CVP is elevated Your perfusionist lowers the CPB flow to protect the level of venous reservoir. What are some of the maneuvers to manage inadequate venous drainage?"
- Check for air locks

- Ensure good position of the venous cannula
- Elevate the level of the patient in relation to the reservoir if relying on gravity
- Use suction drainage
- Increase cannula size
- Reduce flows as long as still within ideal MAP range (may need to cool 32-34° C)
- Exclude other sources of blood flow into the heart especially in the setting of distention (aortic regurge - vent, azygous vein - adjust snares, left sided SVC - snare or cannulate)
- Consider other sites of volume loss (i.e., retroperitoneal or peritoneal hemorrhage) - check abdominal girth, H/H

"In this case the IVC right angle cannula has rotated before snaring the caval tapes and is now pointing towards the right atrium occluding the IVC drainage. You release the snare and reposition the cannula solving the problem. You also noticed that the SVC cannula was inserted into the azygos and reposition accordingly."

"After re-instituting CPB, your perfusionist cannot get the mean blood pressure above 40 mmHg. The anesthesiologist tells you the patient was on a high dose of ACE inhibitor preoperatively. What do you do next?"
Vasoplegia can be seen in patients on numerous antihypertensive medications, in particular ACE Inhibitors. In this situation, phenylephrine, norepinephrine, vasopressin or even methylene blue are options that can be used to increase the systemic pressure. This scenario may arise in the postoperative period as well.

"You placed a coronary sinus catheter for retrograde cardioplegia because the patient has moderate aortic regurgitation. As you start your retrograde infusion, the pressure within the coronary sinus seems to be very low. You inspect the inferior aspect of the heart to make sure there has been no rupture of the coronary sinus or malposition of the catheter. You take out the catheter and the balloon is intact. You place the catheter in again and confirm its position by palpation. Despite this, the pressure remains low and the heart is not arresting. What are the causes of this problem?"
Inadequate retrograde cardioplegia delivery may be due to:
- Catheter displacement into the right atrium
- Rupture of coronary sinus
- Balloon rupture
- Persistent left sided superior vena cava (LSVC)

"You lift the heart to the right and discover a LSVC. You place a snare to occlude it since there is a large innominate vein and you are now able to arrest the heart."
If there is not a persistent innominate vein you can cannulate the LSVC separately.

"You finished your mitral valve repair and wean the patient off bypass. After a few seconds, the blood pressure drops, there is ST elevation on the EKG and the right ventricle distends. You suspect air has entered the right coronary artery. What are some of the maneuvers you use to overcome this problem?"
The right coronary ostium is anterior and susceptible to air embolism. It can be seen after valvular or other cardiac surgery and usually causes transient right ventricular dysfunction and distention. In this case, re-instituting CPB with a high perfusion pressure will help to support cardiac function and push the air through the coronary artery into the venous circulation. De-airing the heart through an aortic root vent will prevent further air migration into the coronary arteries. Consider evacuating air through the apex with a large bore needle if there is a large collection of air at the apex.

"The patient is now off bypass and you and the cardiologist are assessing the mitral valve repair with transesophageal echo (TEE). Your assistant points out to you that the aorta suddenly developed a bluish discoloration. Upon inspection, you notice there is an expanding hematoma in the ascending aorta. On TEE there is a dissection flap in the ascending aorta and the aortic valve is competent. What do you do now?"
The patient has developed an iatrogenic Type A dissection. Establish arterial access within the true lumen (axillary), cool, circ arrest, replace the ascending, resume flow (see Chapter 47, Iatrogenic aortic dissection).

"You are doing a mitral valve repair in a 42 yo woman with asymptomatic severe mitral regurgitation. You performed aortic and bi-caval cannulation, instituted CPB and cooled to 32° C. After placing the aortic cross clamp and arresting the heart, the perfusionist alerts you of poor venous drainage. You notice a large amount of air in the aortic cannula. You are certain air has entered the aorta and suspect it has embolized to the brain. The level of the venous reservoir has gone down too low and air has been pumped into the arterial line. What do you do at this point?"
Even though massive air embolism after initiation of cardiopulmonary bypass is a rare complication (incidence less than 0.2% of cases), it has a high mortality and high incidence of neurologic injury. It most commonly happens if the blood level in the venous reservoir and

oxygenator gets too low allowing air to be introduced into the arterial circuit. Rapid implementation of an algorithm may save the life of the patient or prevent significant neurologic damage.

A useful algorithm in this situation includes:
- Perfusionist
    - Discontinue CPB
    - Clamp arterial and venous lines
    - De-air bypass circuit
    - Add necessary volume to the reservoir
- Anesthesiologist
    - Steep trendelenburg
    - 100% oxygen
    - Steroids/Barbiturates/Mannitol
    - Support circulation with vasopressors
- Surgeon
    - Aspirate air from aortic root
    - Retrograde brain perfusion
- Reinstitute CBP and cool the patient down for brain protection
- Massage coronary arteries to displace air
- Complete surgical procedure and de-air heart in usual fashion
- Consider hyperbaric chamber postoperatively
- ICU
    - Consider deep sedation for brain protection
    - Consider hyperbaric chamber

"You ask your perfusionist to stop the pump and clamp both the aortic and venous lines. You place the patient in trendelenburg, and aspirate the air from the ascending aorta. Next you disconnect the arterial line from the cannula, de-air the line and connect it to the SVC cannula to start retrograde brain perfusion. 300 mL/min of flow directed up to the vena cava is started and after two minutes of perfusion you start seeing bubbles at the ascending aorta which are removed by an aortic root vent you have placed. You then reinstitute CPB and cool the patient down to 28° C for brain protection. You complete your aortic valve replacement quickly. The patient is weaned off bypass after 50 minutes and transferred to the ICU. The anesthesiologist gives steroids and barbiturates to the patient and keeps him in deep anesthesia for two days. A CT scan is performed and is negative for any intracerebral injury. The patient is discharged neurologically intact after 10 days in the hospital."

- Patients undergoing CPB require a comprehensive workup to minimize the risk of end organ injury.
- *Phases of CPB are Induction > Maintanence > Seperation*: be familiar with critical elements of each of these phases.
- Target MAP is roughly equivalent to the patient's age (i.e., 63 yo = 60 mmHg, 83 yo = 80 mmHg).
- Air embolism, dissection, and venous perforations are major adverse events that can occur during CPB. Be prepared to anticipate, prevent and deal with these complications if they occur.
- Poor drainage can result from air locks, inappropriately positioned cannulas, persistent LSVC. An empty heart and poor drainage suggests loss of blood volume (i.e., retroperitoneal or peritoneal hematoma).

Suggested readings

- Bojar RM. Cardiopulmonary Bypass. Chapter 5. Manual of Perioperative care in adult cardiac surgery, 4th Edition 2005.
- Millls NL, Ochsner JL. Massive air embolism during cardiopulmonary bypass: causes, prevention and management. J Thorac Cardiovasc Surg 80:708-717, 1980.
- Svensson LG and Crawford ES. Cardiovascular and Vascular Diseases of the Aorta. WB Saunders Company 1997.
- Brodie JE, Johnson RB. The Manual of Clinical Perfusion, 2nd Edition 1997.
- Kincaid EH, Hammon JW. Cardiopulmonary bypass. John Hopkins Manual of Cardiothoracic Surgery. 2007.

Notes

28. Cardioprotection pitfalls

Robert C. Neely, MD, Linda Mongero, CCP, James Beck, CCP, and Michael Argenziano, MD

Concept
- Cardioprotection strategies for the arrested heart during cardiopulmonary bypass
- Common errors and troubleshooting techniques
- Cardioplegia solutions

Chief complaint
"You are doing an aortic valve replacement on a 65 yo man for severe aortic stenosis with moderate aortic insufficiency who has a history of previous triple vessel CABG (LIMA-LAD, SVG-PDA, SVG-OM). Discuss your options for cardioprotection."

In general, options for cardioprotection for an arrested heart include antegrade and retrograde delivery, continuous or intermittent. Types of cardioplegia include crystalloid or blood based solutions that can be warm or cold. The most common practice is to use a solution that has a 1:4 blood to crystalloid ratio and is cooled to a temperature of 4° C and infused intermittently every 15-20 minutes.

This patient has important issues that influence the approach, namely a reoperation with prior LIMA conduit and the presence of moderate aortic insufficiency. Standard re-operative measures should be taken, including external pacing pads and prepped groins bilaterally in the event that emergency peripheral cannulation is needed for bypass (see Chapter 32, Redo coronary artery bypass surgery).

In order to achieve adequate cardiac arrest with sufficient cardioprotection, one must ensure 4 things in this scenario - #1 excellent drainage through standard atrial, groin or bicaval cannulation (this can be augmented by an LV vent if needed) #2 ability to cross clamp the aorta - need enough room on the ascending for the placement of a cross clamp, axillary cannulation may be needed if the proximals are patent and high on the aorta #3 Identify the LIMA conduit - prior to arresting the heart, the LIMA should be clamped to prevent continuous perfusion during aortic cross clamping (NOTE: could avoid clamping LIMA in favor of cold bypass flow). #4 retrograde and antegrade cardioplegia access. Antegrade would perfuse the OM and PDA territories but not the LAD. Retrograde would perfuse the LAD territory. Adjunctive measures include moderate hypothermia (28-32° C) and direct cardioplegia down the vein grafts but again that would not supply the LAD territory.

In the setting of aortic insufficiency, a retrograde cardioplegia catheter should be inserted in order to ensure cardioplegia delivery. The downside of this approach is incomplete right heart protection when the tip of the retrograde cannula is distal to the middle cardiac vein. Direct retrograde insertion can circumvent this issue. The other downside is that if you get a perforation of the sinus during insertion you are in a difficult situation as the posterior part of the heart is likely to be stuck from the prior operation. On the other hand any dissection that you do to facilitate retrograde insertion risks damage to the grafts. Do what you are most comfortable with but demonstrate thoughtfulness in either direction.

Index scenario (additional information)

"After cross clamping and delivering 500 mL of antegrade cardioplegia, you note poor distension of the aortic root, incomplete arrest, and left ventricular distension on transesophageal echocardiogram (TEE). How would you proceed?"
Switch to retrograde and turn on the aortic root vent. An aortotomy would also allow decompression. Another option is placing an LV vent in order to decompress the left heart as cardioplegia crosses the incompetent aortic valve and fills the LV. However, it may be difficult to get the vent in during a redo.

"You place an LV vent. The LV is decompressed but electrical activity persists. As planned you give retrograde cardioplegia, but you note persistent activity and your perfusionist notes inadequate line pressure. You are unable to reliably palpate the retrograde catheter in the coronary sinus. Transesophageal echocardiography suggests the catheter is not in the coronary sinus. How would you proceed?"
Remember that this is a redo situation. Open the aorta (if you haven't already) and deliver additional antegrade cardioplegia directly down the vein grafts to get the best arrest that you can and cool to moderate hypothermia. Get around the cavas if you can and insert the retrograde catheter directly to get perfusion of the LAD distribution. The other alternative to getting excellent cardioplegia down the LAD territory is to cool to 20° and leave the L-LAD open.

"How do you ensure adequacy of retrograde cardioplegia delivery?"
Look for cessation of electrical and myocardial activity by checking the EKG and looking at the heart. Additionally, confirm with the perfusion team that you have adequate line pressure and flow. Most retrograde cannula tips have pressure monitor probes that report the pressure in the coronary sinus. A conservative upper limit of appropriate pressure is approximately 40 mmHg. This reflects a flow of 50-100 cc/min. Observe flow through the coronary veins and arteries during retrograde cardioplegia. Check the RCA and LCA ostia after the aorta is opened and

retrograde is running to ensure adequate distribution of the retrograde to the right and left circulations. The myocardial temperature can also be a guide to the adequacy of cardioplegia delivery. You should note decreasing myocardial temperature assessed either manually or with a direct temperature probe.

Operative steps

Antegrade cannula placement

- Identify a favorable area on anterior curvature of ascending aorta with adequate room for aortic cross clamp cephalad and proximal anastomosis or aortotomy—if needed—caudad.
- Can check for plaque by palpation or evaluate with epiaortic ultrasound.
- Antegrade needle and cannula should be snared securely.
- After securing the line in place it must be flushed to deair. After cross clamping, run your induction dose and inspect the root for evidence of dissection and inspect the LV for distention. A fast arrest is a good sign.

Retrograde cannula placement

- A purse-string suture is placed in the inferolateral aspect of right atrium.
- Retrograde cannula is placed with an gentle L shaped curve and directed toward the orifice of the coronary sinus with guidance from the operator's opposite hand.
- The final placement is confirmed by palpation and/or transesophageal echocardiographic imaging, and further substantiated by distal pressure readings during infusion.
- Some cannulae have self-inflating balloons; others must be inflated manually. These balloons are rarely completely occlusive. This lack of complete occlusion is helpful in avoiding edema during CABG procedures when giving simultaneous cardioplegia down the retrograde catheter and a saphenous vein graft.
- If indirect retrograde placement is problematic then direct retrograde placement can be used. This requires bicaval cannulation, caval snares for atrial isolation, small atriotomy, hand held retractor, identification of the coronary sinus ostium, purse string and direct placement of the coronary catheter. This is usually done with the clamp in place on the aorta.
- The standard catheters may be used for direct retrograde although an 8 mm flexible polystan catheter may be less traumatic. The purse string is secured which leads to occlusion of the coronary sinus. Thus, giving direct retrograde and cardioplegia down a vein graft simultaneously may theoretically lead to myocardial edema.

- Direct retrograde is a good way to ensure delivery down the right and left since the catheter is not advanced beyond the middle cardiac vein.

"How does the presence of a left sided Superior Vena Cava (LSVC) change your approach to cardioprotection?"
The presence of a left sided SVC poses an issue of volume returning to the right side of the heart (directly or via the coronary sinus) that is not drained by a venous cannula. This volume of blood then enters the pulmonary circulation and returns to the left atrium and ventricle and may cause distension. In addition this blood is warmer than the cardioplegia solution and may negate cooling effects on the myocardium. The other issue is that in cases in which the LSVC drains into the coronary sinus, it is difficult to administer retrograde cardioplegia. In these cases, the LSVC can be occluded or cannulated directly and added to the venous drainage circuit. The latter technique is advisable if the LSVC is very large and is mandatory if there is an interrupted innominate vein.

"Upon infusing antegrade cardioplegia, the perfusionist notes high line pressure. What are your next steps in management?"
This raises concern for a dissection. Stop your antegrade flow. Check for kinks or clamps obstructing flow along the line, ensuring that the cardioplegia is flowing down the appropriate path to the aortic root. Also check to make sure that the pressure monitoring line is connected correctly. With regard to a potential dissection, visualize the aortic root and look for distension or discoloration/bruising around the cannula. Ask the anesthesiologists to visualize the ascending and descending aorta with transesophageal echocardiography. If dissection is confirmed start cooling with your original aortic cannula which is distal to the clamp (assuming the dissection is contained within the root. Prepare for a dissection repair (see Chapter 47, Iatrogenic aortic dissection).

"After unclamping the aorta during a case with retrograde cardioplegia, you notice the myocardium is slow to regain electrical activity. Prior to placing pacing wires, what should you check?"
Check that the retrograde catheter is removed and/or that the balloon is down (if not automatically deflated after infusion) in order to allow for adequate coronary sinus flow.

"While sewing the distal anastomosis on a coronary artery bypass graft, you notice increase bleeding from the coronary arteriotomy, how do you proceed?"
The concern is that the arrested myocardium is getting perfused. First

check that the aortic cross clamp is occlusive and the aortic root vent is on. A possible explanation for mild bleeding at the arteriotomy site is the presence of collateral circulation. If unable to identify a correctable cause, monitor for signs of electrical activity and consider cold topical saline, cooling the patient (mild hypothermia - 32° C), reducing flows as tolerated or more frequent administration of cardioplegia solution.

"Discuss the principles of cardioplegic arrest, how this is achieved by components of the cardioplegia solution, and name some common types of cardioplegia."

Minimizing myocardial oxygen demand is the primary principle of cardioplegic arrest. This is best achieved by rapid diastolic arrest after the aortic cross clamp is applied, thereby minimizing time of high ventricular work against a fixed afterload. Potassium is the most common electrolyte employed to produce diastolic arrest, and there are several common additional components, including sodium, citrate, and magnesium. Magnesium has been associated with decreased ventricular arrhythmias and improved cardiac performance in some studies. Histidine, Tryptophan, and Ketoglutarate (HTK) also comprises commonly used cardioplegia formulas. The cardioplegia solutions are cooled to 4° C which decreases myocardial oxygen consumption and diminishes contractile activity. Dextrose is used for glucose uptake and control of myocardial edema. Lastly, there are several iterations of blood and crystalloid ratios, but no evidence to support superiority, and preferences tend to be surgeon and/or institution specific.

"After placing the retrograde catheter you encounter some dark blood emerging from behind the heart. You check and notice a perforation of the coronary sinus."

The rigid catheter can perforate the sinus especially in older and frail patients. If this happens, initiate cardiopulmonary bypass, cross clamp and arrest with antegrade. Repair the perforation directly with prolene suture or with a pericardial patch (see Chapter 29, Vascular injuries.)

Pearls/pitfalls

In general there are a few things to consider when thinking about persistent activity which can be broadly grouped under "Access," "Collateral flow," and "Myocardial mass."

Access
- Are your retrograde and antegrade cannulas in place and properly connected?
- Is the retrograde too far and not protecting the RV despite antegrade?

Collateral flow
- Is the cross clamp completely occlusive?
- Is the right sided drainage adequate or do you need an additional cannula?
- Is there a persistent left sided SVC filling the right atrium?
- Is the left sided drainage adequate (is the root vent on or additional basket suckers in place; is there so much collateral flow that you need an LV vent)?
- Once drainage is optimized do you need systemic moderate hypothermia to 28-32° C to keep the residual collateral flow cool?

Myocardial mass
- Is the heart so hypertrophied that myocardial delivery of cardioplegia is inadequate—if so, address all of the above and try topical hypothermia?

Suggested readings
- Chambers DJ and Fallouh HB. Cardioplegia and cardiac surgery: Pharmacological arrest and cardioprotection during global ischemia and reperfusion. *Pharmacology and Therapeutics*. 2010. Issue 127 (41-52).
- Levitsky S and McCully J. Myocardial protection. Sellke FW et al (ed). *Surgery of the Chest*. Saunders. 8th Edition.
- Mentzer RM, Salik Jahinia M, Lasley RD. Myocardial Protection. Cohn L (ed). *Cardiac Surgery in the Adult*. McGraw Hill. 2008.
- Sa et al. Is there any difference between blood and crystalloid cardioplegia for myocardial protection during cardiac surgery? A meta-analysis of 5576 patients from 36 randomized trials. *Perfusion*. 2012. July.

Notes

29. Vascular injuries
Alykhan S. Nagji, MD, and John A. Kern, MD

Concept
- Recognition and control of venous injuries
- Strategies for repair of venous injuries

Chief complaint
"An 82 yo man with previous mitral valve repair presents after extensive cardiology work-up which revealed severe mitral regurgitation (MR) with plans for mitral valve replacement. He has no significant medical comorbidities and his only surgical history is a previous mitral valve repair. He is symptomatic from his MR and a holosystolic murmur is heard radiating to the axilla. His TTE demonstrates an ejection fraction (EF) of 30%. What are his options and how would you proceed?"

Differential
Both the diagnosis and surgical need have been established. (See Chapter 40, Reoperative mitral valve replacement for details of work up, management and operative steps.)

Tests
- Venous injuries related to mitral repair include AV groove disruption, injury to venous structures during sternal reentry, and coronary sinus tear with retrograde insertion. Some of these issues can be predicted ahead of time by reviewing the CT and cardiac catheterization.
- *CT scan*: determine the anatomy below the posterior table of the sternum (i.e., location and proximity of the innominate vein, vein grafts, atria, ventricle aorta, etc.).
- *Cardiac catheterization/plain films*: evaluate the mitral valve for MAC or crossing grafts.

Potential questions/alternative scenarios
"While performing your sternotomy, you encounter a significant amount of dark blood from the sternomanubrial junction."
- Remember this is a redo sternotomy and that by being higher up near the manubrium, this would be indicative of an innominate vein injury. Though you may be able to successfully control the innominate vein injury with direct pressure or sponge stick, the safest approach would be packing of the area along with having the sternum re-approximated so as to tamponade the bleeding.

- Cannulate peripherally (i.e., groin) and initiate cardiopulmonary bypass (CPB). This should decompress the heart and reduce the amount of bleeding from the injured innominate vein. Use of the pump suckers will help to capture any remaining blood. Once on CPB, reopen the chest and identify the injury. Carefully dissect out the innominate vein to achieve an adequate length without tension. This is key. Trying to repair it under tension will not work. Perform a repair with a Bovine or autologous pericardial patch using 5-0 or 6-0 Prolene suture (conservative approach). If the defect is small, a primary repair may be performed transversally without narrowing the vein. In a situation where the innominate vein is irreparable, it is safe to divide and oversew both ends of the vein. If the injury is far laterally this can be a big problem. Ligate the innominate vein down the middle to relieve tension. Try to repair the tear. If you cannot and the exposure is poor, consider a trapdoor incision (superior clavicular incision, anterior-thoracotomy into the 3rd intercostal space across the sternum to meet with the median sternotomy, elevate the hemithorax to expose and repair the injury (ligate or primary).

"Let us say that you enter the chest without incidence. The previous repair used cannulation through the right atrial appendage. However, during this reoperation you decide to cannulate the superior vena cava (SVC) directly. While dissecting the SVC you create a large hole. You do not have any purse string sutures in yet."

- Initial management should be to tamponade the SVC injury. Proceed with inferior vena cava (IVC) and aortic cannulation and initiate CPB with vacuum assisted venous drainage so as not to get an air lock. This, along with the use of pump suckers through the SVC injury will help to clear the field. If the injury is visible, it may be possible to cannulate through the injury and fix the injury at the end of the case.
- If still unable to view the SVC injury, the injury may be more severe and would necessitate more proximal control on the SVC using a Rummel tourniquet. You should also consider placing a pump sucker in the azygos vein to help drain upstream of the injury. An alternative is to ligate the azygos vein.
- Once able to view and evaluate the extent of the SVC injury, repair either primarily (as described previously) or with a Bovine or autologous pericardial patch. Then replace your SVC cannula away from the injury or through the RA.

"You were able to successfully cannulate through your SVC injury and proceed with the remainder of your mitral valve repair. You decide to use standard retrograde cardioplegia, but have difficulty placing your coronary sinus catheter. When administering your first dose of cardioplegia, you notice bright red blood pooling in the pericardial well. You lift the heart and see the end of your coronary sinus cannula."

At this time, you should pull the coronary sinus catheter out and protect the heart using antegrade cardioplegia during the course of your mitral valve replacement. You may need to place a few horizontal sutures prior to proceeding with the case to control the bleeding. But once the procedure is completed, if the injured area is still bleeding or friable place a Bovine or autologus pericardial patch using 5-0 or 6-0 Prolene in a running fashion.

"Changing the scenario completely, you now have a 64 yo female who is currently undergoing lead extraction. You are called urgently to the cath lab as the patient has just arrested and become hypotensive."

- Given that this was done under fluoroscopy, you should glean as much information from the cardiologist to help localize the injury in question. With these leads usually being heavily incorporated in the intima of the vessel wall there is a high likelihood of venous injury (in this case the SVC).

- Being that the chest is not open, you should cannulate via the groin and initiate CPB with vacuum assisted venous drainage. Once on CPB, open the chest and pericardium in the usual fashion. With the heart decompressed, identify the SVC and dissect enough length so as to obtain proximal and distal control from the site of injury. When identified, repair either primarily or patch as previously described.

- An alternative might be to open the chest right off the bat which decompresses the tamponade, apply manual compression of the injured vein, cannulate the aorta and RA and go on bypass.

"Taking another route, you have a 60 yo man who underwent a CABG and AVR just 4 months ago and has presented to the emergency room with chest pain and was found to have a Type A dissection. The patient crashes and a decision is made to percutaneously cannulate using the femoral artery and vein. You decide to use a 25 Fr Multi-stage venous cannula. During your venous cannulation the wires and dilators pass easily. However, you have difficulty passing your venous cannula, but it passes and you do have blood return. You complete your femoral cannulation and initiate CPB. When doing so, the patient continues to become hypotensive and you find there is decreased venous perfusion and low volume."

Goals are identifying the location of the injury, cannulating beyond it, and repair. Venogram if available for location otherwise rely on the history. At this time, you should be concerned about iliac vein injury. There are no clearly defined strategies to deal with such an injury. If the chest were open (not in this case) then you could centrally cannulate and repair the injury with aid of sucker bypass. Otherwise, gain access in the contralateral femoral vein and use this as your venous cannulation. Make sure to confirm placement and use a stiff wire. You should be beyond the injured iliac. Initiate CPB and decompress the heart. Repair the injured vein. If you have flouro you could try to get a wire across the injured vein and then a canula.

Bear in mind that the injury may be higher than the common iliac arteries (e.g., infrahepatic IVC). In this case you can try to cross the injury with a wire from the contralateral limb under fluoroscopy and stent the injury with your cannula. You would later need to explore the IVC through the abdomen for definitive repair. If you cannot cross the injury with a wire, then cannulate centrally to maintain distal perfusion while decompressing the venous system and plan for an abdominal exploration with local control and repair of the IVC injury. Sucker bypass can be used as an adjunctive maneuver. If you cannot or do not have time to cannulate centrally or peripheraly then explore and repair the injury directly. This is obviously a very bad situation in the setting of an aortic dissection.

"You are called to the cardiac cath lab for an SVC rupture during balloon dilation for SVC syndrome."

Ensure an airway, IV access, and blood transfusion. Heparinize and perform an emergency median sternotomy. Aortic and bicaval cannulation with the SVC cannula placed through the RA and carefully traversing the injury. Initiate CPB and empty out the heart. Inspect the defect. Large defects require patch closure while smaller ones are amenable to primary repair as long as the SVC is not narrowed. In this patient with SVC syndrome a patch with autologus pericardium is ideal. Other strategies for dealing with a high or large SVC injury include clamping the SVC and establishing distal drainage for the head vessels (i.e., upper SVC or innominate vein). Autologous or porcine pericardium can be used to repair the injury. A large tube conduit with a dacron graft can also be considered. Also as noted above, you can certainly cannulate peripherally prior to opening the chest but it depends on the degree of hypotension. In this scenario the patient was essentially tamponading. Always inquire about any contraindications to femoral arterial cannulation prior to going down that route.

"An 81 yo female patient is undergoing a mitral and tricuspid valve repair. Her tissues are noted to be very thin and frail. During bicaval cannulation the IVC purse string results in a large tear extending down below the diaphragm. How would you proceed?"

These injuries are not easy to control. The first step is to complete venous access and go on CPB as soon as you can. You can carefully pass the IVC cannula distal to the tear if you can see the distal extent. An occluding tape circumferential to the IVC and inferior to the injury may provide adequate exposure if there is room. Initiate CPB. Use fine prolene sutures or even a patch to repair the injury if you can see the distal extent from the mediastinum. Otherwise, go on with the SVC cannula and sucker bypass in the inferior pericardium. Have an assist manually control the bleeding in the IVC while you cannulate the femoral vein. You can try to traverse the injury with the femoral guide wire and then stent across with the cannula. If not at least establish drainage inferior to the tear. You can incise the diaphragm a bit from the mediastinum to expose the distal IVC but ultimately you may need to extend your midline incision into the abdomen and down along the right subcostal margin to expose and mobilize the liver infero-medially. This will allow exposure and repair of the retrohepatic IVC. Once the repair is done, readjust your drainage lines to ensure adequate exposure for your mitral and tricuspid repair.

"You are called to the cath lab because a patient who you were scheduled to perform a CABG on has had his RV punctured during an RV ablation. The pericardial drain placed in the cath lab is showing significant bloody drainage."

Transfer to the OR, emergency median sternotomy, place on CPB, arrest the heart and identify the puncture. Even if small, wide patch repair over the defect (autologous pericardium or other commercially available product). Bypass the orginal coronary lesions (usually with vein in emergency situations).

"You come off pump and are drying up after an ascending aneurysm replacement. You notice some continuous drainage from the left of the aorta. You retract the graft towards you and identify a 3 mm hole on the right pulmonary artery. What would you do?"

An injury to the PA can be lethal especially with a non-decompressed PA which has a paper thin wall. Have a pump in the room. Identify where you will cannulate if needed. Since this injury is small you can attempt a small figure-of-8 or purse string suture (fine) to oversew.

"When taking the bite through the PA it tears and there is significant bleeding. You had previously cannulated with right femoral vein and right axillary."

Have an assistant hold gentle pressure over the tear. Give heparin and cannulate for CPB. In this case, sew an end - end graft to the prior axillary graft. Cannulate the atrium or femoral vein and go on CPB. The PA will decompress. Dissect the PA off the underside of the aorta and ensure it is well mobilized without tension. Close the hole primarily with adventitial reinforcement or sew a pericardial patch. You can tack the PA to the underside of the aorta for extra hemostasis.

"You are cannulated and ready to go on CPB for an AVR. After cross clamping and beginning antegrade cardioplegia you notice some bleeding under the arch of the aorta but are unable to localize a source. You check all your cannulation sites which are fine and there is still bleeding. You dissect further along the posterior backside of the arch and notice bleeding opposite to the aortic cannula."

To address what appears to be a perforation of the backside of the aorta from the cannula you will almost certainly need circulatory arrest. If the bleeding is under control and the forward flow is good then cool with the existing cannula. Otherwise you might consider weaning off CPB and establishing axillary artery access. A small aortotomy and local repair should suffice to address the injury.

"After 20 mintues of cooling the temperature is 20° C. You stop the circulation, release the cross clamp and perform a transverse aortotomy near the injury which reveals a pinpoint tear opposite the aortic cannula. TEE showed no dissection and there is no grossly evident flap. You and are able to locally repair the tear with a horizontal mattress prolene stitch. You close the aortotomy, clamp distal to it and resume bypass. Circ arrest time was 6 minutes and you complete an uneventful AVR."

Pearls/pitfalls

- Perform the appropriate maneuvers to decompress the venous system in the presence of an injury.
- Consider peripheral cannulation when central cannulation would further exacerbate the problem or cannot be safely achieved.
- Have a low threshold to use Bovine or autologous pericardial patch to repair venous injures not amenable to primary repair.

Notes

30. Stable angina

Mark Kearns, MD, and Richard C. Cook, MD

Concept

- Indications for coronary artery bypass grafting (CABG)
- Preoperative evaluation
- Conduit selection and considerations
- Operative management
- Potential complications
- Alternative management strategies

Chief complaint

"You are asked to consult on a 72 yo man with a history exertional chest pain. Following a highly positive exercise treadmill test in the community, he was referred for coronary angiography. This reveals 3-vessel CAD with moderately depressed left ventricular (LV) function."

Differential

In this case, the diagnosis is established. It is still relevant, however, to broadly consider the cardiac and non-cardiac causes of chest pain and dyspnea.

History and physical

Patients with stable angina commonly present with exertional chest pain symptoms. The chest pain is usually gradual in onset and offset, reported as a diffuse chest discomfort that may radiate to the neck, lower jaw and arms, and is typically provocable with exercise, anxiety, cold, and after meals. Exertional dyspnea is a common associated symptom, reflecting pulmonary congestion from ischemia-mediated systolic and diastolic dysfunction. Canadian Cardiovascular Society Functional Class 3 (less than a block of walking) and 4 (mild activity) angina are typically indications for intervention. Other associated symptoms may include nausea, diaphoresis, fatigue, dizziness, and presyncope among others. Angina may present atypically, or be clinically silent in certain individuals, most notably in diabetics, elderly, and women. Comorbid conditions are sought out, particularly those that will impact outcomes and surgical treatment decisions (cerebrovascular disease, smoking, COPD, cardiovascular risk factors, renal disease, peripheral arterial and venous disease, peptic ulcers and gastrointestinal bleeding, bleeding diathesis, active infections, and alcohol use). Physical exam findings in stable angina are often nonspecific. Therefore, screening neurologic and head/neck exams (with attention to carotid bruits) should be performed in addition to focused cardiac, respiratory, abdominal and peripheral vascular exams. Evidence of previous chest, groin, and lower extremity surgery should be noted. An assessment should be made of the availability and quality of peripheral conduits. Assess arm dominance and plan to use the opposite hand for the radial artery if possible. Check an Allen's test in each hand and use a duplex-modified Allen's test for any uncertain cases. The ideal hand would be non-dominant, complete arch, good ulnar flow, and minimal artherosclerotic disease. Check for varicosities which make it unfavorable to use the vein.

Tests

- *Laboratory investigations.* Routine preoperative blood work. Check cardiac enzymes for evidence of acute coronary syndrome.
- *EKG.* Routinely performed to establish a baseline assessment of rate/rhythm, axis, complex morphologies, the presence of conduction system disease, left ventricular hypertrophy, and evidence of prior infarction. Note that acute coronary syndromes including unstable angina, STEMI, and NSTEMI are covered in Chapter 31, Acute myocardial infarction/unstable angina.
- *CXR.* Particular focus is on cardiac and pulmonary irregularities. Note should be made of cardiac or great vessel enlargement, cardiac and great vessel calcifications, the presence of pulmonary interstitial fluid and pericardial or pleural effusions.
- *Angiography.* Selective coronary angiography provides an assessment of coronary anatomy, stenoses, and flow. In addition, aortography can delineate aortic dimensions and calcification, and the presence of aortic valve pathology. Left ventriculography defines left ventricular size, function, and the presence of mitral valve pathology. Attention should be paid to the presence of coronary, epicardial, intra-cardiac, and great vessel calcifications. Lesions $\geq 70\%$ are significant and should be bypassed as long as the target vessel is at least 1.5 mm in diameter. Concomitant lesions > 50% may be "reasonable" to revascularize according to the 2011 AHA/ACC guidelines. LM lesions $\geq 50\%$ are significant. Physiologic studies may be used for questionable lesions. Fractional Flow Reserve (FFR) ≤ 0.8 is considered "significant." Syntax scores are being increasingly used to determine the complexity of the lesions. A score ≤ 22 is considered low and these lesions are reasonable candidates for PCI. A score ≥ 33 is high risk and benefits more from CABG.
- *Echocardiogram.* Routine preoperative echocardiogram to assess ventricular size and function, and to rule out concomitant valvular and aortic disease is reasonable.
- *Myocardial viability studies.* Used in patients with multivessel disease, low EF (< 50%) or extensive areas of akinesis to ensure that the bypass is to viable and salvageable myocardium. This is

especially helpful in high risk patients if there is any question about the utility of revascularization. PET scanning is the most common method used for this. Patients may already have had a PET scan prior to their angiogram. If the PET shows decreased perfusion with preserved F-fluorodeoxyglucose (FDG) uptake then this patient has viable myocardium that will benefit from revascularization. If there is extensive scar tissue as evidenced by decreased perfusion and decreased uptake then the benefits of revascularization are questionable. MRI is another viability study that is sometimes used.

- *Additional investigations.* Dictated by the presence of comorbid conditions. For example, carotid ultrasound in the patient with carotid bruits, or in symptomatic or high risk patients. If the CXR or angiogram raised suspicion for extensive cardiac or great vessel calcification, a computed tomography (CT) scan of the chest is justified, as their presence may impact operative strategies. PFTs for any evidence of pulmonary disease. These tests not only help with planning but also to better risk stratify the patient and provide a better sense of expected morbidity and mortality.

- *Conduit studies.* Venous mapping may be used to assess the suitability of saphenous veins for bypass. The mammary can be assessed by either chest duplex or direct injection during the angiogram.

Index scenario (additional information)

"This patient is a Type II diabetic (on oral agents) with hypertension, dyslipidemia, and a remote smoking history. There is a six-month history of retrosternal chest pain and dyspnea on exertion (CCS/NYHA II), which has worsened in the last month, prompting a visit to his primary care provider. Angiography reveals severe 3-vessel CAD, with high-grade proximal left anterior descending (LAD) and circumflex (Cx) stenosis (left-main equivalent) and a high-grade mid-distal right coronary artery (RCA) stenosis. Echocardiogram demonstrates hypokinetic antero-lateral wall segments with a resting LV ejection fraction of 40%. His EKG is negative for ST elevations and cardiac markers are negative."

Treatment/management

The major domains of treatment for chronic stable angina involve non-pharmacologic and pharmacologic measures, and revascularization. These are reviewed in the 2007 focused update of the 2002 ACC/AHA guidelines for management of patients with chronic stable angina. Briefly, non-pharmacologic measures include smoking cessation, limitation of alcohol intake, regular physical activity, dietary modification and weight loss. Pharmacologic measures aim to reduce symptom burden, and prevent myocardial infarction (MI) and death.

Antiplatelets (ASA), beta-blockers, and lipid lowering agents are routinely used in stable angina patients who are capable of tolerating them. Angiotensin converting enzyme inhibitors (ACEIs) are indicated in diabetics, or in patients with LV systolic dysfunction. Additional medications may be indicated in selected patients. Revascularization options depend on symptom burden, coronary anatomy, left ventricular function and coexisting conditions. Percutaneous coronary intervention (PCI) or CABG in patients with stable angina are considered for: a) highly symptomatic patients despite maximal medical therapy, b) patients desiring an improved quality of life (those not tolerating medical therapy, or who wish to increase their activity level), and c) patients with anatomy for which revascularization has a proven survival benefit. Cardiothoracic trainees should be familiar with indications for surgical revascularization, and the revascularization guidelines endorsed by the major international cardiovascular associations.

The main class I and class IIa indications for CABG (from the 2011 ACC/AHA guidelines for CABG) are as follows:

To improve survival
- Left main disease (> 50% stenosis) (I/B)
- Significant stenoses (> 70%) in 3 major coronary arteries, or in the proximal LAD and 1 other major coronary artery (I/B)
- Survivors of sudden cardiac death with presumed ischemia-mediated ventricular tachycardia (VT) caused by significant stenosis in a major coronary artery (I/B)
- Significant stenoses in 2 major coronary arteries with severe or extensive ischemia, or target vessels supplying a large area of viable myocardium (IIa/B)
- Mild-moderate LV systolic dysfunction and significant multivessel CAD or proximal LAD stenosis when viable myocardium is present in the region of intended revascularization (IIa/B)
- CABG with left IMA (LIMA) in patients with significant stenosis of the proximal LAD especially if supplying a large region of viable myocardium (IIa/B).

To improve symptoms
- CABG or PCI for 1 or more significant stenoses and disabling angina despite guideline directed medical therapy (GDMT) (I/A)
- CABG or PCI for 1 or more significant stenoses and disabling angina in cases where GDMT cannot be implemented (IIa/C)
- CABG is preferred over PCI for complex 3V Dz

In the United States, more than 80% of CABG cases are performed with the use of CPB. Off-pump CABG may be preferred in certain settings, although its capacity to reduce morbidity and mortality is controversial.

The patient in this scenario meets criteria for a CABG given the chronic symptoms and extensive CAD. In addition, he meets anatomic criteria for deriving a survival benefit with CABG over PCI. His low EF and diabetes also support this survival benefit. Given the low EF and hypokinetic myocardium he may benefit from a viability study. Choice of conduits would include a mammary and 2 vein grafts.

Operative steps

Goals – complete myocardial revascularization, while protecting head, heart, and body, and minimizing cardiopulmonary bypass (CPB) time.

- General anesthesia with endotracheal intubation, invasive arterial monitoring, central venous access, Swan-Ganz catheter.
- It is reasonable to routinely use trans-esophageal echocardiography (TEE) for pre and post-CPB cardiac assessment.
- Standard skin prep; draping of chest with groins and both legs exposed; arm(s) prepped and draped if radial arterial harvest is necessary.
- Median sternotomy, harvest of internal mammary artery (IMA) (left +/- right), harvest of other conduits concomitantly.
- Administration of heparin, with a goal activated clotting time (ACT) of greater than 480 seconds.
- "Inverse T" pericardiotomy, pericardial stay sutures, palpation of aorta.
- Aortic cannulation, right atrial (RA) cannulation with a two-stage venous cannula, and root cannulation for antegrade cardioplegia/aortic root vent +/- retrograde via coronary sinus.
- Initiation of CPB when target ACT achieved.
- Cross-clamp with antegrade cardioplegic arrest; consider retrograde as well if severe proximal
- disease. Intermittent maintenance doses of antegrade or retrograde cardioplegia throughout the cross-clamp
  period often augmented with cardioplegia down the vein grafts.
- Final preparation and review of conduits.
- Identification of epicardial coronary targets, assessment of quality and feasibility for grafting.
- Begin with the distal right. Deair and size the graft to the proximal aorta with the heart engorged. Hook up a caridoplegia line to the graft if desired. Move onto the circumflex then the L-LAD. The order may be institution specific.

- Performance of distal and proximal anastomoses -pay attention to anastomotic quality, lie of conduits, and adequacy of territorial perfusion via new grafts.
- For the proximals use running prolene suture, full thickness bites on the aorta, deair after the last proximal.
- Removal of cross-clamp, reperfusion.
- Placement of temporary epicardial pacemaker wires and chest drains.
- Weaning from CPB, de-cannulation, administration of protamine (mg) to heparin (mg) administered 0.5:1-1:1 , aiming to normalize ACT.
- Assessment of operative sites for hemostasis.
- Chest closure and transfer to cardiac surgery intensive care unit.

Potential questions/alternative scenarios

"What are the landmark trials comparing CABG to alternative therapies?"

The Veterans Administration Coronary Artery Bypass Surgery Cooperative Study (VA study, 1972-1974), the European Coronary Surgery Study (ECSS, 1973-1976), and the Coronary Artery Surgery Study (CASS, 1975-1979) were randomized controlled trials comparing CABG to medical therapy. The studies are divergent in terms of their patient cohorts, inclusion and exclusion criteria, and findings. The studies have several limitations and their generalizability to the current era, when medical therapy is markedly different, is also limited.

Numerous studies have compared CABG with plain old balloon angioplasty, and PCI (bare metal stents and drug-eluting stents). The patient cohorts differ in terms of anatomy, symptomatology, and left ventricular function. Cardiothoracic trainees should be familiar with the landmark studies, including contemporary studies such as the SYNTAX trial. Critical analysis of these studies is important to distinguish populations of patients who would be expected to derive a survival benefit with CABG, from those who would be expected to derive only symptomatic benefit, or no net benefit.

"What are the commonly used bypass conduits, and what are their expected long-term patency rates?"

Venous conduits

- Greater saphenous vein (GSV) is the most commonly used conduit in CABG surgery. It has a 10-year patency of between 50-60%. GSV grafts have different modes of failure over time. Other venous conduits include the lesser saphenous vein and the cephalic vein, which should be reserved for cases where no other conduit is available. The lesser saphenous and cephalic veins have markedly reduced patency rates compared with other CABG conduits.

Arterial conduits
- The left and right IMAs (LIMA and RIMA) have 10-year patency rates of > 90%. IMAs have a predilection to spasm and atrophy when grafted to targets without flow-limiting upstream stenoses. When grafting of the LAD is required, the LIMA should be used unless it is unavailable or of poor quality. The LIMA-LAD anastomosis is associated with an improved survival irrespective of age, sex, extent of CAD and LV systolic function. RIMA-LAD is reasonable when the LIMA is unavailable. Bilateral IMA grafting may be beneficial in selected patients (< 70 years old), but doing so in obese and/or diabetic patients is not recommended due to an increased risk of sternal wound complications. In order of preference, the RIMA should be considered to the LAD if LIMA not available, circumflex,or the RCA if the RCA has > 90% stenosis (critical stenosis).
- The radial artery has reported 5-year patency rates in the range of 83-95%. It is also susceptible to spasm and atrophy, and appears to have improved durability when grafted to targets with high-grade upstream stenoses and a reasonably large outflow territory. It is reasonable to use the radial artery to graft circumflex lesions with severe (> 70%) stenosis and right coronary lesions with critical (> 90%) stenoses, especially when supplying LV muscle.
- The gastroepiploic artery (GEA) has reported patency rates of 91, 80, and 62% at 1, 5, and 10 years respectively. It is most commonly used to graft right-sided target vessels, and should only be done in the context of critical upstream stenoses.
- The inferior epigastric artery (IEA) has a patency rate in the range of 90% at 1-year. It should only be used to graft targets with critical upstream stenoses.

"In which scenarios would you consider using all arterial, rather than venous conduits?"
Primarily in younger (60 years or younger according to the ACC/AHA CABG guidelines) patients, who stand to benefit from the longer patency rates associated with arterial grafts. Some surgeons prefer a more aggressive arterial revascularization strategy. Specific conduit, target vessel, and patient considerations related to the individual arterial graft are mentioned above.

"A patient is 75 yo and has 4 vessel disease involving the right, LAD, and 2 OMs. You are making your final assessment of the conduits and realize you do not have sufficient vein for all the anastomosis."
You can always sequence the 2 obtuse marginal branches using a vein

graft. Sequencing allows you to reach 2 different targets with a single conduit. Generally, you would like to make the venotomy and atriotomy on the distal most anastomosis slightly larger than the proximal target of the sequence to prevent steal into the proximal target.

"Upon transferring your 3 vessel CABG patient to the transport bed he has a cardiac arrest."
The most likely diagnosis is air into the graft or occlusion of a graft from a mechanical issue. Begin CPR according to ACLS guidelines while transporting the patient back to the OR table. Give heparin, perform an emergency re-entry, re-cannulate, and initiate CPB. Once you confirm good flows and drainage, assess the lie of your grafts. make any adjustments to the position of the grafts that is necessary. Check the TEE for air and function.

"Using a commercially available flow probe you realize that the vein graft to the PDA is occluded."
You will need to get more vein if available or begin harvesting the radial artery. Arrest the heart, expose the distal PDA and examine for any mechanical complications. If an obvious complication is identified you may be able to salvage the vein graft by re-doing it. Otherwise, redo the entire anastomosis with a new graft.

"While harvesting the mammary the patient becomes hypotensive and unstable."
Stop the harvest, give full dose heparin, replace your retractor with the standard sternal retractor, open the pericardium, cannulate the ascending aorta (if not calcified) and atrium. Initiate CPB. You can carefully complete your mammary harvest after securing your lines and replacing the retractor on bypass. (Note: have the pericardium open and lines available prior to mammary harvest in any high risk CABG with severe proximal disease ie 90% LM and occluded RCA.)

Pearls/pitfalls
- Know the presenting features of stable angina.
- Know which patient comorbidities impact treatment selection, operative planning, and anticipated risks/benefits in the short and long-term.
- Understand the treatment options for patients with stable angina (lifestyle, medical, interventional, surgical).
- Understand the key operative steps for CABG surgery, and the various options that exist for surgical revascularization (e.g., On-pump, OPCAB, MIDCAB, etc.).

Suggested readings

- Kouchoukos NT, Karp RB, Blackstone EH, et al, (eds). *Kirklin/Barratt-Boyes Cardiac Surgery*. 3rd ed. Philadelphia, PA: Churchill Livingstone; 2003.
- Hillis LD, Smith PK, Anderson JL, et al. 2011 ACCF/AHA Guidelines for Coronary Artery Bypass Graft Surgery. *J Am Coll Cardiol*. 2011;58 (24):e123-210.

Notes

31. Acute myocardial infarction/ unstable angina

Basil S. Nasir, MBBCh, and James E. Davies, Jr., MD

Concept

- Initial management of patients with acute myocardial infarction (MI)/unstable angina (UA) with a focus on patients in cardiogenic shock
- Define roles for percutaneous coronary intervention (PCI) and coronary artery bypass grafting (CABG)
- Perioperative anticoagulation strategies
- Critical steps for CABG
- Potential pitfalls and alternate scenarios

Chief complaint

"A 63 yo woman presents with acute onset crushing, substernal chest pain and dyspnea at rest lasting 1 hour. Her past medical history is significant for insulin-dependent diabetes mellitus, hypertension, and hyperlipidemia."

Differential

The initial distinction to make in these patients is stable angina versus acute coronary syndrome (ACS). The later includes unstable angina (UA) or non-ST elevation MI (NSTEMI) [often grouped together for management purposes] and ST elevation MI (STEMI). This further distinction is made on the basis of EKG tracing and cardiac markers. Symptoms occurring at rest rule out stable angina. Other potential diagnoses include acute aortic dissection and pulmonary embolism. In the event that all the above are ruled out, other pulmonary or gastrointestinal causes for the pain may be sought, including cholecystitis, pneumonia, peptic ulcer disease, etc. The initial management, including confirmation of the diagnosis as well as ruling out other pathology will be reviewed below.

History and physical

A full history should be undertaken with a focus on symptoms of chest pain, dyspnea or heart failure, and the chronicity of these symptoms. Assessment of past medical and social history to illicit risk factors for cardiac ischemia should also be performed. A full physical examination should be performed with attention to vital signs, neurological, cardiovascular and respiratory systems to help support the diagnosis and identify potential complications of MI or UA.

- *Laboratory studies.* Cardiac biomarkers are used to confirm the diagnosis of myocardial infarction. Complete blood count (CBC), coags, LFTs, blood gas, lactate and electrolyte panel including creatinine level should be obtained.
- *EKG.* EKG leads are placed in all 4 extremities with the ground typically in the right leg. Six precordial leads wrap around left thorax. Assessment for EKG abnormalities including ST changes, Q waves or T wave inversions may help delineate the myocardium at risk and the culprit vessel. EKG abnormalities in the inferior leads (II, III, aVf) and posterior findings (reciprocal changes in V1-2) suggest RV or RCA territory ischemia (or left dominant PDA disease). EKG abnormalities in the antero septal (V1-2), anteroapical (V3-4) or anterolateral (V5-6, I, aVL) suggest LV or LAD/LCx territory ischemia. Categorization of the myocardial infarction is based on ST changes and the initial clinical evaluation. Patients who present with angina-type symptoms for greater than 20 minutes with ST elevation > 1 mm in 2 contiguous leads or a new left bundle-branch block are diagnosed with an ST elevation myocardial infarction (STEMI). These patients are at greatest risk of transmural ischemia and are most often approached with PCI initially rather than CABG. Patients presenting with chest pain at rest lasting at least 10 minutes with elevated cardiac biomarkers or ST elevation of 0.5 to 1 mm or ST depression greater than 0.5 mm or T wave inversion greater than 1 mm are categorized as having non-ST elevation myocardial infarction (NSTEMI). These patients are more likely to have subendocardial ischemia rather than transmural. NSTEMI and UA patients are often grouped together for management purposes. The goal of management in UA/NSTEMI is prevention of a transmural MI (ST elevations +/- Q waves). The EKG is also helpful in assessment of arrhythmias.
- *CXR.* Evaluate for pulmonary edema, congestive heart failure, or other pulmonary pathology. A widened mediastinum may be a clue to a diagnosis of aortic dissection/aneurysm. Look for calcification of the aorta which should then prompt a CT for further evaluation.
- *Transthoracic echo.* Evaluate global LV and RV function (EF%), regional wall motion abnormalities, valvular dysfunction, septum (VSD), and pericardium (effusions). Regional wall motion abnormalities may reveal the coronary territories involved in the infarct (i.e., posteroseptal/posterior/inferior/diaphragmatic free RV wall - RCA or left dominant PDA; anteroseptal/apical - LAD; lateral wall - LCx). Type of wall motion abnormality may suggest the stage of infarction (i.e., hypokinetic - early, akinetic - old, dyskinetic - could be either).

- *Myocardial viability studies.* These will rarely be obtained in a patient with STEMI but may be useful in patients with chronic stable angina or history of prior infarct. A reasonable indication for a viability study would be a history of ischemia with low ejection fraction (< 50%) and extensive akinesis on echo. This is especially true in a high risk patient when it is unclear if revascularization will improve function or symptoms. Positron emission tomography (PET) scanning is the most common method used for this. If the PET shows decreased perfusion with preserved F-fluorodeoxyglucose (FDG) uptake then this patient has viable myocardium that will benefit from revascularization. If there is extensive scar tissue as evidenced by decreased perfusion and decreased uptake then the benefits of revascularization are questionable. MRI is another viability study that is being used.
- *Computed tomography (CT).* If the initial work-up for cardiac ischemia is negative, CT angio can be used to rule out pulmonary embolism, aortic dissection or other intra-abdominal pathology. CT is useful for ruling out ascending calcification if the CXR suggests excessive calcium.
- *Coronary angiogram*: gold standard for evaluating coronary lesions. Any lesion ≥ 70% is significant and thus a candidate for revascularization. Concomitant lesions > 50% may be reasonable to revascularize during open heart surgery for other issues. LM lesions ≥ 50% are significant. Physiologic studies may be used for questionable lesions. Fractional Flow Reserve (FFR) ≤ 0.8 is considered "significant."

Index scenario (additional information)
"History reveals similar episodes of chest pain in the past, but lasting less than 10 minutes. Physical exam shows a diaphoretic woman with cool, clammy peripheries. Her heart rate is 120 beats per minute and blood pressure is 80/40 mmHg. The rest of the exam is unremarkable. Serum troponin levels are shown to be 10.2 µg/L (normal is < 0.1) and EKG shows ST elevation (> 1 mm) in leads V2 – V5. CXR is unremarkable."

Treatment/management
The diagnosis is cardiogenic shock secondary to an acute anterior STEMI. Initial medical therapy includes aspirin, nitroglycerin, morphine and supplemental oxygen. Heparin is often used as well especially in UA/NSTEMI patients awaiting surgery. Plavix is used if it is likely that a percutaneous intervention will be performed. If Plavix is given it is advisable to wait 5 days prior to CABG when possible (most applicable to UA/NSTEMI or stable angina). Ask about any other GPIIb/IIIa receptor blockers. Beta blockers, although indicated in patients with

coronary ischemia, are contraindicated in this case due to hypotension. Appropriate venous access, with a central line if needed, is established. Invasive arterial monitoring and pulmonary artery catheters are helpful in guiding resuscitation.

Optimizing cardiac filling pressures should be undertaken by using fluid resuscitation or diuretics depending on the situation. Pulmonary capillary wedge pressures (PCWP) should be kept in the 16-22 mmHg range. Additional medical therapy includes use of inotropic agents such as milrinone, dobutamine or epinephrine to augment cardiac contractility once filling pressures are optimized. Vasopressors, such as phenylephrine or vasopressin, may be indicated, but they should be used with caution as they can cause an increase in afterload and other negative effects.

Intra-aortic counterpulsation
Use of an intra-aortic balloon pump (IABP) is helpful in cases of refractory shock despite initial medical management or in patients with major complications of myocardial infarction such as postinfarction ventricular septal defect (VSD) or acute papillary muscle rupture. It is also helpful for patients with UA/NSTEMI awaiting surgery.

The IABP is inserted via the femoral artery. The tip of the balloon should be positioned in the descending thoracic aorta just distal to the left subclavian artery. The position could be estimated at the time of insertion using the manubriosternal junction (angle of Louis) as an external landmark. Position could be confirmed by CXR, echocardiography or by fluoroscopy if placed at the time of catheterization. The IABP is set to inflate during diastole, just after the aortic valve closes, which is signified by the dicrotic notch on the arterial blood pressure tracing. The balloon deflates as late as possible during diastole, just before the aortic valve opens, which is marked by the onset of the R wave on the EKG tracing. By increasing coronary flow during diastole and decreasing afterload during systole the IABP improves myocardial oxygen supply and demand. Severe aortic insufficiency and peripheral vascular disease are contraindications for IABP.

Reperfusion strategies
Despite initial medical therapy and stabilization of the patient, establishing reperfusion of the ischemic myocardium is most important. Options include thrombolysis, PCI and CABG. In the setting of an STEMI, PCI is first line therapy. The goal should be door-to-balloon time of 90 minutes or less. In hospitals with limited access to interventional cardiology expertise, thrombolysis is a reasonable alternative. CABG has a limited role, and has largely been replaced by PCI as first line therapy.

260

Once the culprit lesion is identified and treated with a balloon angioplasty, the decision has to be made to proceed with PCI and intracoronary stenting or CABG for definitive revascularization. Emergency CABG is indicated in the following situation:

- Patients in whom primary PCI has failed or cannot be performed, AND...
- Coronary anatomy is suitable for CABG, AND...
- Persistent ischemia of a significant area of myocardium at rest and/or hemodynamic instability refractory to nonsurgical therapy is present.

OR...

- Patients with mechanical complication of MI including papillary muscle rupture, post-infarction VSD or left ventricular rupture. Note that these are late complications which typically occur 5 to 7 days following MI.

There are situations where emergency CABG may be preferred over PCI even in the setting of an acute STEMI and they generally revolve around scenarios where the lesions are not favorable for complete revascularization with PCI:

- Left main disease > 50% → PCI has become a reasonable alternative in the setting of an STEMI according to most experts although surgery is still the default option. If the patient's lesion is such that the anatomy is favorable for PCI, with a low syntax score, low chance of periprocedural complications and the patient is at high risk for CABG then PCI is the intervention of choice. Otherwise go to CABG.
- Left main equivalent (> 70% stenosis in the proximal left anterior descending (LAD) and circumflex arteries). Similar considerations to that discussed for LM (high risk patient, good anatomy, low syntax - consider PCI if its faster).
- Severe 3-vessel disease → CABG, especially if diabetic, reduced ejection fraction (EF) < 50%, high syntax score (> 32).

Operative steps
Coronary artery bypass grafting in the setting of acute MI and cardiogenic shock.
Note: Preoperatively, have a sense of the degree of end organ damage that has already occurred. Check lactate, LFTs, creatinine. If the patient has already suffered a significant amount of end organ injury, then stabilizing the patient with mechanical support (IABP versus ECMO versus VAD) may be reasonable until some reversal of end organ effects has occurred prior to surgery. If you decide to go to surgery, bear in mind that there is data suggesting waiting for at least 24 hours after the infarct has occurred prior to CABG unless you can revascularize within

6 hours of the infarct. There is some conflicting evidence regarding this issue and thus, the most prudent decision would be revascularize as soon as possible unless there is severe end organ dysfunction. The official ACC/AHA 2011 guidelines support emergency revascularization "irrespective" of the time from MI to CABG.

- Large bore peripheral intravenous access, radial arterial line, central venous line, pulmonary artery catheter, urinary catheter.
- General endotracheal anesthesia. Pre-induction IABP is recommended, especially in patients with reduced EF. Patients taken directly to surgery from the catheterization lab should have an IABP placed prior to transfer.
- Intraoperative transesophageal echocardiogram. Check for complications including ischemic mitral regurgitation (MR), left ventricular rupture, etc.
- Median sternotomy.
- Choice of conduit: Based on American Heart Association guidelines, use of the left internal mammary artery (LIMA) for LAD bypass is reasonable, even in the urgent setting. If the patient is unstable, and salvage surgery is undertaken, then vein grafts are acceptable because of the reduced time in harvesting the conduit.
- Open the pericardium, check the aorta for plaque and have lines available prior to LIMA harvest.
- Give heparin (400 units/kg).
- Arterial cannulation: Cannulation of the ascending aorta is preferred. Palpate the aorta and look for plaques. Epiaortic ultrasound is an adjunctive measure.
- *Venous cannulation*: two-stage cannula via the right atrial appendage.
- *Myocardial protection.* Place antegrade cardioplegia catheter/aortic root vent in the ascending aorta. Place a retrograde catheter in the coronary sinus. Remember to de-air cardioplegia lines prior to connecting them.
- Check activated clotting time (ACT). If ACT > 480 seconds, initiate CPB at normothermia or mild hypothermia.
- It may be helpful to identify targets for the distal anastomoses prior to cross clamping, as that may be difficult in the arrested heart, especially if targets are small.
- *Prepare for aortic cross clamp.* Reduce arterial flow. Apply cross clamp. Go back up to full flow (2.0-2.5 L/min/m^2). Arrest the heart with antegrade cardioplegia followed by retrograde cardioplegia.

- *Distal anastomoses.* Usually start with the right sided grafts. In the case of vein grafts, instillation of blood cardioplegia down the vein graft after finishing the distal anastomosis is encouraged. In general, 7-0 or 8-0 polypropylene suture is used in a running fashion. For the LIMA graft, make sure the graft is occluded with a bulldog clamp while the heart is arrested to ensure adequate myocardial protection.
- *Proximal anastomoses.* Make sure that the vein grafts are not twisted and there is enough slack to allow for distension of the heart when it fills. Create aortotomy. In general, 5-0 polypropylene in running fashion is used.
- Remove aortic cross clamp. Consider terminal infusion of warm blood cardioplegia or "hot shot" in patients with left ventricular dysfunction prior to removing cross clamp.
- Check for hemostasis and wean from CPB.
- Give protamine.
- Place temporary atrial and ventricular pacing wires. Place chest tubes and close.

Potential questions/alternative scenarios

"Patient with acute NSTEMI, hemodynamically stable and meets indications for CABG."

Maximize the patient medically with heparin, ASA, oxygen, and IABP if refractory angina or low EF. Plan for urgent CABG. As mentioned above for revascularization in the setting of acute STEMI, some studies recommend waiting 1-3 days but ACC/AHA 2011 guidelines recommend revascularization irrespective of the timing between MI and CABG. Thus, in general proceed to the OR ASAP although you can afford a short delay of 24 hrs if the patient remains exceedingly stable. Outcomes may be better with the later approach.

"A 70 M patient is resuscitated from a witnessed cardiac arrest. Coronary angiography shows 3 V disease."

Urgent CABG is indicated for patients who have suffered a sudden cardiac arrest or life threatening arrhythmia due to ischemic disease.

"Patient with inferior infarction and right ventricular involvement."

In general, similar considerations regarding timing of OR apply here as well. The assumption is that PCI has failed, or the patient has severe three vessel disease that is more amenable to CABG. Thus, CABG should be considered in an urgent fashion. The one caveat is that outcomes are poor in the setting of severe right heart failure, despite adequate revascularization and myocardial protection. In this setting, it may be preferred to delay CABG until the RV is optimized with inotropes, diuretics, or even mechanical support as needed depending on the degree of shock.

"Patient with recent MI and drug-eluting stent (DES), now presents for CABG."

The question of what do with a recently stented artery is controversial. If the stent is compromised, then it is reasonable to place a vein graft distal to the stent. If the stent is wide open without stenosis, any graft placed distal to it is likely to fail due to competitive flow. It is reasonable to leave that vessel alone, and just graft other compromised vessels.

"The above alternative patient is less than 1 year out from his DES placement. He is currently on clopidogrel and presents for urgent CABG 2 days after a NSTEMI."

Stopping the clopidogrel for 7 days carries a high risk for in-stent thrombosis since the DES is less than 1 year old (30 days in the setting of a bare metal stent). Performing surgery < 24 hrs after stoping plavix increases the risk of bleeding. The best scenario is to discontinue the plavix for 5 days in the elective setting or at least 24 hrs in the urgent setting. Short-acting antiplatelet agents, such as eptifibatide or tirofiban should be discontinued for at least 2 to 4 hours before surgery and abciximab for at least 12 hours before surgery. Clopidogrel is resumed shortly after surgery (usually the next day). If there is concern about in stent thrombosis due to an inability to resume plavix for any reason then it may be reasonable to place a vein graft distal to the stented vessel, regardless of patency.

If you find yourself operating urgently on clopidogrel, there are no good options to reduce the risk of bleeding. Antifibrinolytic agents, such as aminocaproic acid, should be used. There is a higher risk of postoperative bleeding and increased transfusion requirements. Platelet transfusion is helpful in this setting, even if the platelet count appears adequate, as native platelets are dysfunctional.

"Patient with history of MI. Echocardiogram shows akinetic myocardium."

In this setting dobutamine echocardiography, thallium imaging or positron emission tomography (PET) are useful. If hibernating myocardium is identified, then that region will benefit from revascularization. Infarcted myocardium will not.

"Seven days post-CABG, a patient complains of pleuritic chest pain and a fever. There is an associated lymphocytosis."

This likely represents postpericardiotomy syndrome, or if following an AMI, Dressler's syndrome. A pericardial rub may be present. The associated leukocytosis is predominated by lymphocytes or eosinophils. It is important to rule out other infectious complications, especially pneumonia. The diagnosis is one of exclusion. The treatment includes non-steroidal anti-inflammatory agents for 1 to 3 months. If this fails, then a course of steroids should be started. Colchicine has also been described in cases with persistent symptoms.

Pearls/pitfalls

- Distinguish between STEMI and NSTEMI/UA. The former is almost always treated with PCI while the later is more likely to be considered for CABG if anatomy is suitable (LM, 3V Dz).
- CABG is indicated in STEMI for failed PCI, mechanical complications of MI and cardiogenic shock if anatomy is unfavorable for PCI.
- If urgent CABG is indicated and the patient can be stabilized medically, it may be beneficial to delay surgery for 1-3 days.
- Pre-induction IABP placement is recommended for emergency CABG.
- If possible, stop plavix at least 24 hours prior to surgery and preferably 5 days before surgery.

Suggested readings

- Geroge I and Oz MC. Myocardial revascularization after acute myocardial infarction. Cohen LH (ed). Cardiac Surgery in the Adult. 2008;669-697.
- Hillis LD, et al. 2011 ACCF/AHA Guideline for Coronary Artery Bypass Graft Surgery: Executive Summary. Circulation. 2011;124:2610-2642.
- Antman EM, et al. ACC/AHA Guidelines for the Management of Patients With ST-Elevation Myocardial Infarction. Circulation. 2004;110:e82-e292.
- Jneid H, et al. 2012 ACCF/AHA Focused Update of the Guideline for the Management of Patients With Unstable Angina/Non–ST-Elevation Myocardial Infarction (Updating the 2007 Guideline and Replacing the 2011 Focused Update). Circulation. 2012;126:875-910.

Notes

32. Redo coronary artery bypass surgery
Eric Griffiths, MD, and Gorav Ailawadi, MD

Concept
- Indications for redo coronary artery bypass grafting (CABG)
- Preoperative considerations
- Conduit choices
- Critical steps of redo CABG
- Pitfalls and alternative solutions

Chief complaint
"A 73 yo man with history of CABG 12 years prior now has recurrent chest pain for 3 months and multivessel disease of both native arteries and vein grafts on repeat catheterization. He is referred to you for possible repeat surgical revascularization."

Differential
Recurrent CAD versus other non coronary etiologies. Reoperation is indicated in symptomatic patients with ischemia who have evidence of myocardial viability or who demonstrate large areas of myocardium at risk from progression of their disease.

History and physical
Confirm presence of symptoms, evaluate functional status. Identify comorbidities that may affect surgical risk: chronic obstructive pulmonary disease, end stage renal disease, peripheral vascular disease, stroke, or arrhythmias. On exam, evaluate carotid artery/bruits, quality of potential conduits such as vein and radial arteries, and signs of congestive heart failure. Obtain prior operative report.

Tests
- *EKG*: evaluate for arrhythmias, prior MI (Q waves), Bundle branch blocks indicating damage to conduction system.
- *Echo*: evaluate LV function, wall motion abnormalities, valvular function.
- *Cardiac catheterization*: review prior angiograms if possible.
  - Identifies location and degree of stenosis in native coronary, saphenous vein graft (SVG) and arterial conduits.
  - Injection of internal mammary arteries bilaterally should be performed to eval patency or for use as possible conduits.

- *Myocardial viability studies*: restored perfusion to ischemic or underperfused myocardium may lead to improved contractility. Revascularized scar tissue will not provide improvement.
    - Thallium scintigraphy.
    - Dobutamine stress echo.
    - *Positron emission tomography (PET)*: evaluates uptake of FDG as marker of cardiac metabolic activity.
    - Cardiac MRI.
- *CT chest*: evaluate relationship of sternum and underlying mediastinal structures including bypass graft locations, degree of aortic calcification.
- CT abd/pelv to evaluate femoral vessels for possible peripheral bypass.
- *Potential conduit studies*. Venous duplex and mapping for presence and adequacy of saphenous vein, Allen's test/arterial Doppler for radial conduit, cardiac catheterization to inject the mammary arteries and chest wall mammary duplex studies.

Index scenario (additional information)

"The patient has hypertension, moderate COPD. Echo shows EF of 45% with inferior and lateral wall motion abnormalities, and no valvular disease. Cardiac catheterization shows occlusion of SVG to PDA, 80% stenosis of SVG to OM, and patent LIMA to LAD, and 80% stenosis of proximal circumflex. Cardiac MRI shows viable myocardium in the inferior and lateral walls. How would you proceed?"

Treatment/management

The patient appears to be a candidate for surgical revascularization. Percutaneous coronary intervention (PCI) is an option for patients with discrete, focal disease with minimal myocardial areas at risk. This patient has an occluded SVG to an area with viable myocardium. This lesion is typically not accessible via PCI making it necessary for him to undergo redo CABG. Additionally he has large areas of myocardium at risk and is a functional/active patient. Redo CABG has higher risk than primary revascularization with operative mortality rates ranging from 6.9-11% mostly due to increased risk of perioperative myocardial infarction (MI). Causes include incomplete revascularization, atheromatous emboli from diseased SVGs or aorta, damaged grafts, hypoperfusion through new grafts, or early graft occlusion.

Operative steps

- *Redo sternotomy*: increase risk due to adhesions to underlying structures including right ventricle, innominate vein, right atrium, aorta, lung and patent coronary bypass grafts.

- *Evaluate need for possible peripheral cardiopulmonary bypass*: closely adherent right ventricle, pulmonary artery or aorta (see Chapter 36, Redo aortic valve replacement for alternative cannulation strategies).
  - If so place femoral arterial and venous lines.
  - Axillary artery cannulation with end to side tube graft if warranted.
- Proceed with division of the anterior table of the sternum using oscillating saw, posterior table divided using Mayo scissors.
  - Avoid excessive traction on underlying structures.
  - Separate mediastinal structures from chest wall.
- Harvest the internal mammary artery (left, right, or both), if not previously used, may be performed after sternotomy, cannulation, or once on bypass depending on the stability of the patient.
- Intra-pericardial dissection.
  - Avoid excessive manipulation of venous bypass grafts "no touch technique." Avoids embolization of debri.
- Cannulation.
  - Once aorta dissected out, palpate or use epiaortic U/S for safe cannulation site as well as sites for proximal grafts.
  - Consider axillary or femoral bypass for excessive atherosclerotic disease.
  - Venous cannulation through right atrium using multi stage cannula. If unable to clear safe site on atrium due to prior vein grafts or if adhesions to the right atrium are extensive, consider femoral venous cannulation or bicaval cannulation.
- Initiate CPB, dissect out the aorta to make sufficient room for antegrade and cross clamp.
- *Myocardial protection strategy*: combination of antegrade and retrograde cardioplegia. Antegrade cardioplegia alone may not protect areas supplied by patent pedicled internal mammary artery grafts and may dislodge debri in SVGs. Retrograde allows possible washout of coronary debri as well as access to myocardial areas of occluded arterial grafts. Protection of the right ventricle may not be complete with retrograde only cardioplegia. Clamping of patent arterial grafts ensures uniform cooling. If safe, the LIMA can be clamped in tissue between left side of the aorta and medial surface of the left lung (check its trajectory on the CT scan). If this area is difficult to dissect, consider leaving LIMA patent. Do not risk injuring a patent LIMA. If intend to keep LIMA patent, use frequent antegrade and retrograde cardioplegia and consider cooling the patient to 28-30° C.

- *Revascularization strategy*: determine vessels/conduits to be bypassed and conduits to be used. Consider replacing older (> 5 yr) SVG when high degree of atherosclerosis is present. Must be individualized based on degree of stenosis, availability of conduit, and patient risk.
  - Avoid manipulation of SVGs to avoid embolization of atheroma.
  - Stenotic SVGs can be left in place or divided and replaced with new SVG .
  - When replacing stenotic SVG with arterial graft, should leave SVG in place in order to prevent hypoperfusion syndrome (worsening myocardial ischemia or infarction).
  - If possible place left internal mammary artery (LIMA) graft to left anterior descending artery (LAD) or other large vessel perfusing a large ischemic region.
- *Distal sites of anastomosis*: may consider reusing prior distal site when replacing SVG with another depending on degree of disease present there. Otherwise consider "landing" on native coronary distal to prior anastomosis.
- Sites for proximal anastomosis may be limited due to prior involvement on the reoperative aorta.
  - Consider sequencing vein grafts to minimize number of proximal anastomoses.
  - Arterial free grafts can be anastomosed to the hood of new or old SVG due to lack of atherosclerotic involvement there, or can be sewn to other arterial grafts for a "Y" type anastomosis.
- Arterial grafts.
  - LIMA to LAD if not previously performed.
  - Right internal mammary artery (RIMA) to right coronary artery/posterior descending artery or through transverse sinus to circumflex/proximal obtuse marginal. Transverse sinus is typically adherent and requires dissection. Also consider utilizing the RIMA as a free graft.
  - *Radial artery free graft*: affected by competitive flow, best if stenosis > 70% and used to a large vessel/large runoff territory.

Potential questions/alternative scenarios
"Patient fails to wean from bypass."
Check ABG, electrolytes (K+), assess degree of inotropic support, adequate volume and heart rate. Transesophageal echo (TEE) useful for assessing for old/new wall motion abnormalities, volume status of the

heart, presence of unrecognized valvular dysfunction, and possible air in the aortic root. For visible air in the bypass graft, the vein can be clamped and deaired with a small 27g needle. A balloon pump may be necessary. These are longer operations on chronically ischemic hearts and patients are prone to myocardial dysfunction postoperatively. Myocardial protection has to be as optimal as possible (see Chapter 27, Cardiopulmonary bypass pitfalls).

Assess all grafts for adequate positioning (no kinks). Doppler assessment of new constructed graphs to check for patency. If poor flow with associated regional abnormality on TEE, grafts to that area should be reconstructed immediately. Revision can be performed by clamping and arresting the heart. Alternatively, if familiar with off-pump CABG techniques, can use cardiac stabilizer while on full cardiopulmonary bypass and revise the distal anastomosis (but be cautious, it went down for a reason so you want to have optimal conditions the second time). If low cardiac output or regional abnormalities persist, then proceed to intra-aortic balloon pump placement (IABP). If IABP and inotropes fail, then consider placing mechanical ventricular support (ECMO, Abiomed, CentriMag, Impella, or other).

"No room on the aorta for proximal anastomosis."
Other locations for proximals include end- to- side anastomosis to patent arterial grafts, using the hood of patent old or new SVGs. Even occluded SVGs may have a patent hood that can be used. Consider using the RIMA in situ such that a proximal aortic site is not needed.

"You are doing the redo sternotomy and encounter bright red blood before sternum is open. You now see EKG changes."
Suspect coronary/graft injury. Heparinize and urgently place the patient on femoral bypass, open the sternum and expeditiously continue your dissection. If you can identify the injured coronary you can either repair it or place a coronary perfusion catheter in the lumen to perfuse the area with warm blood. Continue operation. Replace injured vein graft.

"You heparinize, cannulate and dissect out the ascending aorta making enough room for cross clamping and antegrade access. The ACT is 480. Unfortunately, you injure the patent mammary while attempting to dissect it near the lung. Almost immediately you notice hemodynamic changes and regional wall motion abnormalities."
Initiate CPB, clamp and arrest the heart. Try to repair the injured mammary. If not it will have to be replaced. Note that this illustrates the importance of being ready to clamp and arrest prior to dissecting out a patent mammary.

- Review cath films, ensure myocardial viability in areas with diseased grafts.
- Thorough preoperative planning including op note, cannulation strategy and conduit assessment.
- Minimize manipulation of old SVGs.
- Make every effort to place LIMA on LAD if not done previously.
- SVGs that are bypassed by arterial conduit should be left in place.
- Be prepared to clamp and arrest when dissecting out a patent mammary.

Suggested readings

- Barreiro CJ and Bansal A. Reoperative coronary artery bypass surgery. Yuh D, Vricella LA, and Baumgartner WA (eds). *Johns Hopkins Manual of Cardiothoracic Surgery* 2007.
- Lytle BW. Re-do coronary artery bypass surgery. Little AG (editor). *Complications in Cardiothoracic Surgery: Avoidance and Treatment.* 1st ed. Blackwell Futura. 2004.

Notes

33. Post-infarction ventricular septal defect

Aaron J. Weiss, MD, and Joanna Chikwe, MD

Concept
- Presentation of post-infarction VSD and LV aneurysm
- Diagnosis and workup
- Operative timing and approaches
- Pitfalls and alternative solutions

Chief complaint
"A 65 yo man was admitted to the hospital with chest pain, and diagnosed with an acute anteroseptal myocardial infarction for which he underwent percutaneous coronary intervention. He was recovering on the floor four days later when he developed new chest pain and breathlessness."

Differential
Post-myocardial infarction ventricular septal defect, free wall rupture, tamponade, acute papillary muscle rupture, pulmonary embolism, aortic dissection/rupture, and ongoing ischemia/infarction

History and physical
If patient is stable and alert, a short and focused history to elicit chest pain and dyspnea, calf or leg pain (possible deep vein thrombosis leading to a pulmonary embolism). Focused physical exam should include vital signs, a full neurological, cardiac with attention to new murmurs, lung, and extremities exam. In addition, one should focus on signs of right-sided heart failure (jugular venous distention (JVD), peripheral edema, etc.).

Tests
- *EKG.* Rule out ongoing or additional ischemic events, any arrhythmias.
- *Echo.* This is diagnostic. Color flow Doppler echocardiography shows the size and location of the VSD, ventricular function, mitral regurgitation, pulmonary artery and right-sided pressures, and rules out free wall rupture/tamponade.
- *Right heart catheterization.* Right heart catheterization shows a step-up in oxygenation between the right atrium and pulmonary artery (> 9% is diagnostic). Other information obtained includes an elevated pulmonary-to-systemic flow ratio (ranges from 1.4:1 to 8:1 and correlates with size of defect).

- *Left heart catheterization.* Most patients undergo this at the time of their initial presentation with acute myocardial infarction. In stable patients without a recent cardiac catheterization left heart catheterization will guide the decision to perform concomitant surgical revascularization. In unstable patients it is reasonable to omit this diagnostic modality.

Index scenario (additional information)

"On physical exam, patient is found to be hypotensive. There is a new harsh holosystolic murmur most prominent at the left lateral sternal border that radiates to the axilla and is associated with a thrill. Coarse breath sounds heard bilaterally. No JVD or peripheral edema noted. EKG shows no new changes from the EKGs performed since admission. Emergency echocardiogram performed at the bedside shows a large new anterior VSD."

Treatment/management

The natural history of untreated postinfarction VSD is poor (25% mortality rate within 24 hours, 50% mortality rate within one week, 80% within one month, 97% at 1 year). Postinfarction VSD is therefore an indication for urgent surgery.

Preoperatively, management should include reducing afterload to decrease the left-to-right shunt, maintain cardiac output and peripheral perfusion so as to avoid end-organ damage, and increase coronary perfusion pressure. These goals can be accomplished through the use of an intra-aortic balloon pump (IABP) as well as pharmacologic therapy with inotropic agents. As surgical mortality is directly proportional to duration of cardiogenic shock and multi-organ failure pre-operatively, current emphasis is on early surgical intervention. A small percentage of patients severely compromised by multi-organ failure may benefit from mechanical assistance such as biventricular support or ECMO for temporary salvage before more definitive surgery can be performed.

Operative steps

Repair of anterior septal rupture

- Arterial line, general endotracheal anesthesia, central line with large bore access (no pulmonary artery catheter), urinary catheter, transesophageal echocardiography (TEE).
- Median sternotomy, conduit harvest (saphenous vein, and left internal mammary artery in stable patients if coronary revascularization is planned), heparin 400 mg/kg, ascending aorta cannulation, bicaval cannulation, antegrade cardioplegia cannula, retrograde cardioplegia cannula, left ventricular vent through the right superior pulmonary vein, +/- systemic cooling to 25° C, once

ACT is 480 initiate cardiopulmonary bypass (CPB), CO_2 insufflation.

- Deair antegrade line and run antegrade induction, followed by retrograde perfusion via the coronary sinus. Additional myocardial protection can be obtained by running cold blood cardioplegia during the VSD repair via retrograde coronary sinus catheter.
- Perform coronary bypasses: cardioplegia can be administered via the grafts prior to completion of the proximal anastomoses.
- Left ventricular transinfarct incision with infarctectomy is performed. Debride necrotic septal myocardium even enlarging the defect if needed. Place pledgeted interrupted horizontal mattress sutures around the defect. Pass the sutures through a felt strip then through the septum from right to left and then snap. Continue along the posterior rim. Along the anterior rim, pass the sutures from epicardium to endocardium. Then pass all the sutures symmetrically through a Dacron prosthetic patch. All sutures are pledgeted again and then tied down. Reapproximate the edges of the ventriculotomy with a double layer closure buttressed with Teflon felt or glutaraldehyde-preserved bovine pericardium.
- If used, biological glue is most effective if applied on dry myocardium in the decompressed, arrested heart i.e., prior to cross-clamp removal.
- Deair, wean from CPB, intraoperative TEE to assess for any residual VSD/shunt/left ventricular function/mitral regurgitation, if not already in place, an IABP may be necessary to help wean off bypass.

Potential questions/alternative scenarios
"On intraoperative TEE, the VSD appears to be apical. How would your operative technique differ?"
The same basic set-up as for an anterior septal rupture. Incision is made through the infarcted ventricular apex and the surgeon should debride any necrotic myocardium involving the left ventricle, right ventricle, and septum. Reapproximate the remaining apical portions to the apical septum using interrupted mattress sutures of 1-0 Tevdek passed sequentially through a buttressing strip of Teflon felt, the left ventricle, a second strip of felt, the septum, a third strip of felt, the right ventricle, and a fourth strip of felt. Tie these sutures down and then reinforce the closure with an over-and-over suture to ensure hemostasis.

"On intraoperative TEE, the VSD appears to be posteroinferior. How would your operative technique differ?"
Place the patient on CPB and arrest the heart. Retract the heart out of the pericardial well as you would for a bypass graft to the PDA. Trans-infarct incision is made through the left ventricle 1 cm lateral to the PDA.

Debridement of necrotic left ventricular septal myocardium is performed. Inspect the mitral apparatus for any papillary muscle infarct. Less aggressive debridement of the right ventricle is performed as you only want to resect as much as necessary to achieve adequate visualization of the defect. If the posterior septum has separated from the free wall, it can be re-approximated primarily using a double-layered buttressed closure. Larger defects require patch closure as described earlier with the only difference being that the sutures are placed from the right side of the septum and from the epicardial side of the right ventricular free wall. Afterwards, a separate patch closure of the infarctectomy using Dacron graft maybe required versus a buttressed double layer primary repair depending on the size of the free wall defect. Primary closure of a large tissue defect has historically resulted in very poor outcomes. Check for hemostasis, deair, and wean from CPB.

"Is preoperative left heart catheterization necessary? And if CAD is found that necessitates bypass grafts, when should this be performed?"
It is controversial whether or not preoperative coronary catheterization is necessary. In patients with multivessel coronary disease, bypass grafts may increase both early and long-term survival. However, often the patient is too unstable to undergo a catheterization prior to surgery and thus necessitates an individual assessment of patient's hemodynamics and clinical situation. If bypass grafts are performed, they should be done before the repair of the VSD so as to optimize myocardial protection.

"Are there any other surgical techniques that might warrant consideration for repair of a VSD?"
Endocardial patch repair with infarct exclusion involves intracavitary placement of an endocardial patch to exclude infarcted myocardium while maintaining ventricular geometry. This technique excludes the VSD from the highly pressured left ventricle instead of closing it. Proponents of this approach argue that maintaining ventricular geometry enhances or at least preserves ventricular function.

"When would delayed repair of a VSD be acceptable?"
Patients with severe end-organ damage deemed too sick to undergo operative repair may be candidates for a delayed repair. Interval treatment may involve placement of a left ventricular assist device (LVAD) that theoretically will help improve end-organ dysfunction and allow for maturation of the infarcted tissue. A biventricular mechanical assist device may be necessary if the LVAD worsens the right-to-left shunt.

"What interventions may help a difficult wean from CPB following VSD repair?"

If an IABP was not inserted preoperatively, one should be inserted at this time to help reduce the afterload and improve coronary perfusion pressure. Pharmacologic adjuncts such as epinephrine and milrinone may help to augment contractility. Milrinone also improves diastolic function and reduces afterload. Other afterload reducing agents may be used as needed. If the patient is having decreased right heart function, the patient may benefit from inhaled prostaglandin or nitric oxide to help dilate the pulmonary vasculature and decrease the work of the right ventricle. A small percentage of patients may require a temporary ventricular assist device.

Pearls/pitfalls

- Discovery of a new onset post-infarction VSD requires urgent surgery.
- The greatest predictor of post-operative mortality is the length of time patients spend in cardiogenic shock pre-operatively.
- Echocardiography is the diagnostic test and is essential to adequately plan the surgical approach.
- The chances of successfully weaning from CPB are improved by expeditious institution of CPB with meticulous myocardial protection.
- The VSD should be approached via a transinfarct incision with meticulous debridement of necrotic myocardium to prevent delayed rupture.
- Inspect the mitral apparatus for any coexisting dysfunction or infarct of the papillary muscles.
- A tension-free closure is important, and therefore patch closure techniques are required for larger defects.

Suggested readings

- Mangi AA and Agnihotri AK. Postinfarction Ventricular Septal Defect. Spencer and Sabiston - Surgery of the Chest. 2010; 1449-1456.
- Gazoni LM. Mechanical complications of coronary artery disease. Mery CM and Turek JW. TSRA Review of Cardiothoracic Surgery. 2011. 282-289.
- Madsen JC and Daggett WM Jr. Repair of postinfarction ventricular septal defect. Semin Thorac Cardiovasc Surg. 1998. Apr;10(2):117-127.

- Arnaoutakis GJ, Zhao Y, George TJ et al. Surgical repair of ventricular septal defect after myocardial infarction: outcomes from the Society of Thoracic Surgeons National Database. Ann Thorac Surg 2012; 94: 436-44.

Notes

34. Aortic stenosis

Gabriel Loor, MD, and Douglas R. Johnston, MD

Concept
- Indications for aortic valve replacement (AVR) in the setting of AS
- Confirmation of severity
- Options for annular enlargement
- Preoperative considerations
- Valve choices
- Surgical options and pitfalls

Chief complaint
"A 75 yo man is referred to you by a primary care physician diagnosed with severe aortic stenosis by echo after presenting with a 3 month history of intermittent chest pain."

Differential
Diagnosis has been established. Confirmation as detailed below is important as well as ruling out concomitant pathologies that often coexist.

History and physical
A focused history to elicit symptoms of angina, syncope or congestive heart failure (CHF) as well as focused questioning to elicit a history of fatigue or decreased exercise tolerance which often precede more overt symptoms. Comorbidities which may affect treatment algorithms [end-stage renal disease (ESRD), bleeding disorders, stroke, peripheral vascular disease]. Focused physical exam with emphasis on vitals, neuro exam, bruits, pulses, edema, heart and lungs. A classic crescendo-decrescendo (diamond shaped) systolic murmur heard best at the right 2nd intercostal space may be appreciated.

Tests
- *EKG*: arrhythmias, LVH.
- *Echo*. Technical note for echos - gradients are determined by continuous wave doppler peak gradient = $4(\text{velocity})^2$. Mean is the area under the velocity curve. Aortic Valve Area (AVA) is determined by continuity equation Area = $[(\text{LVOT area})(\text{LVOT velocity})]/$continuous wave velocity at the aortic valve. Note that velocity is also influenced by cardiac output. Thus, patients may have low gradients because of low cardiac output. In these patients, a dobutamine stress echo may be helpful. Look for intracavitary gradients that may affect the operative plan. Septal hypertrophy

278

may require a myectomy and possibility of intervention on the mitral valve (see Chapter 55, Hypertrophic obstructive cardiomyopathy). One can anticipate a small root from the echo. Severe hypertrophy may pose challenges for cardioplegic arrest. In general it is imperative to ensure that the echo is of excellent quality or have it repeated by a cardiologist you trust.

- Cardiac catheterization (concomitant CAD).
- *CXR +/- CT scan.* CT scan may be warranted if a calcified aorta is evident on CXR or the patient has evidence of aneurysmal disease on the echo. CT is especially important for bicuspid aortic valve patients who may have aortopathies. Also patients with strong atherosclerotic risk factors should have a CT.

Index scenario (additional information)
"This patient is a diabetic, no syncope or CHF. Echo shows a valve area of 0.8 cm² and mean gradient of 40 mmHg with a tricuspid valve. CT scan shows no aneurysm or ascending calcification. What are his options and how would you proceed?"

Treatment/management
This patient meets AHA Class I indications for an aortic valve replacement (angina, severe stenosis). Valve choices include bioprosthetic and mechanical. Patients younger than 60 years of age may benefit from mechanical valves given the lower reintervention rate (90% freedom from reintervention at 20 years) compared with tissue valves. Also, mechanical valves are associated with greater survival in the younger age group in some studies. However, they are associated with a 2%/year thromboembolic rate and 2.5%/year bleeding rate. For patients > 60-70 years old a bioprosthetic offers excellent long term durability with minimal thromboembolic and bleeding risks (80-90% freedom from structural valve deterioration [SVD] within 10-15 years). Bioprosthetic valves should be considered in younger patients with a desire to avoid long-term anticoagulation provided reoperation can be performed with a low mortality rate. In patients who are inoperable with an STS score greater than 15%, transcathether aortic valve replacement (TAVR) is a reasonable option and has improved mortality benefit compared to medical therapy. For patients at high operative risk (i.e., STS 11%-15%), surgery and TAVR had similar 1 year mortality at 1 year, 26.8% and 24.2%, respectively, while TAVR was associated with higher incidence of stroke. The role of TAVR in the intermediate risk category (STS 4%-11%) is unknown and is currently undergoing investigation in the PARTNER IIA Trial.

Aortic valve replacement
Goals – relieve obstruction, replace the valve, protect the heart and coronaries and prevent embolization.

- Large bore IV, arterial line, general endotracheal anesthesia (GETA), pulmonary artery catheter, foley – watch for v-fib on induction.
- Intraop TEE to confirm/re-evaluate AI or other unexpected pathology.
- Median sternotomy, pericardial stay sutures, palpate the aorta for calcifications.
- Heparin (400 mg/kg), aortic cannulation, 2 stage venous cannula, retrograde cannula, once ACT is 400 initiate CPB, dissect aorta from PA, insert antegrade.
- Deair antegrade line, insert, clamp and run antegrade induction, follow with retrograde. Intermittent doses of retrograde with occasional doses directly down the right coronary (depending on duration and whether good retrograde flow is noted coming from the RCA).
- +/- LV vent through right superior pulmonary vein (RSPV).
- Aortotomy – define the RCA, small transverse aortotomy anterior midline 1 cm above the RCA. Extend laterally towards the LCA ostium, then medially in an oblique fashion towards the middle of the noncoronary sinus. Place stay sutures as needed.
- Inspect and resect the valve along the annulus.
- Debride the calcium, patch or primary closure of any defects with autologus pericardium, irrigate copiously and size the valve.
- Place horizontal mattress sutures along the annulus (usually 2-O braided pledgeted).
- Pass them through the valve ring, seat the valve.
- Check the pledgets, LCA ostium, RCA ostium.
- Tie, irrigate, check LCA and RCA ostium again and close the aortotomy with a running prolene suture.
- Deair by valsalva and compressing the heart prior to closing the aortotomy, assess rhythm, pacing wires, wean from CPB, assess the valve by TEE.

"The patient has v-fib on induction."
Secure the airway and ventilation, initiate CPR immediately, assistant preps while you scrub. Drape, give heparin, and perform an emergency median sternotomy. Aortic and venous cannulation. Initiate cardiopulmonary bypass (CPB), assess flows and drainage, and proceed with AVR.

"You are unable to arrest the heart."
A slow arrest is not uncommon in a hypertrophied heart. Go systematically down your algorithm for persistent activity – check the cross clamp to ensure you are completely across, check your drainage (distention, elevated pulmonary artery pressures) and improve it if necessary. AI may be underestimated by echo. When in doubt or if AI is suspected open the aorta and give ostial cardioplegia. Add topical ice, consider systemic cooling to mild-mod hypothermia (30° C).

"The TEE shows a moderate perivalvular leak."
Define the anatomy on TEE carefully, clamp, arrest, open the aorta and reassess the valve, if you identify an obvious gap you can place a horizontal pledgeted suture or be prepared to remove and replace the valve. Consider the patient's condition. A trivial leak in an 85 yo patient should probably be left alone.

"When you release the cross clamp the heart distends."
Most often this occurs in the setting of paravalvular leak. With a mechanical valve the washing jet AI may be enough to distend the heart if it fibrillates. Turn flow down, compress the heart, defibrillate, or place a vent and defibrillate. If unable to obtain a rhythm the possibilities include, electrolyte abnormality such as hyperkalemia or poor protection. If unable to restore rhythm with the heart empty, clamp and rearrest the heart (see Chapter 27, Cardiopulmonary bypass pitfalls).

"You determine that only a 19 mm St Jude Biocor will fit into this patient. The EOAI assuming a BSA of 2.2 m^2 is 0.59. What are your options?"
One can determine the EOAI (cm^2/m^2) by sizing the valve, checking the EOA for that valve using a published manufacturer chart and dividing by the patients BSA. An EOAI < 0.8 suggests a small aortic root with the risk of patient prosthesis mismatch (PPM). Options include implantation of a mechanical valve, stentless tissue valve (if familiar with this technique), root enlargement, root replacement or acceptance of PPM with a valve that yields the greatest EOA. In this patient with relatively good quality tissue and few comorbidities the longer clamp time may be worth the added EOA.

- *Annulus-enlargement procedure - Nick's procedure*: extend the aortotomy into the nadir of the noncoronary sinus and base of the anterior mitral leaflet with the goal of obtaining a size that is 1 or 2 increments larger than the original. Use autologous pericardium (or other commercially available products ie. CorMatrix, Perigaurd) to patch and enlarge the opening. Place sutures along the left and right coronary sinuses as usual. Seat the valve. Pass non-pledgeted sutures inside out through the sewing ring and patch for the non-coronary portion and tie over a strip of felt. Complete the aortic closure with the patch.

- Another annulus enlargement alternative is the Manouguian procedure whereby the aortotomy is extended posteriorly to the commissure of the non-coronary and left coronary cusps and carried into the anterior leaflet of the mitral valve. The left atrium is opened in this process and must be closed as well.
- *Alternatives.* Root replacement with a homograft or a stentless bioprosthesis and coronary reimplantation. You can usually place a larger homograft/stentless root than a standard bioprosthetic/mechanical valve and the hemodynamics are better.

"Patient is 78 yo, ESRD, inactive, and the EOAI is 0.8 with a highly calcified root."
Use an alternative valve that will yield a slightly greater EOAI and accept some degree of PPM. The harm of a longer cross clamp time, and technically more challenging and tenuous root procedure is not worth the minimal symptomatic benefit of a greater EOAI in this patient. Studies have shown that while 30 day mortality is affected by PPM, long term survival is not. This would also be a patient to consider transcatheter valve, when available.

"A 70 yo female undergoing workup for 3V CABG is found to have moderate AS on echo – would you replace the aortic valve at the time of the CABG?"
This scenario represents a Class IIa indication (i.e., weight of evidence is in favor of usefulness). The decision to replace the valve hinges on the risks involved with the added procedure and the benefits of a longer reintervention free interval. The average rate of valve decrease is 0.12 cm^2 per year. Some patients are likely to progress faster such as those who have already shown fast progression (> 1 mmHg/year) or those with excessively calcified valves. While long term survival is not affected by the addition of AVR, the reintervention rates are lower. In general, it is prudent to replace moderate AS at the time of CABG for reasonable candidates with minimal comorbidities especially in the setting of a highly calcified valve, fast progression or patients younger than 70 years of age.

"Patient is 75 yo asymptomatic with severe aortic stenosis on echo. How would you determine the timing of surgery?"
The prognosis for patients without symptoms is excellent but it falls significantly once symptoms develop. Watchful waiting with medical management including risk factor modification and statin therapy is appropriate for most patients. However, some require surgery based on specific indications and others require additional testing to elicit

symptoms. Immediate indications for surgery in this patient would include low gradient (< 40 mmHg) severe AS with LV dysfunction (< 50%) and contractile reserve; critical AS (AVA < 0.6 cm^2); evidence of severe LVH (LV thickness > 1.6 mm); patients undergoing another open heart procedure (i.e., CABG, mitral valve). Patients with atypical or vague symptoms may undergo a stress echo. Dizziness or chest discomfort signifies a positive test and provides grounds for AVR.

Pearls/pitfalls

- Replace severe (velocity > 4m/s, mean ≥ 40 mmHg, AVA < 1 cm), symptomatic AS.
- Patients older than 70 – generally tissue valves.
- Palpate the aorta for calcifications that may change clamp/CPB strategy.
- Irrigate debris and check the LCA and RCA ostia after seating the valve.
- PPM – EOAI < 0.8 – consider root enlargement procedure.
- Asymptomatic with severe AS – replace if low gradient with < 50% EF, critical AS (< 0.6 cm^2), severe LVH, concomitant cardiac operation, fast progression, severely calcified.

Suggested readings

- Barbour JR and Ikonomidis JS. Aortic valve replacement. Yuh D, Vricella LA, and Baumgartner WA (eds). *Johns Hopkins Manual of Cardiothoracic Surgery* 2007.
- Johnston DR and Sabik JF. Acquired aortic valve disease. Selke FW, del Nido PJ, and Swanson SJ *Surgery of the Chest*. 2010;1195-1207.
- Balckstone EH, et al. Prosthesis size and long-term survival after aortic valve replacement. *JTCVS* 2003; 126:783-96.

Notes

35. Aortic regurgitation

Juan G. Penaranda, MD, and Harold M. Burkhart, MD

Concept
- Indications for aortic valve replacement and repair
- Acute and Chronic aortic valve regurgitation
- Preoperative Considerations
- Operative Strategy
- Pearls/pitfalls

Chief complaint
"A 64 yo man with known aortic valve regurgitation has been followed by his local cardiologist for the last 5 years. On echocardiogram this year there is severe aortic valve regurgitation with an ejection fraction of 45%, a left ventricular end-systolic diameter (LVESD) of 50 mm and a left ventricular end diastolic diameter (LVEDD) of 65 mm."

Differential
The diagnosis has been revealed to you. Rule out other concomitant valvular pathology or coronary artery disease, which may change your approach.

History and physical
Focused history to establish presence of symptoms and functional class is the first step. Ask about symptoms such as exertional dyspnea, syncope, orthopnea, paroxysmal nocturnal dyspnea, angina, and palpitations. Ask about prior history of endocarditis, rheumatic fever, aortic dissection, trauma, congenital valve anomalies such as bicuspid aortic valve to help determine the etiology of the AR. Focused cardiopulmonary physical exam to document the presence of diastolic and systolic murmurs, displaced apical impulse, signs of CHF or pulmonary edema, widened pulse pressure and its classic peripheral signs (water-hammer, quincke pulse, Duroziez sign).

Tests
- *EKG*: will document left ventricular (LV) hypertrophy and arrhythmias among other findings.
- *CXR*: an enlarged cardiac silhouette may suggest LV dilation or aortic root enlargement.
- *Echocardiography*. Confirms the diagnosis, assess the etiology of AR and assess valve morphology, provide semiquantitative and quantitative estimates of AR severity, assess LV dimensions, mass, and systolic function and assess aortic root size. Most commonly

the AI is graded as 1-mild, 2-moderate, 3-moderately severe 4-severe. Evidence of severe AI includes: 1) jet width > 65 percent of the left ventricular outflow tract (LVOT) diameter 2) vena contracta width > 0.6 cm 3) Early closure of the mitral valve 4) regurgitant volume > 60 mL or fraction > 50%.

- *Coronary angiography*: to be done in patients with significant risk factors for coronary artery disease or those older than 40 years of age in whom aortic valve replacement (AVR) is considered. Rule out or identify any coronary anomalies that may alter your cardioplegia strategy (i.e., direct coronary givers) and any root replacement techniques.
- Cardiac catheterization with root angiography and measurement of LV pressures is indicated when echocardiograms are inconclusive or discordant with physical findings.
- *CT scan*: important test to assess the presence of concomitant aortic root pathology namely aneurysmal disease, dissection, porcelain aorta, or endocarditis.
- *Cardiac MR*: evaluation and quantification of aortic regurgitation and its impact on LV function as well as aortic root and ascending aorta pathology. Especially useful in the presence of suboptimal echocardiograms.
- *Exercise testing*: valuable in assessing functional capacity in patients with minimal or equivocal symptoms.

Index scenario (additional information)

"This patient denies any exertional dyspnea, orthopnea, paroxysmal nocturnal dyspnea, chest pain; he revealed a previous syncopal episode 40 years ago. Past medical history is remarkable for hypertension and COPD. On physical exam there is a displaced apical impulse and a grade IV/VI diastolic murmur in the mid left sternal edge and a wide pulse pressure. EKG demonstrates NSR with non-specific intraventricular conduction delay. CXR reveals cardiomegaly. Echocardiogram demonstrates ejection fraction of 45%, severe aortic valve regurgitation with regurgitant volume of 77cc, LVEDD is 65 mm LVESD is 50 mm, mild tricuspid and mitral regurgitation, with max aortic root and ascending aorta dimensions of 40 and 38 mm, respectively. There is no evidence of abscess, vegetation, or dissection. A CT scan was not performed because his creatinine was 1.8 and the echocardiographic findings did not suggest aortic root pathology. What are the treatment options at this time and how do you counsel the patient regarding valve option?"

Treatment/management

Surgical management of AR most commonly involves aortic valve replacement (AVR). In highly selected patients, an aortic valve repair by an experienced surgeon may be an option. Note: See the general recommendations regarding valve choices in Chapter 34, Aortic stenosis. Aortic root pathology is discussed chapters 48 and 50 (aneurysmal disease and dissections). According to AHA/ACC 2006 Guidelines, indications for AV replacement/repair include:

- *Class I*
  - Symptomatic patients.
  - Asymptomatic with LV dysfunction (EF < 50%).
  - Presence of severe AR while undergoing CABG or aortic surgery or other valvular procedure.
- *Class IIa*
  - Asymptomatic patients with LV dilation (LVEDD > 75 mm or LVESD > 55 mm).
- *Class IIb*
  - Moderate AR while undergoing aortic surgery.
  - Moderate AR while undergoing CABG.
  - Asymptomatic with normal EF but dilated ventricles (LVEDD > 70 mm LVESD > 50 mm), progressive ventricular dilation, declining exercise tolerance or abnormal hemodynamic response to exercise.

Operative steps

Aortic valve replacement

The surgical steps for aortic valve replacement for aortic regurgitation are similar to those for aortic stenosis (see Chapter 34, Aortic stenosis), although a few considerations should be mentioned.

- *CPB and myocardial protection.* Any degree of AI carries the risk of distention once CPB is initiated. This is especially true for severe AI. You will rarely get arrest with antegrade. Thus, an LV vent for decompression during CPB, room to clamp the aorta, room for the aortotomy and retrograde cardioplegia access should all be ensured in the event that the heart distends during CPB. The same applies for circulatory arrest cases or any case where a patient has even moderate AI.
- *Exposure.* An LV vent catheter helps to keep the operative field dry and prevent distention as discussed above. Other options include placement of a pulmonary artery vent or simply use a pump sucker across the aortic valve into the left ventricle.
- *Aortotomy.* Usually an oblique aortotomy towards the middle of the non-coronary sinus will provide adequate exposure. It will also allow aortic root enlargement if needed. In the cases where the ascending aorta needs to be replaced, the aorta should be transected just above the sinotubular junction.

"The heart continues to eject and begins to distend shortly after initiating CPB."

Prior to initiating bypass make sure you are ready for the possibility of ventricular distention. If this occurs you will need to arrest the heart immediately. Prior to initiating CPB, establish retrograde cardioplegia access. If there is a question about the location of the retrograde catheter then be prepared for direct retrograde insertion which requires bicaval (IVC and SVC) cannulation from the onset. After establishing retrograde make room for the aortic cross clamp and identify a reasonable site for your aortotomy. Now initiate CPB and place the LV vent. Placement of an LV vent (usually once CPB is started) allows you time while you complete any additional dissection that may be needed to clamp and arrest. It does require exposure of the right superior pulmonary vein. Either a basket sucker directly into the atrium or a vent catheter that crosses the mitral valve can be used. If you distend remove volume through the vent. Next, cross clamp the aorta and give induction cardioplegia through the retrograde catheter. In order to vent during this phase of induction, turn on the aortic root vent (assuming you had time to place it) or make the aortotomy. Once the retrograde is complete, finish the aortotomy, identify the coronary ostia carefully and give induction cardioplegia directly down the coronaries. For the remainder of the case give retrograde every 15-20 minutes or alternate between retrograde and direct ostial perfusion as you wish.

"The retrograde cannot be established or the position is questionable."

Cannulate the IVC and SVC separately. Make room for the aortic cross clamp and identify your aortotomy site. Once CPB is initiated, place the LV vent, clamp, make the aortotomy and give direct cardioplegia down the ostia. With the heart arrested, snare the SVC and IVC, make a right atriotomy and place the retrograde catheter in just past the opening of the coronary sinus. Continue induction cardioplegia through the retrograde. Direct retrograde can also be established prior to cross clamping but the exposure is a bit tricky.

"During placement of the retrograde catheter you get dark blood behind the heart. You confirm a small coronary sinus perforation. How is your cardioprotection scheme altered?"

Retrograde will be unreliable in this setting. The safest option is to initiate CPB, place an LV vent, clamp and give antegrade direct throughout the case. If the operation is lengthy you might consider small coronary catheters for intermittent perfusion without having to pause for the handheld perfusion catheters every 15 minutes. If the sinus injury is small and involving a branch off the sinus, you can consider repairing and replacing the retrograde catheter in direct.

"Intraoperative transesophageal echocardiogram shows a tricuspid aortic valve with prolapse of the right cusp. After making the aortotomy and inspecting the valve you confirmed the TEE findings. What are your surgical options at this time?"
Aortic valve replacement with a mechanical valve or bioprosthesis is the safest answer in this scenario.

Aortic valve repair can be performed in isolated cusp prolapse of tricuspid or bicuspid aortic valves. Techniques such as triangular resection or plication of the free edge of the cusp are well described. Isolated cusp perforations can be repaired with an autologous pericardial patch. Commissures can be re-suspended as in cases of aortic dissection. Sinotubular junction dilation with central regurgitation may be amenable to repair with commissure plication. Valve sparing root replacement is a well known surgical approach for aortic root aneurysms commonly used in patients with annuloaortic ectasia and normal aortic cusps where the regurgitation is due to lack of cusp coaptation.

"Patient fibrillates and arrests while cannulating the right atrium. You attempt to defibrillate but the heart dilates and you are unable to cardiovert back into sinus rhythm."
Quickly institute cardiopulmonary bypass, empty out and defibrillate. If unable to empty out due to severe AI, cross clamp and open the aorta. Decompress the heart with a sucker through the aortic valve and localize the coronary ostia to give antegrade cardioplegia with an ostial cannula. Once heart is arrested, perform the aortic valve replacement.

"After AVR, you are unable to close the aortotomy secondary to the large prosthesis putting tension on the aortotomy suture line."
The aortotomy should be closed utilizing a bovine or autologous pericardial patch to insure no tension on the suture line.

"You remove the aortic cross clamp and immediately notice that the left ventricle dilates. There is significant ventricular ejection while trying to come off bypass and once you are off bypass the pulse pressure is significantly wide. What would you do at this point? The TEE shows severe periprosthetic regurgitation with reversal of flow in the descending aorta, the regurgitant jet is coming from the noncoronary sinus. How do you manage this situation?"
Peri-prosthetic leaks should be dealt with in the operating room. It is important to differentiate prosthetic versus peri-prosthetic regurgitation. It is vital to quantify and localize the leak as this will dictate your approach. Leaks from the non-coronary sinus may be amenable to direct suture repair while other locations may require removing the prosthesis in order to fix the problem.

"You go back on pump, arrest the heart and reopen the aorta. There is a small gap in the non-coronary sinus after probing and inspecting the valve. You are able to place an everting mattress suture from outside of the aorta into the sewing cuff solving the problem. As you finish your case your chief resident calls you from the other operating room. He had done a mitral valve repair with a triangular resection and a complete annuloplasty ring. As he came off bypass he noticed severe aortic valve regurgitation on TEE. The jet appears to be originating from the left coronary cusp on short axis view. He is puzzled and wants your advice."

Aortic regurgitation is an uncommon but known complication from mitral valve procedures. The aortic valve cusps can be entrapped with the sutures used for the mitral repair/replacement. TEE can help diagnose this problem in the operating room.

"You go back on CPB and arrest the heart, you open the aorta with an oblique incision and notice the left cusp has been retracted with an annuloplasty stitch. You then reopen the left atrium, cut the offending suture, and place one more annuloplasty stitch avoiding the aortic valve. Before closing the left atrium, your final inspection of the aortic valve revealed an intact valve. You close the aorta and come off bypass. TEE shows trivial aortic and mitral regurgitation.

As you walk out of the operating room, you get a call from the emergency room. There is 25 yo man who was involved in a motor vehicle collision. He is short of breath, tachycardic and has a loud diastolic murmur. Auscultation of his lungs reveals bilateral basilar rales. CXR show mild pulmonary edema. Trauma work-up so far has been negative except for a non-displaced sternal fracture and small bilateral knee lacerations. You ask them to get an echocardiogram as you make your way to the emergency room. What is your differential diagnosis at this time?"

Cardiac blunt injury after motor vehicle collision is most commonly seen as myocardial contusion with conduction disturbances, dysrhythmias or pericardial tamponade. Rarely the cardiac valves can be affected; the aortic valve followed by the mitral valve are the valves most commonly injured. Acute aortic and mitral regurgitation can be seen. A good differential would include acute aortic or mitral regurgitation, aortic dissection with secondary aortic regurgitation, and a ventricular septal defect.

"Echocardiography shows severe aortic regurgitation with prolapse of the right-coronary cusp. How do you approach this patient?"

Acute aortic valve insufficiency has been described after blunt trauma to the chest. The mechanism seems to be related to a sudden increase in intracardiac pressure during diastole. The aortic cusps can have perforations, tears or can be completely detached from the aortic root. The non-coronary and right cusps are most commonly involved.

"You decide to operate on the patient and upon exploration of the aortic valve, you notice the right cusp has been almost completely detached. What do you want to do?"
The safest and most durable treatment for aortic valve injury with acute aortic regurgitation involves aortic valve replacement in most cases. Highly selected patients may be able to undergo repair.

"What type of valve do you use?"
A bioprosthesis seems to be a good option in the acute setting especially in patients with concomitant injuries where postoperative anticoagulation may be problematic. If there is no hemodynamic compromise and other significant injuries are present, delaying operative repair for few days maybe a reasonable strategy. Patients who present in a delayed fashion, once their acute injuries are over, may be considered for a mechanical prosthesis if indicated.

Pearls/pitfalls

- Replace or repair the aortic valve in the setting of severe AR if symptoms are present or there is evidence of LV dysfunction or LV dilatation (LVEDD 7 cm or LVESD 5 cm). If you wait too long the outcome will be compromised.
- Anticipate how AI can alter your cardioprotection strategy. Ensure retrograde access. Cardioplegia directly down the coronary ostia is an alternative.
- Prior to initiating bypass be prepared for LV distention. Make room to clamp the aorta, identify your aortotomy site, establish retrograde cardioplegia and anticipate the need for an LV vent. Have ostial plegia catheters available.
- Concomitant root pathology (> 4.5-5 cm) should be addressed in good surgical candidates at the time of the operation.
- Symptomatic acute aortic regurgitation should be taken care of expeditiously since the ventricle has not had time to develop any adaptation to overcome the increased volume load. This may lead to rapid clinical decompensation.

Suggested readings

- Bonow Ro, Carabello BA, Chatterjee K et al: ACC/AHA 2006 Guidelines for the Management of Patients with Valvular Heart Disease: a Report of the American College of Cardiology/American Heart Association Task Force on Practice Guidelines. J Am Coll Cardiol 2006;48:e1-e148.

- Zoghbi WA, Enriquez-Sarano M, Foster E, et al: Recommendations for evaluation of the severity of native valvular regurgitation with two dimensional and Doppler echocardiography. J Am Soc Echocardiogr 2003;16:777-802.
- Detaint D, Messika-Zeitoun D, Maalouf J, et al. Quantitative echocardiographic determinants of clinical outcome in asymptomatic patients with aortic regurgitation: a prospective study. J Am Coll Cardiol imaging 2008;1:1-11.
- Dujardin KS, Enriquez Sarano M, Schaff HV et al. Mortality and morbidity of aortic regurgitation in clinical practice: a long term follow up study. Circulation 1999;99:1851-1857.
- Loop FD, Hofmeier G, Groves LK. Traumatic disruption of the aortic valve. Cleveland Clinic Quarterly 1971, 38:187-194.
- Egoh Y, Okoshi T, Anbe J, Asaka T. Surgical treatment of traumatic rupture of the normal aortic valve . Eur J Cardiothorac Surg 1997,11:1180-1182.
- Ducharme A, Courval JF, Dore A, Leclerc Y, Tardiff JC. Severe Aortic Regurgitation immediately after Mitral Valve Annuloplasty. Ann Thorac Surg 1999;67:1487-89.

Notes

36. Redo aortic valve replacement
Leora Yarboro, MD, and John A. Kern, MD

Concept
- Discuss the common indications and preoperative workup for Redo AVR
- Operative Planning
- Potential pitfalls and their management

Chief complaint
"A 78 yo man with history of prior aortic valve replacement now presents with dyspnea on exertion."

Differential
The differential in this patient includes: structural valve disease, coronary artery disease, and primary pulmonary disorders such as progressive COPD. Certain conditions such as bicuspid aortic valve, rheumatic disease and endocarditis can lead to early native valve failure. In patients with previous valve replacements, recent studies examining the 10 year freedom from reoperation for aortic valve bioprosthesis demonstrated a 90% freedom from reoperation in porcine valves vs. 97% freedom from reoperation in pericardial valves. Porcine valves in this study were more likely to demonstrate structural valve deterioration (SVD). Mechanical valves in the aortic position demonstrate a 96% freedom from redo AVR at 15 years.

History and physical
A focused cardiopulmonary history and exam is important. Focus on surgical scars and prior vein harvest sites. Listen for new murmurs, JVD and assess femoral and pedal pulses as this may be important in determining alternative cannulation strategies.

Tests
- Echocardiography
- Cardiac catheterization (look for coronary artery disease as well as the status of the left main and right main)
- CT (with intravenous contrast) of chest if history of CABG, otherwise non contrast would suffice.
- Consider CTA of chest abdomen pelvis if creatinine normal to evaluate vessels for femoral cannulation if required
- Carotid duplex
- Pulmonary function testing (PFT)
- Vein mapping if previous CABG

- UA/Blood cultures
- *CBC, Chemistry I*: LDH (hemolysis), renal insufficiency, type and cross
- Obtain previous operative note
    - When was the last operation?
    - What was the manufacturer and size of the last valve?
    - What exactly was the procedure? Was there a root enlargement or other root procedure performed?
    - History of previous CABG? What were the conduits? Do the conduits cross the sternal midline?

Index scenario (additional information)
"Patient has isolated aortic regurgitation on echocardiography with no significant coronary artery disease."

Operative steps
- Perioperative monitoring
    - Transesophageal echo, PA catheter, cerebral oximetry, Foley with temp probe, arterial line.
    - Review CT scan for areas of concern – proximity of aorta/right ventricle/innominate vein/atrium/grafts. Check for excessive ascending aortic calcification.
    - Prep legs in case of coronary injury and need for vein.
- Cannulation
    - Have a plan for alternate cannulation sites – axillary vs. femoral cannulation. Be sure to expose the right axillary region during draping. While it is not always necessary, it is probably safest practice to have femoral vessels exposed in case of an emergency prior to opening the sternum.
    - Be able to discuss which patients you would go on bypass for prior to opening the sternum (i.e., CT scan demonstrates live grafts in close proximity to sternum or previous aortic injury on entry).
    - A reasonable approach for cannulation is the following:
        - 1 – *structures a safe distance away*: expose the femoral vessels prior to sternotomy (if you injure something you can heparinize, cannulate the femoral vein and artery).
        - 2 – *structures in close proximity*: sew the axillary graft on with 5,000 heparin and have the femoral vein exposed with a wire in place (if you injure something you can heparinize, connect the axillary graft and cannulate the vein).

- o 3 – *critical grafts under the sternum, aorta close to the sternum*: go on bypass through the axillary and femoral vein prior to sternotomy and cool to at least moderate hypothermia (28-32° C) (if you injure something you can empty out and even drop flows as needed) - the main drawback to fully heparinizing and cannulating prior to the dissection is bleeding.
  - o 4 – *calcified aorta*: see Chapter 26, Management of the porcelain aorta.
  - o Other reasons to cannulate peripherally electively prior to or after sternotomy deal with "real estate" - usually the ascending aorta can be safely cannulated distal to the prior cannulation site but if you do not have enough room because of live grafts or it proves too hazardous to expose then cannulate the axillary artery/fem artery. If the atrium is stuck then proceed to femoral venous or bicaval cannulation.
  - – Cardioprotection
    - o *Know whether patient has any degree of aortic insufficiency.* Be prepared with retrograde cardioplegia and left ventricular vent. Cool to 32-34° C.
- Dissection
  - – dissect out the atrium and ascending aorta for cannulation sites.
  - – heparinize, cannulate, clamp, arrest.
  - – Previous aortotomy site may be calcified. Open just proximal or distal to it. Excise valve sharply. Remove all sutures with blade. Use freer elevator to gently remove valve. Vigilantly identify and remove all pledgets.
- Valve
  - – Size annulus after debriding pannus. Place annular sutures and tie down valve.
- Close aortotomy
- Place pacing wires
- Post op
  - – Redo AVR have significantly longer operative, bypass and cross clamp times. As a consequence they may have variable degrees of vasoplegia and cardiogenic shock requiring resuscitation. They also have higher rates of heart block so make sure you have well placed and reliable wires.

"Patient fibrillates during initial dissection."
Know if substantial aortic insufficiency is present. Have external defibrillator pads on the patient prior to prepping. May place LV vent for decompression. If unable may need to clamp and perform aortotomy with vent through valve and direct handheld cardioplegia. The problem arises when the patient distends and defibrillates before you have the heart dissected out. Two things that cause this include bovie and CPB with an incompetent valve. Thus, try to avoid going on CPB until the heart is dissected out. Try to avoid electrocautery near the left ventricle during the initial dissection until you are ready to go on pump and arrest. If you do fibrillate prior to having the heart dissected, shock with external pads at 100-200 Joules. If the patient becomes hemodynamically unstable cannulate (centrally or peripherally) and go on pump immediately. If the heart then distends, do the best you can to decompress manually or with a vent until you are able to clamp and arrest.

"Patient with previous CABG."
Preoperative cardiac catheterization is crucial in these patients. Mobilize previous grafts to allow for aortotomy. If unable to mobilize graft and it is still patent may need to transect and perform bypass. The proximal can be to the aorta or hood of the vein graft and the distal can be to the vein graft or new distal. Ligate the old graft.

"Tear in aorta/outflow tract when removing old valve."
Valve may be incorporated or previous dissection may have been extensive. Be prepared with bovine pericardium or even homograft for reconstruction if necessary.

"Right Coronary ostia injured during excision of valve."
Be prepared by prepping in the legs on all redo operations. Perform bypass. Reference cath to be sure that bypass is distal to any native disease.

Pearls/pitfalls
- Review echo and cardiac catheterization to ensure no other surgery necessary.
- CT scan of chest.
- Obtain previous operative note.
- Have a general idea of what size valve pt needs or can tolerate.
- Discuss mechanical vs. tissue valve preoperatively.
- Be prepared for complications - need for aortic root enlargement/ replacement.
- Plan your cannulation strategy carefully and have blood available prior to starting the sternotomy.

- Injury to coronary vessels - bypass with vein grafts.
- In general any complication that can occur in a primary is more likely to occur in a redo.
- Place pacing wires - increased risk of heart block postoperatively.

Suggested readings
- Potter DD. Operative risk of reoperative aortic valve replacement. *J Thorac Cardiovasc Surg* 2005.

Notes

37. Tricuspid regurgitation

Emmanuel Moss, MD, and Robert A. Guyton, MD

Concept
- Indication for intervention on the tricuspid valve
- Preoperative considerations
- Choice of intervention - repair vs. replace
- Valve choices - bioprosthesis vs. mechanical
- Critical steps of tricuspid valve repair and replacement
- Pitfalls and controversies

Chief complaint
"A 45 yo man presents with a 6-month history of progressive fatigue, shortness of breath and lower extremity edema. Auscultation reveals a holosystolic ejection murmur at the left ventricular apex."

Differential
The clinical scenario mentioned is typical for congestive heart failure. The causes can be several (CAD, MR, MS, AS, etc.). The peripheral edema and murmur raise concern for tricuspid regurgitation. Other diagnoses to consider include: Cirrhosis, constrictive pericarditis, or restrictive cardiomyopathy.

History and physical
This patient may have valvular disease of any type but most likely has mitral or tricuspid regurgitation. Valvular disease can lead to symptoms of congestive heart failure. It is important to determine the onset and duration of her symptoms as well as the character (asthenia, fatigue, weakness, malaise, peripheral edema). Evaluate for signs of right heart failure (ascites, hepatosplenomegaly, pulsatile liver, peripheral edema, pleural effusions). Late findings include cachexia, wasting and jaundice. Atrial fibrillation is common. Look for evidence of coronary artery disease (chest pain, risk factors, etc).

If TR is high on the differential then consider primary and secondary causes:
- *Primary (structural)*. Congenital (e.g., Ebstein, AV canal/cushion defect), rheumatic disease (never isolated), endocarditis (IV drug use and Modified Duke's criteria), myxomatous degeneration, endocarditis, iatrogenic (e.g., permanent pacemaker (PPM) lead, repetitive myocardial biopsies), carcinoid (see below for explanation), trauma (e.g., chordal rupture from anterior leaflet), valvular tumor.

- *Secondary (functional)*. Most common form of TV dysfunction. Leaflets are normal. Caused by left sided lesion (e.g., mitral regurgitation), ischemic cardiomyopathy, dilated cardiomyopathy, cor pulmonale.

Tests
- *CXR*: cardiomegaly, enlarged RA/RV, pleural effusions.
- *TTE*. Transthoracic rather than transesophageal is particularly helpful for evaluating the tricuspid valve. It is used for diagnosis and decisions regarding management PREOPERATIVELY. For functional TR, intraoperative transesophageal echo is unreliable due to changes in vascular tone under general anesthesia, reducing the degree of regurgitation. For regurgitation, a jet that penetrates 2 cm into the RA is mild, 3-5 cm is moderate and systolic flow reversal of the hepatic or caval veins is severe. The grade is often reported as 1-mild, 2-moderate, 3-moderately severe, 4-severe. In addition a jet radius greater than 9 mm, vena contracta > 0.7, ERO > 0.4 cm^2, or regurgitant volume 45 mL indicate severe regurgitation.
- *Annulus size and the gradient:* Annular size > 40 mm is a rough cut off for a valve that needs intervention. Mean gradient of 3-5 mmHg is considered severe. Also need to inquire on the character of the leaflets (tethered, thickened, prolapsed, flail).
- *TEE*. Important for getting more detailed information on the mitral valve. Should also assess pulmonary artery pressure (PAP), right ventricular (RV) function, presence of PFO or ASD (bubble test if there is a doubt), endocarditis (vegetations) or carcinoid lesions.
- *Catheterization*: evaluate for any coronary lesions. TR can be due to or result in RV failure. Obtain the cardiac index, PCWP, PAP, RA/RV end-diastolic pressure and CVP. Cardiac index may be unreliable in the setting of TR and you should rely on the EF for assessment of function. Absent X descent, prominent V wave, and ventricularization of RA tracing all *support tricuspid disease.*

Index scenario (additional information)
"Echocardiogram reveals a left ventricular ejection fraction of 45%, severe mitral regurgitation, moderate pulmonary artery hypertension, and moderate-severe tricuspid regurgitation with normal leaflets and a dilated annulus (45 mm)."

Treatment/management
This scenario addresses combined tricuspid and mitral valve disease. In addition to mitral valve (MV) repair or replacement, this patient meets criteria for tricuspid valve repair with an annuloplasty ring. This patient has several risk factors for persistent and progressive TR following mitral

valve surgery. If the TV is deemed irreparable at the time of surgery, it is reasonable to consider replacement with a mechanical valve, depending on the patient's preference and other anticoagulation concerns. Although bioprostheses deteriorate at a slower rate in the tricuspid position, this patient will likely require a future intervention (whether surgical or transcatheter), while risk of thrombosis with bileaflet mechanical valve is greatly decreased compared to older models (ball-cag, tilting disk).

Indications for surgery: ACCF/AHA guidelines
- Class I
  - – TV repair for severe TR in patients requiring MV surgery (level B).
- Class IIa
  - – TV repair or replacement for severe, SYMPTOMATIC, primary TR (level C).
  - – TV replacement is reasonable when not amenable to repair.
- Class IIb
  - – Annuloplasty may be considered for less than severe TR in patients undergoing MV surgery when there is pulmonary hypertension or tricuspid annular dilation. (level C).
- Other suggested indications for concomitant repair (not AHA): End-systolic annular dimension > 40 mm or intraoperative measurement of anteroseptal to anteroposterior annulus > 70 mm (Dreyfus et al, 2005).
- *Endocarditis*. Not addressed in AHA guidelines. Generally accepted indications include: 1) severe TR with persistent sepsis, 2) vegetation > 15 mm, 3) persistent vegetation or sepsis despite med tx, 4) Recurrent pulmonary embolism.

Operative steps
- *Critical anatomy*: 3 leaflets (septal, posterior, anterior). Septal annulus relatively fixed, annulus dilates posteriorly > anteriorly. AV node contained in triangle of Koch (between coronary sinus, septal annulus, tendon of Todaro).
- Intraop TEE (assess valve function and dimensions, PFO), median sternotomy, aortic and bicaval cannulation with caval snares.
- *Cardioplegia*: cross clamp, antegrade +/- retrograde. For retrograde – after clamping, run antegrade, caval snares are tightened, right atriotomy, hand held retractor, purse string around coronary sinus, insert cannula and inflate balloon, pull back cannula until arrested by purse string (maximize distribution).
- Left sided lesions addressed first.

- Tricuspid valve can be addressed with the aorta clamped or the heart beating (PFO, if present, must be closed before releasing the cross clamp). Advantages of beating heart include assessment of iatrogenic conduction disturbances, reduce cross-clamp time. Concern with beating heart is ejection of air in the presence of an undetected interatrial communication and the added challenge of performing a precise annuloplasty on the beating heart.
- Oblique atriotomy directed posteriorly from appendage toward the right inferior pulmonary vein and inferior vena cava.
- On septal annulus, sutures are placed through the base of the septal leaflet to avoid damage to the AV node.

Annuloplasty techniques
- Ring annuloplasty
    - Interrupted mattress sutures leaving a gap at koch's triangle (roughly 1 cm from the anteroseptal commissure to midpoint on the septal leaflet. Be careful with the sutures near the anteropostero commisure. These can injure the RCA. Several rings available, with semi-rigid incomplete ring being the most commonly used (e.g., Edwards Classic, Edwards physio, MC3). Favored over flexible band.
    - *Methods of selecting ring size*: 1) Using sizer, measuring the septal leaflet and surface area of leaflet tissue arising from anterior pap muscle, or 2) 30-32 mm for female, 32-34 mm for male.
- *Suture annuloplasty (DeVega)*. Simpler and faster, however, may have increased long-term risk of recurrence compared to rings. Both limbs of a pledgeted 2–0 Prolene running from anteroseptal commissure along the RV free wall portion of the annulus to the posteroseptal commissures.
- *Posterior leaflet plication (Kay)*. Obliterates the posterior leaflet.

Replacement
- Preservation of native valve leaflets, similar to mitral valve.
- Sutures near the AV node placed through the septal leaflet.

Endocarditis
- Excise vegetations until healthy tissue. Close gaps primarily or with patch.
- Consider annuloplasty if valve competence is in question.
- Replace valve if extensive destruction.
- 2-stage replacement may be considered in IVDU (intravenous drug users), with normal RV function and PAP.

Intra-operative valve assessment. Fill RV with saline with a bulb syringe and assess coaptation. TEE to assess repair on CPB.

"What elements will influence your decision to address the TV in a patient undergoing mitral valve surgery?"

Decision to operate often a difficult clinical dilemma because improvement with repair of left-sided lesions remains unpredictable. In general, moderate to severe TR or any structural TR should be addressed concomitantly with left sided lesions. LV function, RV function, degree of pulmonary hypertension, tricuspid annulus size, and tricuspid valve morphology must all be assessed. The presence of preoperative right heart failure is a strong indication for addressing TR. Some advocate repair of even mild disease without risk factors for progression. If LV and RV function are near normal, the TV annulus is not dilated, pulmonary vascular resistance is low, and a good result is expected from MV repair, then progressive tricuspid regurgitation is less likely. When weaning from CPB, if TR persists and elevated RAP > LAP is encountered with an underfilled well-contracting LV, TV repair should be performed.

"What type of prosthesis would you use for TV replacement?"

Similar to the mitral and aortic valves, decision is based on age, anticoagulation considerations, and social issues. Incidence of valve thrombosis was considered prohibitive with older mechanical prostheses (ball-cage and tilting disk), but is not the case with bileaflet valves. However, bioprostheses have better freedom from structural valve deterioration than in mitral position, and unlike mechanical valves, they do not limit the implantation of a transvalvular PM lead in the future.

"Under what circumstances can TV excision without replacement be considered?"

In endocarditis and extensive destruction or an active IVDU. PAPs and RV must be near normal. Replacement can be performed months to years later. Early morality 12%, with hepatic failure frequently playing a role. Survival is 60% at 15 years, with 50% of patients having RV failure. Approach has fallen out of favor.

"When coming off pump following TV replacement, the RV dilates, CVP is high, and PAP decrease. How do you manage this?"

Routine checklist of possible causes of RV failure post CPB (metabolic, air embolism…) and TEE for anatomic assessment. Rule out RVOT obstruction due to redundant billowing of anterior leaflet tissue - If this is the case, central portion of anterior leaflet may be excised while maintaining chordal attachments. If ST changes are noted in the inferior leads then consider RCA occlusion with the mattress sutures and perform a bypass to the right with vein. Even when all goes well after TVR, there may be an element of RV dysfunction which is treated in the ICU with inotropes (epinephrine or milrinone), fluid restriction, diuresis and pressors. Chemical unloading of the heart can be achieved with milrinone or nitroglycerin drip. An IABP can further help to unload a struggling RV in more severe cases and improve RCA perfusion. Note that you do not always have the luxury of Swan-Ganz monitoring after tricuspid valve surgery. It cannot be used if placing a mechanical valve. It is not ideal when placing a tissue valve. It can be used after a repair but it would be best if it were manually inserted by the surgeon under direct visualization. This may factor into your selection process as well. A sick patient with poor EF may be better off with 1-2+ residual TR after a repair and a PA catheter for ICU management than no TR with a mechanical valve but no PA catheter.

"What are the risk factors for recurrence of TR following TV repair?"
No ring used, improper placement of the ring (usually by rotation), severity of baseline TR, residual TR at first operation, persistent pulmonary hypertension, residual left sided lesions, transvalvular PPM lead.

"What factors influence operative mortality in TV surgery?"
Preoperative functional class, ejection fraction, prior valve surgery, older age, excision without replacement.

"When should tricuspid valve repair be performed in patients who have undergone a previous mitral valve surgery?"
No consensus exists. Historically, operative mortality for reoperative TV surgery has been relatively high, making the benefit over medical therapy unclear. Waiting for the development of severe symptoms before TV repair in this setting has resulted in poor results, reinforcing the belief that this is a high-risk operation. Some now advocate early reintervention in mildly symptomatic patients, hoping to decrease operative risk. Effectiveness of this approach has not been proven.

"Coming off CPB you notice complete heart block, CHB."
The sutures near the anteroseptal commissure can easily damage the AV node. This can also occur from radial force with the prosthetic valves. If both the mitral and tricuspid were replaced then the chance of recovery is lower. Giving the patient time to recover in the ICU is reasonable but make sure that you have 2 sets of properly functioning ventricular pacing wires as well as a set of atrial wires. Eventually the patient may require an endocardial or epicardial permanent pacemaker. Endocardial pacers

can be placed percutaneously into the atrium and through the coronary sinus to achieve ventricular conduction. If the coronary sinus cannot be cannulated then worse case scenario they can traverse the repaired valve. If the patient had a tissue valve placed this can be harder but is still possible. Epicardial lead placement is another alternative and avoids a foreign object across the fresh repair/replacement. But you need to balance this decision with the risk of returning to the OR and be able to describe how you reoperate for an epicardial lead. If a mechanical valve is in place and you end up with heart block then you will not be able to cross it with endocardial wires and the coronary sinus route or epicardial route may be needed ultimately.

"A patient with tricuspid valve endocarditis and a PPM for heart block undergoes a combined mitral/TV repair. How do you handle the pacer leads?"

The original wires should be removed in the setting of bacteremia and endocarditis. You have no way of knowing if it was the wires themselves that caused the infection or will seed a new infection. Some advocate debriding the wires or inspecting them but the safest thing would be to remove them. Epicardial wires can be placed on the RV. Transvenous atrial wires can be placed later if needed. Place temporary wires as well since you will not be relying on the epicardial lead until it is connected and a formal device check is performed. Be familiar with the procedure for epicardial lead placement (5-O prolene to fasten the RV lead, tunnel the lead through the left intercostal space a safe distance away from the mammary and out to an area in the skin where you make a subcutaneous pocket for the device.). If you are concerned about the degree of bacterial burden intraop and feel that the epicardial lead could get infected then you can wait a few days post op on antibiotics and place an endocardial lead through the coronary sinus, repaired valve or tissue valve.

"A patient with a prior history of brady syndrome and a PPM comes to the OR for a TVR."

Note that in the absence of endocarditis the wires can be left either around the sewing ring or through the valve itself accepting a slightly higher risk of recurrent TR. For a younger patient it may be worth placing the wire in the epicardial position since you would like to minimize the chance of recurrent TR. For a mechanical valve you will need to remove the wire and replace later or use an epicardial wire.

"After replacing the tricuspid valve you feel the need to determine PAP and CI due to worsening hypotension."

You cannot float a swan in the setting of a mechanical valve and it is not advised after a tissue valve. It can be done with caution in the setting of a repair. An alternative is to use the CVP with venous saturations and echo data to help guide your management. It can be placed through a tissue valve carefully if absolutely necessary.

"Coming of CPB you notice 2+ TR. The patient has extensive comorbidities, 4+ MR which you have just fixed and a low EF."
The management must weigh the risks of going back on CPB and arresting the heart against the risks of leaving behind residual TR. For this patient the most prudent course of action would be to leave the regurgitation alone. 2+ residual TR will rarely be a good reason to replace the valve. The exception to this would be a younger patient with primary tricuspid disease and evidence of early right heart failure. For that patient you would want to remove as much of the regurgitant volume as possible.

"What is carcinoid valvular disease and how is the tricuspid valve managed with this disease process?"
Carcinoid tumors are serotonin-secreting tumors of the Kulchitsky cells of the GI tract. They can metastasize to liver where serotonin and other vasoactive hormones are excreted, affecting the right sided cardiac valves and pulmonary bed. Carcinoid syndrome leads to focal or diffuse fibrous tissue deposits on the endocardium of valve cusps and cardiac chambers. White fibrous carcinoid plaques present on the ventricular side of the TV cusps cause adherence to the RV wall, preventing leaflet coaptation. Tricuspid valve replacement is required. Involvement of the pulmonic valve may necessitate its replacement as well. In the absence of an ASD or VSD, left sided heart valves are not affected due
to inactivation by monoamine oxidase as it passes through the lungs.

Pearls/pitfalls
- Decision to intervene should be based on PREOPERATIVE TTE.
- Incomplete rings avoid suture placement near the triangle of Koch.
- For TV replacement, suture near AV node should be placed at base of septal leaflet, not in the annulus.
- Rule out PFO before performing TV repair with beating heart.
- Consider need for epicardial pacemaker lead at the time of surgery, particularly if implanting a mechanical valve.
- Risk of PPM following TV replacement is 6-10%, commonly following combined TV and MV procedures.

Suggested readings
- Bonow RO, Carabello BA, Kanu C, et   al: ACC/AHA   2006 guidelines for the management of patients with valvular heart disease. *Circulation* 2006; 114:e84-e231.

- Chikwe J, Ayanwu AC. Surgical Strategies for Functional Tricuspid Regurgitation. *Semin Thoracic Surg* 2010;22:90-96.
- Dreyfus GD, Corbi PJ, Chan KM, Bahrami T: Secondary tricuspid regurgitation or dilatation: Which should be the criteria for surgical repair?. *Ann Thorac Surg* 2005; 79:127-132.
- Duran CMG. Surgical Treatment of Tricuspid Valve Disease. Selke FW, del NIdo PJ, Swanson SJ (eds). Sabiston and Spencer - *Surgery of the Chest.* 2010; 1241-1258.

Notes

38. Ischemic mitral regurgitation

Kenan W. Yount, MD, MBA, and Gorav Ailawadi, MD

Concept

*   Coronary artery disease (CAD) and myocardial infarction (MI) can lead to mitral regurgitation (MR) as a consequence of left ventricular (LV) remodeling.
*   The result can be ischemic MR (IMR), a type of functional MR (FMR). Unlike other forms of MR, these are not diseases of the leaflet.
*   Myocardial revascularization alone may not be enough for some of these patients. Ignoring certain degrees of IMR at the time of CABG may limit the potential benefit obtained from surgery and compound an already poor prognosis.

Chief complaint

"A 68 yo woman presents with progressive shortness of breath and limitation of activity over the past six months. Her past medical history is significant for stent placement in the left circumflex (Cx) and right coronary artery (RCA) four years ago after an inferior STEMI. A transthoracic echocardiogram (TTE) at that time showed inferior and lateral wall hypokinesis with mild-to-moderate MR and a LV ejection fraction (EF) of 40-45%."

Differential

Acute coronary syndrome, CHF, pulmonary edema, ischemic or structural MR.

Differential for MR with normal leaflets: functional mitral regurgitation (FMR)

*   Pronounced global LV dilation resulting in annular enlargement. These patients may have severely depressed LV function (usually EF < 30%).
*   *IMR (ischemic MR)*: a form of FMR caused by *asymmetric* ventricular remodeling, most often affecting the inferior and lateral LV wall. Although it can be seen with global LV remodeling, the distinguishing feature usually involves substantial disruption of the subvalvular apparatus, especially downward and lateral (i.e., apical) displacement of the posteromedial papillary muscle leading to leaflet tethering.

- In reality, these two entities lie along a clinical spectrum given the heterogeniety of ischemic heart disease. Although they cannot be completely separated, clarifying the mechanism will help determine surgical management because the degree of LV dysfunction, chamber remodeling, and valvular complex disruption differ with each.
- Carpentier's classification system describes the mechanism of MR. Type I involves normal leaflet motion—MR results from LV enlargement and subsequent annular dilatation (e.g., chronic FMR). Type II involves leaflet prolapse. Type III involves leaflet restriction and is further subdivided into IIIa (restriction during systole and diastole, e.g., rheumatic disease) and IIIb (restriction during systole alone). Chronic IMR is classically Type IIIb and acute IMR due to papillary rupture is Type II.
- *Other diagnoses to consider*: acute postinfarction ischemic mitral regurgitation (with or without papillary muscle rupture; see "Alternative Scenarios"); ischemic CAD with concomitant MR as a result of other etiologies (e.g., degenerative mitral valve disease, rheumatic disease, endocarditis).

History and physical

A focused history and physical should clarify any recent history of acute coronary syndrome (ACS) or angina. Most patients have symptoms of congestive heart failure (CHF) due to worsening LV function and moderate-to-severe MR in the setting of known or unknown prior MI. Consequently, it is necessary to obtain a history of prior cardiac interventions, prior imaging, and progression of current symptomatology. Comorbidities, such as diabetes, pulmonary disease, kidney disease, cerebrovascular disease, and peripheral vascular disease impact surgical outcomes. These patients tend to be high-risk with surgical mortality approaching 5%.

Tests

- CXR may show pulmonary edema and an enlarged cardiac silhouette. Also assess for calcification of the aorta and arch which would warrant a CT.
- EKG may show changes of a prior inferior MI.
- Transthoracic echo (TTE) may show evidence of prior MI and LV dysfunction. Given the primary mechanism is leaflet tethering, the regurgitant jet will be directed *toward* the restricted leaflet; annular dilatation, however, will cause the jet to appear central. Grade – 1 = mild, 2 = moderate, 3 = moderately severe, 4 = severe.
- Transesophageal echo (TEE) is the study of choice to clarify the mechanism of regurgitation. The grade of MR may be lower intraop due to anesthesia and ventricular unloading. Rely on the estimated

degree of regurgitation preoperatively by TTE or TEE but ensure that you have a TEE at some point to give the best anatomical detail and clarity.

- Coronary angiography may show significant multivessel CAD; look for an occluded vessel with inferior wall motion abnormality on LV gram. Clarify right versus left dominance.
- Viability testing may identify patients who could benefit from surgical repair. MR in the setting of inferior scar tissue will not improve with CABG alone while MR in the setting of a lot of viable myocardium may only require bypass.

Index scenario (additional information)
"A more recent TEE now reveals a EF of 40% and severe MR (4+). A subsequent coronary angiogram demonstrates patent Cx stent but a 70% RCA stenosis along with interval development of other significant stenoses (70% OM2, 80% LAD)."

Treatment/management
This patient has severe MR and thus there is no debate that some procedure to address the MR is warranted in addition to the CABG. Although the existence of a survival benefit is controversial, patients with moderate-to-severe IMR with symptomatic CAD have lower rates of postoperative MR and increased functional status after combined CABG-MV repair with fewer patients having postoperative New York Heart Association (NYHA) functional class II or greater (15.5% vs. 43.7%).

Reduction annuloplasty with a slightly undersized, complete ring along with coronary revascularization represents the best surgical approach for this patient. A complete (rigid or semi-rigid) ring is used since both the fibrous and muscular portions of the annulus dilate in IMR and FMR. Annular reduction with a slightly undersized ring (28-30 mm) reduces LV curvature, thus decreasing wall stress and improving LV function. However, this may show more clinical benefit in patients with FMR from global dilatation since symmetric annular dilation predominates. For patients with papillary muscle tethering, this approach may ultimately be insufficient due to the more localized pattern of geometric deformation, possibly explaining their higher rates of recurrent MR postoperatively. Subvalvular interventions to reposition the posterior papillary muscle toward the septal annulus may be of specific benefit for patients with IMR but be sure you have good experience with these procedures if describing them. Most practitioners do not perform ancillary subvalvular interventions in the setting of IMR.

- Swan-Ganz catheter placement should be considered if LV dysfunction and/or pulmonary hypertension are present.
- Intraoperative TEE will help clarify the mechanism of MR and determine the quality of the repair, but it is *not* reliable in judging the severity of MR. Go by the preoperative grade.
- Median sternotomy is the classic approach for combined mitral valve-CABG.
- Bicaval cannulation is routine. Consider femoral venous cannulation in re-do's.
- Myocardial Protection: After the aorta is cross-clamped, antegrade cardioplegic arrest followed by continuous or intermittent retrograde cardioplegic infusion is routine. When significant RCA disease is present, consideration should be given to first anastomosing a vein graft to enable periodic antegrade delivery to the RV.
- After completion of the CABG, expose the mitral valve via left atriotomy.
- Segmental valve analysis with two nerve hooks helps identify P2-P3 leaflet restriction and posterior papillary muscle displacement. Try to rule out any alternative structural leaflet pathology that may explain the MR. For truly IMR the leaflets should be normal but posteriorly restricted.
- Place 2-0 braided non-pledgeted sutures through the annulus in a horizontal fashion. The anterior portion is usually approached last as it is the most difficult to expose. Closely spaced or overlapping sutures will prevent dehiscence when performing restrictive annuloplasty. Size according to both inter-trigonal and anterior leaflet size using the manufacturers sizer. Downsize by roughly one size (usually 28-30 mm), but note that over downsizing increases the risk of dehiscence and stenosis. Sutures are then placed through the ring and tied down to secure the ring to the annulus.
- Cold saline test with forceful ventricular injection to test the valve and/or determine the degree, site, and direction of any residual MR. An alternate method is to give antegrade cardioplegia with the mitral retractors in place rendering the aortic valve partially incompetent.

Potential questions/alternative scenarios

"A 75 yo male presents with 2+ MR, and 3 vessel CAD each with > 70% stenosis. Would you perform a CABG or CABG MVR? He has a history of poorly controlled diabetes, COPD and ESRD."

This patient has moderate IMR with multivessel CAD. Options include surgical revascularization alone versus concomitant mitral valve repair or replacement. Overall, retrospective studies comparing the two approaches have been inconclusive. Although surgical revascularization alone may solve mild IMR, it may be less likely to address moderate-severe disease. To clarify the appropriate management of moderate IMR, an ongoing prospective randomized NIH trial is studying outcomes between the two approaches for patients found to have moderate MR at the time of a planned CABG. Surgical correction introduces a longer cardiopulmonary bypass (CPB) time and combined procedures have an operative mortality of 3-5$^+$%. In a patient who has this many comorbidities you would certainly be justified in doing the most expeditious procedure with least risk which in this case is a CABG alone. For a healthier individual who can tolerate a ring, doing so may decrease the incidence of worsening MR in the future. A viability study may help give this decision. Judgement always comes into play with 2+ MR. As a rule of thumb, 3-4+ should get a mitral ring/replacement unless you have a really good reason to want to limit your pump time and the patient just barely makes 3+ MR.

"A 68 yo male presents with worsening chest pain that began acutely 2 days ago. He had some improvement initially and did not come into the hospital. He now presents with worsening chest pain and increasing shortness of breath. A coronary angio shows a 70% mid circumflex lesion and a 80% RCA lesion. He is left dominant with the circumflex giving off the PDA. His echo shows a ruptured posterior papillary muscle. He is on moderate doses of epinephrine and levophed with PAP of 50/20 and cardiac index of 2.0. His EF is estimated at 50%. His blood pressure is 80/40 mmHg. Physical exam reveals bilateral crackles and a new holosystolic murmur. His CXR shows acute pulmonary edema. How would you proceed."

At least 25% of patients develop either a new mitral murmur or have TTE evidence of MR after an acute MI. Usually, these are transient alterations that ultimately resolve, but MR can be persistent in approximately 1-5% of patients as a result of papillary muscle ischemia. Papillary muscle rupture, in particular, is increasingly rare with today's focus on rapid revascularization after acute STEMI. Nevertheless, it still carries a mortality approaching 50-75% without surgical intervention and 20-25% with surgical intervention. Major contributors to mortality are advanced age, the duration of preoperative shock, the presence of other cardiovascular comorbidities, and operative delay. Postoperative morbidity can result from peripheral organ failure and stroke. Acute IMR occurs 2-7 days (mean 4 days) after MI. Patients present with acute dyspnea due to pulmonary edema and cardiogenic shock. A new holosystolic murmur with the above history could be seen in either an acute VSD or acute IMR. Unlike an acute VSD, MR is best heard at the apex rather than the left sternal border and does not have an associated thrill.

The posteromedial papillary muscle is more vulnerable because of its single blood supply (RCA for right dominant or circumflex for left dominant) compared to the dual blood supply of the anterolateral papillary muscle (LAD and circumflex). Papillary muscle rupture results in flail leaflet. Unlike acute VSD, acute IMR is more commonly associated with acute inferior STEMI.

- *Tests.* EKG may show signs of inferior MI whereas an acute VSD may show conduction abnormalities. A bedside TTE may demonstrate flail mitral leaflets and a mass attached to the chordae, representing the ruptured papillary muscle.
- *Preoperative Stabilization.* Acute IMR can rapidly result in pulmonary edema and multisystem organ failure from reduced forward flow. Inotropes (e.g., milrinone), and vasodilators (e. g., nitroprusside) can stabilize the patient's hemodynamic status; by contrast, volume overload or increased afterload would worsen the patient's MR. Intubation and mechanical ventilation may be required for respiratory failure. Diuretics may reduce pulmonary edema but caution should be taken not to create prerenal azotemia. Other options in unstable patients with evidence of severe end organ damage include intra-aortic balloon pump (IABP) or circulatory support with ECMO or Tandem Heart insertion.
- Pre-operative cardiac catheterization is often performed at the time of diagnosing the MI. This may occur a few days prior to the papillary rupture in which case a stent or angioplasty was likely performed or the cath may be done at the time of diagnosing the IMR if the patient presented in a delayed fashion. If the patient's coronary lesions have not already been addressed then a CABG and MVR should be done. Otherwise proceed to the MVR alone unless there is suspicion for stent thrombosis (EKG with evolving infarct) in which case the cath should be redone.
- *Operative Repair.* Mitral valve repair for papillary muscle rupture is rarely possible. Re-implanting a ruptured papillary muscle into recently infarcted LV tissue can result in repair failure, prolonging bypass time in a patient who has already been in shock. Consequently, mitral valve replacement with chordal preservation if possible is preferred.

"A patient experiences recurrent 3+ MR 1 year after a combined CABG, mitral repair for IMR."
If the patient is symptomatic he is a candidate for a redo mitral valve replacement after re-evaluating his coronary anatomy. Preoperative predictors of annuloplasty failure include larger MV annular diameter (> 3.7 cm), higher tethering area (> 1.6 cm^2), and greater MR severity (3.5+).

"What is the role of mitral valve replacement in ischemic MR?"
Repair typically results in superior LV function, avoidance of a prosthetic valve or the need for long-term anticoagulation, and less distortion of ventricular shape. Thus, while replacement solves the problem of recurrent MR, it is generally reserved for 1) inability to address leaflet tethering or severe leaflet tethering 2) an unclear or combined mechanism (e.g., degenerative or rheumatic disease with IMR), 3) papillary muscle rupture and 4) re-operative settings. Repair does not appear to offer better survival over replacement in subset of patients with eccentric and complex jets, NYHA III-IV, or severe shock with multiple comorbidities. These "sicker" patients can do just as well with a replacement which gives you the best chance of leaving the operating room with a single pump run and no MR. In reality, both approaches are widely performed and much of the literature comparing repair vs. replacement in advanced IMR has been derived from retrospective studies, which have produced conflicting results. A currently ongoing prospective randomized NIH trial for patients with severe IMR comparing the two strategies may provide further guidance.

If replacement is chosen, complete chordal preservation leads to better postoperative LV function and survival compared to complete excision. A bioprosthetic valve is logical given that a majority of patients in whom replacement is favored in these settings will not experience valve degeneration in their lifetime.

"What is the current role of percutaneous therapy for IMR?"
While the MitraClip may not provide comparable results to a standard surgical repair in the reduction of MR severity, patients at high surgical risk *may* be good candidates. MitraClip achieved reduction of MR by 2 grades in 65% of patients and clinical improvement in 90% of patients. Ongoing studies (e.g., the COAPT trial) will help determine the efficacy of this therapy in functional MR patients.

"Is there any role for cardiac re-synchronization (CRT) in IMR?"
The MIRACLE trial revealed that CRT not only induced reverse remodeling but also reduced the degree of IMR at 12 months, likely by correcting dyssynchrony between the posterior papillary muscle and the lateral LV wall. This therapy should also be considered as an adjunct to surgical correction in
patients with MR and heart failure.

- Mild-to-moderate MR with symptomatic CAD: Sometimes the association can be incidental. Concomitant repair in these settings is more controversial. Combined CABG-mitral valve repair will decrease MR severity more than CABG alone, but it may have no effect on survival. Consequently, preoperative risk factors should help guide the decision to add mitral valve repair to a CABG (e.g., mitral annular calcification, extensive aortic calcification warranting off-pump CABG, etc.). 3-4+ MR gives more justification for a combined procedure.

- *Intraoperative TEE.* The decision to perform mitral valve repair ideally should be made prior to the OR, as intraoperative TEE may downplay the degree of MR as a consequence of the unloading effect of general anesthesia.

- *Residual MR.* Preoperative predictors of annuloplasty failure include larger MV annular diameter (> 3.7 cm), higher tethering area (> 1.6 cm^2), and greater MR severity (3.5+).

- Adjunctive therapies to address the subvalvular apparatus: Consider posterior leaflet extension, papillary muscle repositioning using a pledgeted suture from the papillary head to the annulus, resection of secondary chordae, or septolateral "cinching."

- If the LV is markedly enlarged, a Dor procedure can stabilize the position of the papillary muscles and prevent late apical migration of the subvalvular apparatus.

Suggested readings

- Adams DH, Filsoufi F, Aklog L, Salzberg SP. Mitral Valve Repair: Ischemic. Kaiser LR, Kron, IL, Spray TL (eds). Mastery of Cardiothoracic Surgery 2nd edition. 2007.

- Anyanwu AC, Aklog L, Adams DH. Ischemic mitral regurgitation. Selke FW, del Nido PJ, Swanson SJ (eds). Surgery of the Chest 8th edition. 2010.

- Atluri P, Gorman RC, Gorman JH, Acker MA. Ischemic Mitral Regurgitation. Cohn L (ed). Cardiac Surgery in the Adult 4th edition. 2011.

- Cohn L. Mitral valve repair. Kaiser LR, Kron, IL, Spray TL (eds). Mastery of Cardiothoracic Surgery. 2nd edition. 2007.

- LaPar DJ, Kron IL. Should all ischemic mitral regurgitation be repaired? When should we replace? Curr Opin Cardiol. 2011 Mar;26(2):113-7.

Notes

39. Non-ischemic mitral regurgitation

Jennifer M. Worth, MD, and Chittoor B. Sai-Sudhakar, MD

Concept

- Indications for mitral valve intervention in the setting of non-ischemic regurgitation
- Preoperative considerations
- Repair and valve choices
- Critical steps
- Pitfalls and alternative solutions

Chief complaint

"A 68 yo woman is referred to you with a 4 month history of shortness of breath after being diagnosed with severe mitral regurgitation by echocardiography."

Differential

Differentiate functional versus organic etiology. Functional mitral regurgitation (normal leaflets) is often ischemic in origin. Organic mitral regurgitation (intrinsic valve abnormality) is often non-ischemic. Degenerative causes for the later include primary myxomatous disease, flail leaflets and annular calcification. Endocarditis and rheumatic disease each account for about 5% of mitral regurgitation cases.

History and physical

Important to elicit any symptoms of angina or heart failure in addition to comorbid conditions which all affect survival. Focused physical exam including vitals, neuro exam, carotid bruits, heart/lung sounds, peripheral exam including pulses and edema. Murmur of MR best heard in the left lateral decubitus position at the apex. The murmur will be holosystolic, radiating to the axilla.

Tests

- *EKG*: look for evidence of previous infarcts, cardiomegaly; may see left atrial (LA) enlargement or atrial fibrillation.
- *CXR*: may see cardiomegaly or LA enlargement.
- *Echo*: severe MR documented by a vena contracta width of ≥ 0.7 cm, effective regurgitant orifice (ERO) ≥ 0.4 cm^2, regurgitant volume (RV) ≥ 60 mL, regurgitant fraction (RF) $\geq 50\%$ and an effective regurgitant orifice/jet area (ERO) $> 40\%$ of LA area. 3D echo is a useful modification to enable better visualization of functional and anatomic relationships to help plan operations.

Table 39-1. Mitral regurgitation severity.

	RV	RF	ERO
Mild	< 30 mL	< 30%	< 0.2 cm²
Moderate	30-59 mL	30-49%	0.2-0.39 cm²
Severe	> 60 mL	> 50%	> 0.4 cm²

- More commonly the MR is graded on a scale of 1-4: 1 = mild, 2 = moderate, 3 = moderately severe, and 4 = severe.
- *Cardiac catheterization*: look for evidence of coronary artery disease.

Index scenario (additional information)
"The patient is not diabetic, has shortness of breath with moderate activity and vena contracta of 0.6 cm, EF 55-60% with mild dilation of the LA, and prolapse of the P2 leaflet. The MR is graded as 3-4+. What are her options and how would you proceed?"

Treatment/management
This patient has moderate-severe symptomatic MR and thus meets criteria for mitral valve intervention. Options include repair vs. replacement with repair yielding the most favorable survival profile. Criteria favoring mitral valve repair include chordal rupture in a limited portion of the posterior leaflet with normal anterior leaflet, or simple prolapse of the posterior leaflet. In addition, ruptured chordae to the anterior leaflet, myxomatous degeneration, or leaflet perforation/chordal rupture from endocarditis are often amenable to repair as well.

Operative steps
Goals – Repair valve if technically feasible, otherwise replace with mechanical valve if less than 60 yo (needs to be explained to the patient preoperatively). Use a bioprosthetic valve in patients > 60 yo, women of childbearing age, or if contraindication to warfarin exists.

- Place a large bore IV, arterial line, GETA, PA catheter, foley catheter.
- Check intraoperative TEE for mitral anatomy. Confirm the direction and complexity of the jet, the presence of flail or prolapse. Anteriorly directed jet - think posterior prolapse, and vice versa. The TEE gives you a sense for the feasibility of repair. Also bear in mind your tolerance for a second pump run if the repair fails. For this you need to consider comorbidities, age, etc.
- Median sternotomy, pericardial stay sutures, palpate the aorta for calcifications.

- Heparin (400 mg/kg), aortic cannulation, bicaval venous cannulation, antegrade and retrograde cardioplegia catheters placed. Initiate CPB once ACT is 480. Deair antegrade line, run antegrade induction, follow with retrograde. +/- Cool to 28-32° C. Dissect the IVC and SVC free and encircle and snare with Rummel tourniquets.
- The exposure is a matter of choice but make sure that the exposure is excellent. The suturing needs to be precise and thus you need to be able to describe or conduct an exposure that you are most comfortable with. Also you may need to conform to the patients anatomy. Deep chest with wide AP diameter favors transseptal while Sondergaard's groove is favored otherwise. If the transseptal needs to be extended you carry a risk of damaging the artery to the SA node which lessens the chance of sinus rythm. The following describes the LA approach (Sondergaard's groove):
  - Stab wound is placed in the LA at the base of the RSPV. LA is opened to the level of the inferior pulmonary vein and superiorly towards the SVC. A pump sucker or basket is placed into the LA to keep the operative field dry. Self retaining or hand held retractors are used to aid the exposure.
- Examine the valve anatomy: note the annulus (dilated, calcified - atrial versus ventricular calcification), note the leaflet tissue (prolapse - which segment?, flail, redundant myxomatous tissue or limited fibroelastic degenerative tissue), examine the chordal attachments (primary-margin, secondary - underside, tertiary - annulus), and the height of the posterior leaflet (ideal is 2/3 anterior and 1/3 posterior, or less than 1.5 cm posterior leaflet).

Valve repair
- A ring annuloplasty is considered a necessary adjunct to reinforce most repair techniques. Some surgeons place the annuloplasty sutures first to aid the exposure. Start with the posterior trigone (right - surgeons view), and work clockwise towards the other side using non-pledgeted braided horizontal sutures. Make sure you get the fibrous trigones. Care with the coronary sinus along the right, the circumflex along the base and the aortic valve along the left vertical surface (surgeons view).
- Often helps to place a silk suture around the healthy chordae that flank a diseased segment.
- *Posterior leaflet prolapsed.* Depending on the amount of redundant leaflet tissue and height of the leaflet, either a simple triangular resection or quadrangular resection can be performed. Excessive, myxomatous tissue with high posterior leaflet = quadrangular resection of the prolapsed leaflet with or without sliding annuloplasty depending on the degree of height reduction that you

need. Cut edges of leaflets are approximated using interrupted or running non-absorbable suture.

- Not much redundant tissue, fibroelastic degenerative, elderly patient with reasonably sized height, isolated ruptured chordae with flail = triangular resection with reapproximation.
- Anterior leaflet prolapsed = artificial chordae or chordal transfer of primary and secondary chordae from posterior to anterior leaflet.
- Adjunctive maneuvers include closure of strained clefts, lateral resection and sliding annuloplasty for prolapsed lateral segments, artificial chordae (especially for prolapsed anterior leaflet) etc.
- Size the annuloplasty band to the anterior mitral leaflet or intertrigonal distance and upsize if possible. In general you are placing a 30-34 mm band. The larger band helps prevent systolic anterior motion (SAM).
- Sew the band and tie the sutures.
- Assess the valve on TEE with low threshold to convert a repair to a replacement if left with 2-3+ MR. Use judgement, 1-2+ MR in a frail elderly patient is likely to be ok. Incidentally, the older the patient and the more the comorbidities, the more you might consider a replacement with a tissue valve.

Valve replacement
- Resect the valve leaflets 2-3 mm from the anterior annulus. If the posterior leaflet is thin and pliable, leave it in position and only resect the anterior leaflet. There are methods to preserve the anterior leaflet including suturing it to the posterior annulus with the valve stitches or resecting an anterior rectangle and suturing the two halves to their respective lateral or posterior annulus. The more you can preserve, the better the postoperative function, however, do not sacrifice a wide open LVOT especially in a small hyperdynamic LV cavity.
- If calcium is encountered in the subannular space, debride only if necessary for the valve to lie flat and well apposed to the annulus. Atrial decalcification can be done safely but the more you debride the ventricular calcification the greater the risk of AV groove disruption or circumflex injury. If you debride the calcification extensively including the ventricular calcium then you need a pericardial patch that saddles the annulus circumferentially. If you do not need much debridement an option is to take your suture bites such that the pledgets remain on the ventricular side. Otherwise, suture using interrupted horizontal mattress sutures with pledgets on the atrial side.

- Bioprosthetic valves should be oriented with the post well out of the outflow tract. Mechanical valves are sutured in an anti-anatomic arrangement.
- Close atriotomy with running prolene suture, irrigate, deair and wean from CPB.

Potential questions/alternative scenarios

"A 60 yo woman presents for follow up of her known mitral regurgitation. She has minimal symptoms which in no way disrupt her activities of daily living. She is fairly active. When would you offer an asymptomatic patient an MVR."

According to the guidelines, patients with chronic severe MR (3-4+) should be offered surgery if the patient experiences mild-moderate LV dysfunction with an EF less than 60%, moderate PHTN (PAP > 50 mmHg at rest), new onset afib, or a left ventricular end systolic diameter (LVESD) greater than or equal to 40 mm. Asymptomatic patients with preserved EF and > 90% likelihood of successful repair may be offered surgery for chronic severe MR.

"Your patient being evaluated for a mitral repair had a previous AVR complicated by a wound infection and mediastinitis requiring flap closure."

Right anterolateral thoracotomy approach - 4th intercostal space centered in the anterior axillary line. Femoral venous and arterial cannulation. Be familiar with alternative strategies to arrest the heart since you may not be able to clamp and deliver antegrade so easily in this case. Options include hypothermic fibrillatory arrest or endoballoon.

"Patient is obese with a very deep chest and you anticipate difficulty exposing the mitral valve through the left atrium."

Transseptal approach. Limited transseptal requires a stab incision into the fossa ovalis that is extended inferiorly towards the IVC. For an extended transseptal, extend this incision superiorly towards the dome of the LA. Make the RA incision meet the septal incision and extend onto the dome. If you were already in the LA (Sondergaard's groove approach) then your options are to extend the incision superiorly and inferiorly as much as possible or close the incision and convert to a transseptal. The SA node artery can be injured with this approach but the exposure is excellent. This is helpful in patients with deep chests, redos, small LA or previous atriotomy.

"Anesthesia gives the patient nipride to make room for more volume when coming off the pump. The patient becomes hypotensive and 3+ MR is noted with encroachment of the anterior leaflet onto the LVOT. What is the treatment?"

This patient has systolic anterior motion (SAM) of the mitral valve which was accentuated by the increased ventricular systolic contraction in the setting of an underfilled ventricle. The treatment of choice here is to wait while the the volume rolls in. May also consider adding a beta blocker to reduce the vigor of the systolic contractions once the volume is optimized.

"Describe SAM and options for correcting it after an attempted mitral repair."

The line of coaptation after a reduction annuloplasty and leaflet resection/repair typically gets displaced just a bit more anterior (towards the LVOT) than it did before. The anterior leaflet can obstruct the LVOT during systole creating a gradient. As the anterior leaflet gets sucked into the LVOT during systole (Venturi effect), the posterior leaflet prolapses towards the atrium causing an anteriorly directed jet. Thus, the 2 main worrisome components of SAM are regurgitation and high LVOT gradient. If the posterior leaflet is left > 1.5 cm in height after repair the risk for SAM is greater. If the patient has a small hyperdynamic ventricle the risk for SAM is greater. If the ring is undersized too much then the risk of SAM is also greater because the line of coaptation bulges anteriorly. First ensure that you are not simply underfilled as described in the prior scenario. Otherwise, treatment strategies aim to reduce the posterior leaflet height if it is clear that that is the culprit. Folding valvuloplasty of the edge of the posterior leaflet with interrupted horizontal pledgeted sutures, changing a triangular resection into a quadrangular with sliding annuloplasty, and placement of a larger ring are all options for reducing the posterior leaflet height. A more aggressive maneuver is to replace the valve. Another simple fix in a frail high risk patient that may not tolerate a second pump run is an Alfieri stitch.

"After a mitral valve replacement a significant amount of bright red blood is seen welling up behind the heart once the cross clamp is released!"

Atrioventricular dissociation after mitral valve replacement. Often occurs after completion of CPB or a few hours after procedure. Patients have massive intrapericardial hemorrhage which can be a lethal event. Rupture occurs in the LV near the AV groove posteriorly. Tends to occur more in women with small LVs. Generally considered to be a technical error from a) too much traction on the annulus during excision of the valve or insertion of prosthesis; b) tearing of the annulus after the new valve is in place when the heart is lifted manually; c) penetration of stitches in the posterior left AV groove; d) perforation from papillary muscle excision; e) perforation of AV groove during calcium debridement (especially with ventricular calcium). Go back on CPB and arrest. Re-open the LA, remove the prosthesis and inspect the ventricle. An appropriately sized pericardial patch is secured over the area of perforation with a running prolene suture and interrupted pledgeted sutures as needed. The valve is re-inserted through the patch and the operation is completed as previously described.

"ST changes are noted along the lateral leads and the patient becomes hypotensive requiring high dose epinephrine and levophed. What has happened?"
The differential may include postcardiotomy syndrome with cardiogenic shock from reperfusion or poor protection. However, the most likely culprit in the setting of a valve replacement is damage to the coronary especially with the isolated lead changes. Go back on, harvest a segment of vein, arrest and bypass to a distal OM.

Note that a valve causing excessive traction on the circumflex can lead to delayed myocardial ischemia and even LV rupture secondary to erosion of the strut through an infarcted LV free wall. This is seen most often in women with a small LV or when the LV is weakened after an infarct. Special care needs to be taken to ensure the safety of the circumflex artery and if any question is raised, a marginal branch should be bypassed using a SVG prior to coming off cardiopulmonary bypass.

Pearls/pitfalls
- Know the indications for mitral valve surgery - symptomatic 3-4+; asymptomatic 3-4+ with PHTN, afib, ESV > 40 mm, EF < 60%, high likelihood of repair in severe 4+ MR.
- Know the different exposures for the mitral valve and when you would choose one over the other. ie. transseptal for deep chest or redo, lateral thoracotomy for hostile mediastinum.
- Know the major complications of the procedure - circumflex injury, AV disruption.
- Recognize SAM and its treatment (medical - volume, betablocker, and surgical - leaflet valvuloplasty, quadrangular resection with sliding annuloplasty, upsizing the band).
- Know how to deal with a calcified mitral annulus.

Suggested readings

- Kouchoukos NT and Kirklin JW. Kirklin/Barratt-Boyes *Cardiac Surgery: Morphology, Diagnostic Criteria, Natural History, Techniques, Results, and Indications.* Philadelphia, Pa: Churchill Livingstone, 2003.
- Yuh, DD, Vricella LA and Baumgartner WA.*The Johns Hopkins Manual of Cardiothoracic Surgery.* New York: McGraw-Hill Medical Pub, 2007.

Notes

40. Redo mitral valve replacement

Cynthia E. Wagner, MD, and Gorav Ailawadi, MD

Concept

- Indications and outcomes for reoperative mitral valve surgery
- Considerations for re-repair vs. primary replacement
- Considerations for bioprosthetic vs. mechanical valve replacement
- Operative details specific to redo mitral valve surgery
- Complications of mitral valve surgery

Chief complaint

"A 70 yo woman with a 3-month history of dyspnea on exertion is referred by her cardiologist after a TTE showed severe MR due to leaflet prolapse, mitral annular calcification, mild pulmonary hypertension, and EF 55%. The patient underwent mitral valve repair for leaflet prolapse ten years ago."

Differential

The diagnosis has been established and should be confirmed with a detailed H&P and appropriate tests. In the absence of an echo report, the differential diagnosis for these symptoms in a patient s/p valve repair would include recurrent MR, MS, AS, AI, cardiomyopathy, CHF, pulmonary hypertension, stable/unstable angina, or primary pulmonary disease.

History and physical

A thorough history to establish functional status, assess for comorbidities (HTN, HLD, DM, AF, CAD, carotid disease, PVD, CKD), and determine all prior surgeries or procedures. Detailed operative reports from all prior cardiac surgeries should be obtained. Some patients will not recognize stent placement (cardiac or aortoiliac) or pacemaker placement as surgery and should be asked directly about these procedures, as they will guide further work-up and may impact plans for cannulation. A history of trauma to the right chest should be inquired about if a right lateral thoracotomy is planned. Medications should be reviewed and indications for anticoagulation should be questioned, as this may impact choice of valve prosthesis if mitral valve replacement (MVR) is planned. Social factors, including family planning in younger female patients, occupation, and hobbies, should be identified that may increase bleeding risk from anticoagulation for a mechanical valve. All patients should be asked about prior stroke and residual deficits prior to cardiac surgery. A focused physical examination should follow, assessing for heart rate and rhythm, murmurs, bruits, bibasilar rales, and lower extremity edema, and noting all prior surgical incisions. In select patients, assess fall risk and frailty with grip strength and 15 ft walk test.

Tests

- EKG to assess for AF.
- CXR to assess number of sternal wires, may show cardiomegaly and cephalization of pulmonary blood flow.
- Non-contrast chest CT to assess distance between posterior sternum and anterior RV as well as extent of aortic calcification and mitral annular calcification, and CTA chest to identify course of patent grafts if patient has undergone prior CABG.
- CTA abdomen/pelvis to assess vessel caliber and tortuosity if femoral cannulation is planned.
- Preoperative TEE to better visualize mitral valve pathology is essential in determining mechanism of MR, especially if re-repair is planned, and may identify thrombus in the LA appendage if patient has AF.
- Cardiac catheterization should be routine, as undiagnosed CAD may result in perioperative morbidity or the need for further reoperation, and is essential in determining patency of grafts in patients who have undergone prior CABG.
- Consider right heart catheterization in patients with severe LV or RV dysfunction or symptomatic patients in class III-IV CHF.
- Carotid duplex in high-risk patients.
- PFTs in select patients.
- Obtain prior operative report to include year of surgery, details of operation, valve exposure, possible location of grafts, manufacturer of valve.

Index scenario (additional information)

"The patient has had progressively worsening MR and LV function on annual TTE, and has been asymptomatic on a diuretic and an ACE inhibitor until recently. She does not have AF and does not require anticoagulation for any pre-existing disease. She has HTN, hyperlipidemia (HLD), and DM, and a preoperative cardiac catheterization shows severe multi-vessel CAD. This prompts a carotid duplex prior to cardiac surgery. A chest CT shows a mildly dilated RV immediately posterior to the sternum and an ascending aorta with minimal atherosclerotic disease. A CTA abdomen/pelvis is done in anticipation of femoral cannulation prior to redo sternotomy."

Treatment/management

This patient meets criteria for a reoperative mitral valve surgery according to current ACC/AHA guidelines.

Table 40-1. Indications for intervention in mitral valve disease.

Symptomatic patients with moderately severe to severe MR (3-4+) or moderate to severe MS
Asymptomatic patients with severe MR with any of the following conditions: • EF < 60% • LV end-systolic diameter > 40-45 mm • PHTN with PASP > 50-60 mmHg New-onset AF

Mitral valve repair eliminates the risks associated with MVR, including bleeding, thromboembolic events, and prosthetic valve endocarditis. Re-repair is associated with lower mortality compared to replacement at reoperation, and may be attempted on previously repaired mitral valves unless severe calcification of the leaflets, annulus, and subvalvular apparatus or extensive leaflet destruction from endocarditis is present. However, this requires a high comfort level with redo repair strategies - it is never wrong to replace especially during a redo. Etiology of valve disease dictates durability of repair. After primary mitral valve repair, freedom from reoperation at 10 years is 95% in patients with degenerative valve disease vs. 53% in patients with rheumatic valve disease. Early failure after repair (< 2 years) is often the result of technical failure, while late failure after repair (> 2 years) is often due to progression of native valve disease. Repair without ring annuloplasty is a predictor of recurrent MR and need for reoperation. The majority of first-time reoperations after mitral valve repair result in replacement, for which preservation of the subvalvular apparatus should be attempted as this has been shown to reduce operative mortality and preserve EF. Major factors to consider in discussions regarding bioprosthetic vs. mechanical MVR include patient age, life expectancy, comorbidities, and bleeding risk from anticoagulation. Bioprosthetic valves will deteriorate, and the rate of structural valve deterioration and need for reoperation are inversely related to patient age at implantation. Mechanical mitral valves require lifelong anticoagulation (INR goal of 2.5-3.5), and the risk of hemorrhagic stroke is 2-4% per patient per year. The rate of thromboembolic complications (1-3% per patient per year) and the risk of prosthetic valve endocarditis are similar between bioprosthetic and mechanical valves. Although mechanical valves do not structurally deteriorate, they are prone to paravalvular leaks and undergo nonstructural dysfunction (pannus formation). The average time to reoperation after primary MVR is similar between bioprosthetic and mechanical valves (mean 11.5 years), though the durability of a mechanical valve can extend years beyond that of a bioprosthetic valve. The majority of bioprosthetic valves are replaced for structural deterioration and the majority of mechanical valves are replaced for paravalvular leak. The operative mortality of redo MVR is approximately 4.7%. There is no significant difference in operative mortality after redo MVR in patients receiving bioprosthetic vs. mechanical valves (5% vs. 4.4%). Mortality rates have decreased in recent years due to earlier intervention prior to significant LV dysfunction and advances in operative techniques and perioperative care.

Operative steps

- Consider femoral or axillary arterial cannulation and femoral venous cannulation prior to redo sternotomy if RV is adherent to chest wall. (See Chapter 36, Redo aortic valve replacement for cannulation algorithm).

- Redo sternotomy is the most common approach for reoperative mitral valve surgery and demands preoperative identification of patent grafts from prior CABG, proximity of heart to posterior sternum, and RV dilatation. A median sternotomy is necessary in the setting of concomitant CABG or AVR. However, a right lateral thoracotomy is an alternative approach in select patients undergoing exclusive mitral valve surgery (tricuspid valve may also be visualized with this approach).

- Myocardial protection is commonly achieved with cardioplegic arrest with antegrade and/or retrograde cold blood cardioplegia. Strategies for myocardial protection will need to be altered in patients with a patent LIMA-LAD from prior CABG. DHCA or ventricular fibrillatory arrest may be feasible in select patients undergoing exclusive mitral valve surgery without significant AI.

- Standard left atriotomy is begun in Waterston's interatrial groove and extended inferiorly to provide optimal exposure of the mitral valve. A transeptal approach through a right atriotomy is a common alternative in patients with significant adhesions undergoing reoperative mitral valve surgery.

- In patients undergoing MVR after repair, all attempts should be made to preserve native leaflet tissue and associated chordae tendineae during MVR, as disruption of the continuity between the mitral annulus and LV apex has been shown to result in decreased LV function postoperatively. This can be accomplished by imbrication of the leaflet tissue to the annulus.

- Care must be taken when resecting valve sewing rings to avoid removal of excess annular tissue and subsequent disruption of the atrioventricular junction. There are several options for mitral annular reconstruction, including bovine vs. autologous pericardial patch reconstruction or suture placement across the atrioventricular junction to restore a fibrous mitral annulus.

- In patients presenting with a paravalvular leak after MVR, consider percutaneous closure devices or open repair with pledgeted reinforcing sutures or a bovine pericardial patch prior to excision of a competent valve (though most often these patients require redo MVR). Read the prior operative report carefully. These type of minimally invasive options may be ideal for patients who had a very difficult initial operation with annular reconstruction.

- Determining valve competency with saline test and intraoperative TEE following repair is crucial in identifying need for immediate revision, as residual MR (> 1+) at the completion of surgery is a risk factor for recurrence of moderate/severe MR and need for reoperative mitral valve surgery, and cumulative risk of mortality increases with each reoperation.

Potential questions/alternative scenarios

"The patient requires high-dose pressors as they are weaned from CPB. This pressor requirement persists into postoperative day 1 and a TTE shows a lateral wall motion abnormality. Discuss the complication."

The distance between the posterolateral mitral annulus and the circumflex artery is 2-4 mm. Patients are at risk for postoperative MI if sutures are placed too wide or deep around the posterolateral annulus during MVR or ring annuloplasty.

"The patient is unable to be weaned from CPB without external V-pacing. The monitor shows complete heart block. Discuss the complication."

The AV node is deep to the posteromedial commissure. Care must be taken to avoid placing sutures too deep around the annulus during MVR or ring annuloplasty.

"Discuss the risks, management, and prevention of prosthetic valve endocarditis (PVE)."

Risk of infection is greatest during the first three postoperative months and decreases thereafter to < 1% per patient per year after the first postoperative year. Early PVE (within the first 2 months) is often caused by virulent *Staphylococcus* infections and has a higher mortality than late PVE, often the result of *Streptococcus* infections. Infection is localized to the sewing ring of mechanical valves, resulting in abscess formation and dehiscence, while infection of bioprosthetic valves occurs on the leaflets and leads to vegetations and leaflet perforation. Indications for and timing of surgery should be individualized and based on response to antibiotics and hemodynamic stability (see Chapter 45, Endocarditis). Despite improved outcomes after surgery, PVE continues to carry a high mortality rate, and in patients with prosthetic heart valves, the AHA currently recommends prophylaxis with amoxicillin or cephalexin prior to dental procedures, invasive procedures of the respiratory tract involving biopsy, or excision of infected soft tissues.

"The patient agrees to undergo bioprosthetic MVR. She asks if a third operation will be likely."

In patients receiving bioprosthetic valve replacements, the freedom from reoperation at 15 years is 80%. Bioprosthetic valves in the mitral position are exposed to increased hemodynamic stress during systole compared to bioprosthetic valves in the aortic position and undergo deterioration at a higher rate. Currently, younger patients are receiving bioprosthetic valves due to improvements in valve design and durability and options for transcatheter valve-in-valve implantation.

Pearls/pitfalls

- Considerations in reoperative surgery include alternative strategies for cannulation, surgical approach to the mitral valve, and myocardial protection.
- Mitral valve repair at primary surgery and at reoperation is associated with lower mortality compared to MVR and should be attempted if possible (this requires a high comfort level with redo repair strategies - it is never wrong to replace especially during a redo).
- Choice of bioprosthetic vs. mechanical MVR should be based on individualized risk of reoperation vs. anticoagulation.
- MVR with leaflet/chordal sparing is associated with improved outcomes but do not compromise your outflow.
- The mitral annulus is in close proximity to the circumflex artery and AV node.

Suggested readings

- Acquired disease of the mitral valve. Sabiston and Spencer - Surgery of the Chest, 8th edition. 1207-1240.
- Reoperative valve surgery. Cohn L (ed). Cardiac Surgery in the Adult. 3rd edition. 1159-1174.
- Nardi et al. Survival and durability of mitral valve repair surgery for degenerative mitral valve disease. J Card Surg. 2011 Jul;26(4):3606.
- Suri RM et al. Recurrent mitral regurgitation after repair: should the mitral valve be re-repaired? J Thorac Cardiovasc Surg. 2006 Dec;132(6):1390-7.
- Potter et al. Risk of repeat mitral valve replacement for failed mitral valve prostheses. Ann Thorac Surg. 2004 Jul;78(1):67-72.

Notes

41. Mitral stenosis

Marek Polomsky, MD, and Robert A. Guyton, MD

Concept

- Indications for mitral valve replacement (MVR) in setting of mitral stenosis (MS)
- Preoperative conditions
- Valve choices
- Critical steps of MVR
- Pitfalls and alternative solutions

Chief complaint

"A 53 yo immigrant man presents with a diagnosis of mitral stenosis. His primary care physician heard a diastolic apical heart murmur, and subsequent echocardiogram revealed severe mitral stenosis."

Differential

The diagnosis of mitral stenosis is established. Differential causes of mitral stenosis include rheumatic heart disease (majority), congenital malformation, infective endocarditis (IE), mitral annular calcification, rheumatologic disorders, endomyocardial fibrosis, conditions that obstruct the mitral valve (left atrial myxoma, cor triatriatum), and prosthetic valve complications (thrombosis, calcification).

History and physical

A focused history is performed to elicit symptoms of dyspnea and hemoptysis, as well as chest pain and hoarseness, which occur less frequently. Symptoms are brought on by any situation that increase the transmitral pressure gradient (exertion, stress, exercise, tachycardia, fever, infection, atrial fibrillation (AF), pregnancy). Many patients deny symptoms because progression of disease is very slow, thus there is a gradual decrease in activity and exercise tolerance. MS can present with complications such as AF, pulmonary edema, embolic events, IE, and right heart failure. One should ascertain whether there is a prior history of rheumatic heart disease (if treated and which kind of antibiotics) and if the patient is an immigrant from another country. A complete physical should be performed focusing on the cardiovascular exam with presence of murmur (low-pitched diastolic rumble most prominent at the apex), opening snap of the mitral valve heard at the apex, and signs of right heart failure indicative of advanced disease. Pinkish blue patches on cheeks ("mitral facies") may be present from vasoconstriction due to low cardiac output.

Tests

- *EKG.* An EKG is performed to assess for any arrhythmias (particularly AF). In addition, a broad p-wave that is notched with increased amplitude ("p-mitrale") from left atrial (LA) hypertrophy or enlargement may be present.
- *Echo (M-mode, two-dimensional and color Doppler flow mapping).* Echocardiography is used to assess morphology of the valve apparatus and subvalvular structures (chordae and papillary muscles), measurement of valve orifice, Doppler transvalvular gradient and valve area (calculated from diastolic velocity curve), coexisting mitral regurgitation, pulmonary pressures, systolic function, exclusion of LA thrombus, and size of LA, left ventricle, and right ventricle. Transesophageal echo (TEE) is generally preferred over transthoracic echo (TTE).
- *Cardiac catheterization.* Cardiac catheterization is performed in order to assess the coronaries, mitral valve gradient, and pulmonary artery pressures.
- *CXR.* LA enlargement, a calcified mitral annulus, and pulmonary vasculature congestion or cephalization may be visible on a CXR. If aorta appears calcified check CT.
- *Stress echo (exercise or dobutamine stress echo).* A stress echocardiogram is used to objectively evaluate exercise activity, which is important for provocation of symptoms in inactive patients, and to assess pulmonary artery pressures with exertion.

Index scenario (additional information)
"The patient had history of rheumatic heart disease as child, and after diagnostic work-up was found to have very calcified severe MS (valve area 0.8 cm^2) with severe pulmonary hypertension (70 mmHg). He is mildly symptomatic."

Treatment/management
This patient meets criteria for mitral valve replacement. Surgery (MVR) is indicated (2006 ACC/AHA guidelines) in patients who are found to have moderate-severe MS (MV area < 1.5 cm^2), NYHA class III or IV symptoms, and the valve is not amenable to either percutaneous mitral balloon valvuloplasty (PMBV). In addition, mildly symptomatic patients (NYHA II) with severe MS and pulmonary hypertension (PAP > 50 mmHg at rest, > 60 with exercise) who are not candidates for valvulotomy are considered for surgery. Severe PHTN, however, raises a red flag. It is hard to tell whether this will be readily reversible or not. It is worth a chance but care must be taken in the postoperative setting. PMBV is not appropriate if there is presence of LA thrombus that persists despite anticoagulation, mitral valve is nonpliable or severely calcified, or if there is moderate-severe mitral regurgitation (MR).

Wilkins score > 8 predicts failure with valvuloplasty (leaflet mobility, thickening, calcs, subvalvular apparatus). Mechanical prosthesis is recommended in this patient, and in patients that present young (< 65 yo) especially with long standing AF. A bioprosthetic valve would be indicated in patients who are elderly, who cannot have warfarin, or who are not compliant.

Operative steps

Mitral valve replacement

Goals – relieve obstruction, replace the valve, protect the heart/ coronaries, prevent further clot formation and embolization.

- Place central line with Swan-Ganz catheter, arterial line, general endotracheal anesthesia (GETA), foley.
- Assess mitral valve via TEE.
- Perform median sternotomy. Palpate for aortic calcifications +/- epiaortic US.
- Systemic heparin, aortic cannulation, 3-stage venous or bicaval cannulation, retrograde cardioplegia cannula.
- Initiate cardiopulmonary bypass (CPB) once ACT level appropriate (400-600), +/- cooling (28-32° C).
- Cross-clamp, run cold blood antegrade cardioplegia, followed by retrograde.
- Vertical left atriotomy incision in Sondergaard's groove anterior to the right pulmonary veins (or use exposure of choice).
- Place sump vent into LA in dependent position near left superior pulmonary vein.
- Inspect the mitral valve.
- *Note*: perform any necessary afib procedures such as left atrial appendage excision/ligation/ MAZE at this time to avoid manipulating the heart too much after the prosthesis is in place.
- Excise calcified leaflets leaving 1-2 mm of leaflet tissue along the annular circumference, dividing chordae along tips of papillary muscles (preserve subvalvular apparatus and papillary muscle-chordal-leaflet attachments whenever possible, but not at the expense of outflow tract obstruction in a small ventricle). Usually the posterior leaflet can be salvaged to maintain continuity while the anterior is resected.
- Size the valve, place horizontal mattress sutures 8-10 mm apart (usually with pledgets) around the annulus, everting (atrium–ventricle) for mechanical valve, and non-everting for bioprosthetic valve (ventricle-atrium) or calcified annulus.

- Pass sutures through sewing ring, and seat the valve. Mechanical valve should be in anti-anatomic position, bioprosthetic valve with largest leaflet facing the left ventricular outflow tract (LVOT) avoiding outflow obstruction. Use a dental mirror to double check.
- Tie down sutures, and start rewarming if cool.
- Close left atriotomy with 3-0 or 4-0 prolene, leaving LV vent.
- Give hot shot cardioplegia before releasing the cross-clamp, deair, wean from bypass, and assess valve by TEE, leave pacing wires.

Potential questions/alternative scenarios

"Patient is a pregnant female."

In previously asymptomatic female, elevations in heart rate and cardiac output during pregnancy can increase the transmitral gradient which can lead to symptoms. Medical management should be the first line of therapy, and if fails then anatomically suitable valves can undergo PMBV. Mitral valve surgery during pregnancy is associated with an increased maternal and fetal risk. Females with MS planning to become pregnant should have their MS treated prior to conception.

"Patient has a non-calcified and pliable mitral valve."

The patient is candidate for PMBV or open commissurotomy and valve repair. Patients who have pliable and non calcified valves, with little or no subvalvular fusion and no calcification in commissures, absence of 3+ or 4+ MR (moderate - severe MR), and no LA thrombus are candidates for PMBV or open commissurotomy and valve repair. If there are not any contraindications, PMBV should be performed first. Extent of valve pathology dictates PMBV vs. open commissurotomy and repair ("soft" rheumatic changes without extensive subvalvular pathology are amenable to PMBV). In addition patients who are at high surgical risk from comorbidities to undergo MVR should be considered for PMBV.

"In what order would you proceed with concomitant AVR, TVR, or CABG."

Distal coronary anastomoses are performed first, which avoids lifting of the heart after mitral prosthesis is placed and allows using the bypass grafts for cardioplegia. Aortic valve leaflets are excised, and then perform MVR. Then perform AVR. TVR is performed after MVR, and it can be performed after removing the cross-clamp.

"A 64 yo female with ESRD has severe mitral annular calcification (MAC)."

Patients with ESRD are at increased risk for MAC. The degree of MAC influences the surgical approach. Mild amounts can be handled by placing the sutures in an inverted manner (ventricle → atria) around or even through the calcium (if soft enough). Moderate amounts can be debrided until you have a smooth symmetrical surface for the prosthesis to attach. You can then take the inverted sutures along the posterior half of the annulus and pass them through a pericardial patch or felt strip before going through the sewing ring for additional reinforcement. Greater degrees of MAC may require radical debridement of the calcified annulus down to epicardial fat followed by reconstruction with a pericardial patch (autologous pericardium or glutaraldehyde-fixed bovine pericardium) that saddles/sandwiches the annulus. The patch is attached to LV endocardium on the LV side and atrial tissue on the LA side. Valve sutures would then pass through the patch going from the LV to LA and then the sewing ring. Other alternatives include seating the mitral prosthesis at the intra-atrial level with the aid of a Dacron collar. Be sure you are familiar with these approaches before describing or performing them.

"You discover AV groove rupture."
Atrioventricular groove rupture can occur if the sutures are placed too deep, if there is excessive retraction, if the heart is massaged too vigorously at time of deairing, or if there is overly aggressive debridement or decalcification of the posterior leaflet and annulus. If an AV groove rupture is discovered rearrest the heart if not already cross-clamped, and close the full extent of the tear with a pericardial patch. The patch should be secured by sutures into healthy myocardium for a tension-free repair, with careful placement of sutures near coronary vessels.

"After coming off bypass EKG changes are noted in the lateral leads with lateral wall motion abnormalities and depressed ventricular function."
A circumflex artery injury is suspected which can happen if sutures are placed too deep along the posterior annulus. In order to fix this problem, a RSVG to the circumflex artery distribution will be needed.

"After removing cross-clamp you see increased LV distention."
An aortic valve injury may happen when sutures are placed too deep across the anterior annulus, thus injuring the non-coronary or left aortic valve cusps. It is recognized once one removes the cross-clamp and sees the LV distend due to aortic insufficiency, which can be visualized on TEE as well. Re-arrest the heart, open the aorta and left atrium, and after inspection remove the offending suture or possibly the whole mitral prosthesis. The aortic cusp will need to be repaired or replaced.

"Conduction block post-op."
A conduction block can happen if one takes sutures too deep near the posterior commissure and right trigone where the AV node and Bundle

of His can be injured. Often times with radical debridement there is no other room to place sutures. If the conduction disturbance does not improve after several days post-op, a permanent pacemaker will be needed.

"When coming off bypass you note increased gradients across the left ventricular outflow tract (LVOT)."
LVOT obstruction can occur from the prosthesis if it is a high profile mechanical valve, large stented biologic valve posts, or even from low-profile valves that are not properly seated. Typically one will need to replace the valve with a lower profile valve. In addition if one leaves the mitral anterior leaflet unresected with chordal sparing techniques, systolic anterior motion (SAM) can occur due to retained anterior leaflet and chordae, especially if there is septal hypertrophy. In general SAM usually improves if one stops inotropes, volume loads, adds beta-blockers, and adds vasopressors (increasing afterload). Occasionally one may need to perform an aortotomy with transaortic excision of the offending subaortic mitral tissue, and myectomy.

"Perivalvular leak on the postoperative echo."
Most small leaks will stop after protamine administration. If there is a significant leak, then you will have to go back on bypass and fix or re-implant the valve.

"How would you manage patients postoperatively after MVR."
Close attention should be paid to patient's respiratory status and pulmonary pressures. If a patient develops or has elevated pulmonary artery pressures signifying severe pulmonary hypertension, more aggressive diuresis than usual will be needed. Right ventricular function may be compromised necessitating ionotropic and pulmonary vasodilatory therapy. Be very careful with volume overload on these patients. Run them high (inotropes) and dry (diuretics). Anticoagulation (AC) therapy will need to be initiated for mechanical valves (goal INR 2.5-3.5).

Pearls/pitfalls
- Mitral valve replacement is indicated for moderate-severe MS (MV area < 1.5 cm^2), NYHA class III or IV symptoms, and the valve is not amenable to either percutaneous mitral balloon valvuloplasty (PMBV) or open commissurotomy.
- Mildly symptomatic patients (NYHA II) with severe MS and pulmonary hypertension (PAP > 50 mmHg at rest, > 60 with exercise) who are not candidates for valvulotomy are considered for surgery. Patients with severe MS and new onset afib are also considered for PMBV or replacement.

- Tissue valve in patients > 65 yo, sinus rhythm, and who cannot take or are non-compliant with warfarin.
- *Order of concomitant procedures*: distal coronary anastomosis → debride aortic valve → MVR → AVR → TVR (can be done w ccx removed).
- Overly aggressive debridement or retraction/lifting of the heart can lead to AV groove rupture.
- Deep valve sutures can cause injury to the circumflex artery, aortic cusps, and conduction system.

Suggested readings

- Yun KL and Miller DC. Acquired valvular heart disease: mitral valve replacement. *Mastery of Cardiothoracic Surgery* 2007. 378-390.
- Gallegos RP, Gudbjartsson T, and Aranki S. Mitral valve replacement. *Cardiac Surgery in the Adult* 2012.
- Bonow RO et al. ACC/AHA 2006 Guidelines for the management of patients with valvular heart disease. A report of the American College of Cardiology/American Heart Association Task Force on Practice Guidelines (Writing committee to revise the 1998 guidelines for the management of patients with valvular heart disease). *JACC* 2006. 48:e1.

Notes

42. Combined CABG/valve
Mark Roeser, MD, and Ravi Ghanta, MD

Concept
- Indications for combined valve/coronary artery bypass grafting
- Preoperative considerations
- Critical steps in valve/coronary artery bypass grafting

Chief complaint
"A 64 yo man with chronic exertional chest pain is referred to you with moderate aortic stenosis on a TTE obtained by his primary care physician. On follow up catheterization he is found to have 60% RCA stenosis, 80% LAD stenosis, and a 70% circumflex lesion."

Differential
Either the CAD or the aortic stenosis could be contributing to his symptoms.

History and physical
Ask and evaluate for evidence of syncope, angina, CHF, pulmonary edema, dyspnea, and other comorbidities which may factor into your decision regarding the aortic valve.

Tests
Careful review of the cath, echo, CXR, EKG and baseline labs. Catheterization and exercise testing can be used to clarify aortic valve stenosis.

Index scenario (additional information)
"Exercise testing shows a mean gradient of 45 mmHg with exercise. Review of the echo suggests a highly calcified aortic valve. He denies history of dyspnea or syncope."

Treatment/management
Indications for concomitant AVR in patients who require a CABG
- All patients with moderate to severe aortic stenosis
- All patients with moderately severe to severe aortic regurgitation
- Consider in patients with mild AS and moderate to severe calcification or rapidly progressing disease (decrease in AVA 0.3 cm^2 per year or increase in gradient 15-20 mmHg per year)
- Consider in patients with moderate AI

Indications for concomitant CABG in patients who require an AVR
- Any lesion > 70%
- LM lesion > 50%
- "reasonable" to consider bypassing lesions > 50% (LIMA for LAD)

In the above clinical scenario, the patient's symptoms are most likely due to the coronary disease but he should also have the aortic valve replaced at the time of surgery. The data suggests that he will have a lower freedom from reintervention rate with this approach but not necessarily improved survival. Thus, you need to exercise judgement and balance the risks and benefits of an AVR with moderate AS in the setting of CABG. Frail, older patients with multiple comorbidities may benefit from an expeditious operation that addresses the CAD and leaves the moderate AS behind. On the other hand a younger patient with few comorbidities will benefit from the decreased reintervention rate. You should also factor in the rate of progression of the aortic valve disease (see Chapter 34, Aortic stenosis). Also, patients with moderate AS and low cardiac output should have the aortic valve replaced at the time of CABG to reduce afterload.

Potential questions/alternative scenarios

"A 58 yo woman with history of moderate mitral stenosis secondary to rheumatic fever undergoes a cardiac catheterization for exertional chest pain. She is found to have an 80% lesion in the proximal LAD, 70% RCA and 60% OM2 not amenable to PCI."

Indications for concomitant mitral valve surgery in patients who require a CABG:

- *Mitral stenosis*: there are no uniform guidelines regarding mitral stenosis in the setting of a CABG but in general patients who require CABG should have the diseased mitral valve replaced if they meet criteria for an isolated MVR (see Chapter 41, Mitral stenosis) – i.e., moderate to severe MS with NYHA III-IV, asymptomatic with PAP > 60 mmHg, recurrent embolic events, new onset afib, or evidence of RV dysfunction. If a patient does not meet criteria for mitral replacement but has severe MS it is reasonable to replace. For moderate MS not meeting indications for MVR this is more controversial. The decision should factor in whether the patients coronary induced symptoms are potentially due to MS. You might also consider checking the catheterization to clarify the degree of mitral stenosis according to the Gorlin formula if there is a discordance between the echo and clinical presentation.
- *Gorlin formula*:
  valve area (cm^2) = CO / (HR x systolic ejection period (sec) x 44.3 x sq root mean gradient)

- *Structural mitral regurgitation*: severe or moderately severe mitral valve regurgitation secondary to structural valve degeneration (i.e., ruptured cord, leaflet prolapse, etc..) should undergo repair or replacement at the time of CABG. This would be an unusual presentation since most patients with dominant CAD and concomitant mitral regurgitation have ischemic MR. In the absence of a structural lesion assume ischemic MR (below).
- *In patients with ischemic (or "functional") mitral regurgitation*. Severe MR can get a ring annuloplasty repair or mitral valve replacement. Repair when feasible but replacement is acceptable with similar survival, especially for complex jets or sicker patients. Moderate MR is controversial. Patients may get either a ring annuloplasty, replacement or nothing (NIH trial ongoing). Addressing the MR may improve symptoms and decrease the chance of worsening MR. The decision depends on degree of symptoms attributable to the MR as well as comorbidites that make extra cross clamp time more hazardous.

Indications for concomitant CABG in patients who require mitral valve surgery:
- Any lesion > 70%
- LM lesion > 50%
- "reasonable" to consider bypassing lesions > 50% (LIMA for LAD)

In the above scenario, the patient needs to have her right sided heart pressures clarified. If she has moderate-severe pulmonary hypertension (PAP > 50 mmHg at rest or > 60 mmHg with exercise) then the mitral valve should be replaced. If she does not have pulmonary hypertension, new onset afib, right ventricular dysfunction, or embolic events then you should go back to the history and decide whether the moderate MS is more or less than likely to be contributing to her symptoms. Also factor in her comorbidities to see how well she will tolerate the extended cross clamp. In this scenario, exertional chest pain, as reported by the patient, is most consistent with coronary disease and is less likely to be from mitral disease. If she were older, frail with multiple comorbidities it would be reasonable to leave the mitral valve alone. On the other hand if she could tolerate the extra operative time then MVR would remove the mitral disease as a potential source of her symptoms and source of postoperative problems. Thus, moderate stenosis should be left alone if unlikely to be involved in the patients clinical presentation especially in the absence of an isolated indication for MVR. It can be considered if MS is borderline severe or likely to cause problems in the future in a good surgical candidate.

Combined aortic valve replacement/CABG

- Transesophageal echo (TEE).
- Median Sternotomy.
- LIMA + SVG procurement.
- Aortic and right atrial cannulation.
- Antegrade cardioplegia catheter. Retrograde cardioplegia catheter ideal (especially if tight proximal coronary lesions, significant LV hypertrophy, or significant AI).
- LV vent ideal but not required (institution/surgeon dependent).
- Aortic cross-clamp.
- *Cardioplegia.* It is important to appreciate that a CABG/AVR carries a higher mortality and is longer than any of the component procedures done in isolation. Cardioprotection for this case is critical and you have to think through your protection strategy carefully before you start.
    - *Moderate - severe AI*: retrograde induction and consider LV vent to avoid ventricular distension. Make sure the retrograde is in perfectly. Can try to give some through the antegrade but stop if distention occurs.
    - *High grade proximal coronary lesions*: antegrade is unlikely to be sufficient. Plan on antegrade, retrograde and direct cardioplegia down the vein grafts.
- Along these same lines, it is helpful to get to the distal anastomosis and particularly the right distal done ASAP. This will allow you to deliver extra cardioplegia directly down the coronary conduit and protect the RV. Do the same for the circumflex lesion.
- For the LAD you can do the LIMA to LAD and leave it clamped or do the LIMA to LAD following the AVR.
- Make sure you are administering a full dose of cardioplegia every 15-20 minutes.
- Size up the proximals with the heart distended.
- Complete the AVR and close the aortotomy.
- Proximal anastomosis.
- Wean from CPB.
- *Summary*: distals > AVR > proximals.

Operative sequence for mitral valve repair/replacement/ CABG

- TEE.
- Median sternotomy.
- LIMA + SVG procurement.
- Aortic and bicaval cannulation.
- Aortic root vent, antegrade and retrograde cardioplegia.

- Distal anastomoses.
- Size up the proximals with the heart engorged.
- Left atrial vs. transseptal approach for mitral valve repair or replacement.
- Consider left atrial ablation +/- LA appendage ligation if concomitant atrial fibrillation prior to the mitral replacement due to the higher risk of AV rupture with manipulation of the heart (see Chapters 54 Arrhythmia surgery for further details on management of concomitant AF).
- Mitral repair or replacement.
- Key concept is to perform the distal anastomosis first so that heart manipulation/lifting can be minimized after mitral valve replacement is performed. Additionally, performing distal first could facilitate additional cardioprotection down the grafts.
- Proximal anastomosis.
- *Summary*: distals > mitral repair/replacement > proximals.

Operative sequence for aortic and mitral valve surgeries plus CABG
- TEE.
- Aortic and bicaval cannulation with mild systemic hypothermia 32-34° C.
- This is definitely a longer operation. Systemic hypothermia and excellent cardioprotection increase the chances of getting through it safely.
- *Aortic*: root vent, antegrade and retrograde cardioplegia.
- Distal anastomoses and size up the proximals with the heart distended.
- Aortotomy and debride the aortic valve. The concept is to debride the aortic valve before performing mitral valve repair/replacement since debriding after a mitral valve repair/replacement can be problematic.
- Mitral valve replacement/repair via transseptal or left atrial exposure (do any afib procedures first)!
- AVR.
- Close the aortotomy and perform the proximals.
- Wean from CPB.
- *Summary*: distals > debride aortic valve > mitral > AVR > proximals.

Potential questions/alternative scenarios
"You have performed the CABG AVR but coming off CPB the CI is 1.7 and the heart function is decreased compared to baseline. You are on high doses of inotropes and vasopressors. The echo shows that the valve is well seated with no regurgitation and no significant gradient.

The RCA appears to have flow in it by echo. There are no regional wall motion abnormalities. You assess the position of all your grafts which appear satisfactory and use a flow probe which reveals good flow in all the grafts. Your cross clamp time was 2 hours long but you had considerable difficulty with the position of the retrograde throughout the case. How should you proceed?"

These procedures are longer than usual. Cardioprotection has to be carefully carried out. Note that if you perform the mitral via transeptal approach consider direct retrograde insertion into the coronary sinus. Perform the distals first and deliver cardioplegia directly down the distals. In this case the most likely diagnosis is cardiogenic shock from poor protection. You can rest the heart on full flow for 10-15 minutes (make sure the heart is completely decompressed) and see if you recover but ultimately it may be difficult to leave the OR without the aid of a IABP. If the shock persists or worsens in the ICU over the next 12 hours consider an angiogram to assess the grafts.

Pearls/pitfalls

- In general, combined procedures should be performed when indications for each procedure are met. For example, an AVR plus CABG can definitely be performed if the patient meets the indications for AVR and meets the indications for CABG. When a patient however meets the surgical criteria for one cardiac operation (for example CABG), the threshold criteria for performing an additional procedure (for example AVR for moderate AS) maybe lowered after considering the patients overall state.
- Plan out your cardioprotection strategy carefully - plan on retrograde, antegrade and cardioplegia down the coronary conduits.
- General sequence is distals, aortotomy, MVR, AVR, proximals.
  - *CABG/AVR*: distals > AVR > proximals
  - *CABG/MVR*: distals > MVR > proximals
  - *CABG/AVR/MVR*: distals > debride aortic valve > mitral > AVR > proximals
- Reasonable to bypass coronary lesions greater than 50% at the time of a valve operation; mandatory to bypass LM > 50% or any other reasonable target > 70%.

Notes

342

43. Combined aortic and mitral valve disease
Travis Abicht, MD, and Edwin McGee, MD

Concept
- Indications for combined valve operation
- Preoperative considerations
- Intraoperative considerations
  - Sequence of operation
  - Myocardial protection
  - Valve choices
- Pitfalls
- Postoperative issues

Chief complaint
"A 75 yo man is referred to your office after being diagnosed with a murmur heard by his primary care physician. He had a history of a febrile illness when he was younger. He has been increasingly lightheaded and short of breath with exertion to the point that he cannot walk a full block."

Differential
Given the patient's age, aortic stenosis is a concern. Other conditions that should be considered include mitral valve disease. Certainly the patient could have a combination of aortic and mitral valve disease. Endocarditis is another possibility. As always, etiology such as ischemic heart disease and primary pulmonary issues should be ruled out.

History and physical
The history should focus on symptoms such as angina, syncope or congestive heart failure (CHF). Clarify the febrile illness. One should keep in mind any co-morbid conditions that may affect how treatment proceeds. The physical will emphasize vitals, neuro exam, edema, vascular exam, heart and lungs.

Tests
- *EKG*: rule out arrhythmias.
- *Echo.* This is the most important piece of the puzzle in this scenario. The echocardiogram needs to be of high quality so that all valvular function can be adequately assessed. (Refer to technical note in Chapter 34, Aortic stenosis.) If there is any doubt of the findings or quality of the echo, then have it repeated by a cardiologist you trust or perform TEE. Other things to gain from the echo include the presence/absence of septal hypertrophy and

annular sizes.

- *Cardiac catheterization*: rule out any concomitant coronary artery disease (CAD). Also, right heart catheterization will give insight into resultant pulmonary hypertension from MR/MS.
- *CXR +/- CT scan*: make sure there is no concomitant lung pathology. If there is evidence of calcified aorta, bicuspid aortic valve, or high risk factors for atherosclerotic disease then get a CT.

Index scenario (additional information)

"It turns out that the patient had rheumatic fever as a teenager. He is otherwise healthy. His ejection fraction is 50%. He has what appears to be calcific aortic stenosis and rheumatic mitral stenosis by echo. A valve area of 0.7 cm² and a mean gradient of 45 mmHg were noted for the aortic valve, while a valve area of 1.5 cm² with thickened relatively immobile leaflets and moderate MR were noted for the mitral. TEE confirms these findings and shows a mean mitral gradient of 8 mmHg. Estimated PA systolic pressure was in the 40s. Right heart catheterization shows a PAP of 55 mmHg at rest. What are his options and what, if any, operation would you offer him?"

Treatment/management

This patient has severe aortic stenosis and moderate mitral stenosis. He is symptomatic with NYHA Class III. Operative choices include AVR with mitral valve repair or replacement versus AVR alone. The aortic stenosis meets indications for replacement (severe stenosis, symptomatic) and arguably the moderate mitral stenosis also meets indication for surgery (NYHA III, pulmonary hypertension). This presentation is typical of rheumatic heart disease and both valves can be affected with obstruction of flow. The procedure of choice for the mitral valve is replacement. Thus, a double valve replacement will provide the best results for this patient. The question of valve choice is also present. Given the patients age (75) he will be well-served by bioprosthetic valves in both positions. His freedom from structural valve deterioration (SVD) will be on the order of 85-90% at 10-15 years. Additionally there are minimal thromboembolic and bleeding risks. If the patient were younger (< 60), then a mechanical valve would provide a lower rate of re-intervention (20 year freedom from re-intervention rate of 90%). Note if the patient had severe mitral stenosis and moderate AS then an AVR would still be advised. The reverse is not necessarily true. If moderate MS did not appear to be contributing to the patients clinical presentation (normal PAP, minimal dyspnea, 2+ stenosis) then you might consider aborting the mitral procedure especially if the patient was high risk.

Operative steps
Combined aortic/mitral valve replacement

Goals – relieve obstruction/eliminate regurgitation, replace the valves, myocardial protection, prevent embolization.

- Large-bore IV access, arterial line, general endotracheal anesthesia (GETA), pulmonary artery catheter, foley.
- Intraoperative TEE to recheck valvular pathology and rule out any other unexpected pathology.
- Median sternotomy, create pericardial well, palpate the aorta for calcification. If there is any question of safety of cannulation site, then use the epiaortic ultrasound.
- Heparinize (400 mg/kg), central aortic cannulation, bi-caval cannulation, retrograde cardioplegia cannula. At ACT of 480 CPB can be initiated.
- Dissect Sondergard's groove.
- Insert antegrade cardioplegia catheter. Cross-clamp aorta and run antegrade cardioplegia for induction followed by retrograde. Intermittent doses of retrograde should be given throughout the operation with direct ostial cardioplegia given if poor return flow noted (especially from the RCA). If there is no return flow from the left ostia, then the retrograde catheter is likely not in place. An alternative at this point would be direct retrograde especially if if the approach to the mitral valve was transseptal.
- *Aortotomy*: make sure that you know where the RCA is. Make aortotomy ~1 cm above the RCA and carry it laterally a short distance toward the LCA and then obliquely towards the middle of the noncoronary sinus.
- Inspect the aortic valve. Resect the leaflets along the annulus. Debride the calcium at this point (once the mitral valve has been replaced you run the risk of debriding your mitral annular sutures). Patch or primary closure of any defect. Take care near the membranous septum. The conduction system is particularly at risk with a double valve procedure. An option that allows you to pressurize the left ventricle for testing the mitral valve after repair/replacement would be to do a simple running closure of the aortotomy at this point.
- Make the left atriotomy in Sondergard's groove. Insert self-retaining mitral retractor (i.e., Cosgrove retractor). Inspect the mitral valve. In this instance, both the leaflets and subvalvular apparatus appear thickened.
- Perform a cord-sparing mitral valve replacement. Whether to excise any of the anterior or posterior leaflet is a personal/situational choice – you should do what you know and are comfortable doing. Keep in mind that it is hard to preserve thick cords and dividing the anterior leaflet is usually necessary in the setting of rheumatic

345

disease. Take care near the posteromedial commissure. The conduction system is particularly at risk with a double valve procedure.

- Place horizontal mattress sutures of 2-0 braided polyester with pledgets along annulus (inverting/everting is your choice but if the annulus is calcified, ventricular to atrial sutures are best).
- Pass the sutures through the valve ring. Seat the valve. Check the pledgets and then tie down the valve (beginning at the valve struts). Once the valve is tied down, remove the valve obturator. Remove your self-retaining retractor.
- Check for paravalvular leak by pressurizing the left ventricle with saline. If happy with results, then decompress the left ventricle and close the left atriotomy.
- Reopen the aortotomy. Size your aortic valve.
- Place stay sutures at the commissures – this will help orient the valve. Place horizontal mattress sutures of braided 2-0 polyester with pledgets along the annulus.
- Pass the sutures through the valve ring and seat the valve.
- Check the pledgets, and both coronary ostia. Tie the valve in place. Irrigate and recheck the ostia. Close the aortotomy with a running non-absorbable monofilament suture.
- Deair, and wean from CPB.
- Once off CPB, assess the valves with TEE.

Potential questions/alternative scenarios
"After separating from cardiopulmonary bypass, you note that the patient has a junctional bradycardia (ventricular escape in the 30's). What is a possible cause and how could you have potentially prevented this?"

As in operations for isolated mitral or aortic valve disease, the location of the conduction system needs to be kept in mind. For the mitral portion of the procedure, care should be taken when placing annular sutures around the lateral aspect of A3. When replacing the aortic valve, care needs to be taken with annular sutures around the membranous septum (at the commissure of the right and non-coronary cusps). Furthermore, when replacing both valves, over sizing the valve could potentially cause compression of the conduction system between the new valves.

In this scenario, assuming the valves were not oversized, the etiology of the conduction abnormality likely had to do with overly aggressive placement of annular sutures in aforementioned areas. At this point placement of atrial and ventricular temporary epicardial wires is appropriate. The majority of patients will recover an intrinsic rhythm. The need for permanent pacemaker placement is ~5% for isolated valve surgery (with the risk being 3-fold higher for multiple valve surgery).

"You have trouble defibrillating coming off bypass and the post-bypass TEE shows lateral wall motion abnormality."
The important thing to remember in this situation is the intimate association of the circumflex with the mitral annulus. You have either distorted or injured the circumflex artery. In this scenario, you should re-heparinize immediately and go back on bypass. You will need your PA to get a length of vein adequate to bypass the circumflex. Take care when exposing the lateral wall as you now have a replaced mitral valve, and if you did any annular debridement, then you could potentially disrupt the AV groove. This scenario should be kept in mind for any mitral valve repair/replacement (see Chapter 41, Mitral stenosis for AV disruption).

"Your patient has severe aortic stenosis and severe mitral regurgitation. On induction, the patient arrests. Why did this happen and what are you going to do?"
On induction the SVR drops. Venous return decreases. The mitral regurgitation is accentuated. This leads to decreased coronary flow. The incidence of arrest on induction with these combined lesions is higher than that for isolated severe AS.

In treating this patient, the first step is to secure the airway. Ventilate the patient. CPR should be going on. Heparinize and have the patient prepped/draped while you are scrubbing. Perform emergency sternotomy. Perform aortic and venous cannulation. Initiate cardiopulmonary bypass. Proceed with AVR/MVR as above.

"On preoperative workup, the symptomatic patient has severe mitral regurgitation and an AVA of ~0.9 cm^2, but the gradient across the aortic valve is only 28 mmHg. How would you proceed?"
It is likely that there is low-gradient aortic stenosis in this situation. The calculation of AVA is dependent upon measurements of the LVOT (which can be operator-dependent by echo). As such, if you do not trust the study then repeat it with a cardiologist whom you are confident. The patient may need a TEE to better define calcification of the valve or the measurements of the LVOT (which directly affect the measurement of the AVA). If after these repeat tests there is still discrepancy, then the patient can get some kind of exercise test (treadmill or dobutamine). This should confirm severe AS (keep in mind that patients with contractile reserve benefit more from AVR). Proceed with the operation as indicated from that point forward. Also note that even if the patient has moderate AS and meets an indication for mitral repair due
to severe regurgitation then the aortic valve should be replaced.

"You have an 85 yo otherwise healthy patient who has severe calcific aortic stenosis and 2+ mitral regurgitation. There are no mitral leaflet abnormalities noted. How would you proceed?"

This patient likely has functional mitral regurgitation that is accentuated by his/her severe aortic stenosis. The safest thing to do in this situation is the most expeditious operation possible. It is very likely that once the stenotic aortic valve has been replaced, then the mitral regurgitation will decrease to trace or mild – which in an 85 year old patient can be medically managed without great fear of long term complications. In other patients use the TEE to carefully delineate the mitral valve morphology and it may be worthwhile to "explore the valve" without necessarily committing to repair or replacement. If a definite structural abnormality is noted then it may be repaired.

"A 65 yo female presents with combined aortic insufficiency and mitral regurgitation. The AI is 3+ (moderately severe). She is short of breath with minimal exertion. Her EF is 45% and end diastolic volume is 7 cm². TEE confirms that the MR is severe."

For regurgitation, treat according to the dominant lesion and treat both if both are clearly contributing. In this case either the mitral or aortic could be contributing so both should be addressed by repair/replacement as deemed appropriate. If the MR were moderate (2+) then it is not indicated to repair/replace the valve. However, check the TEE and directly explore the valve if needed to rule out a structural lesion that is contributing to the regurgitation. If flail, chord rupture, or prolapse were noted you may be justified in repairing the valve if feasible but rarely should you replace for moderate MR at the time of AVR. Conversely, if the aortic valve regurgitation were moderate and the mitral severe then treat the mitral valve and leave the aortic valve alone. Very rarely will moderate AI or moderate MR be the dominant lesion. Again, be sure to check the intraop TEE carefully to confirm that the lesions are indeed moderate and consider direct visual inspection if warranted.

Pearls/pitfalls
- When faced with combined valvular disease use TEE to confirm the degree of regurgitation or stenosis.
- Treat according to the dominant lesion.
- Once you are in the OR for at least one valve that meets surgical indication then replace all severely stenotic valves. In this setting, repair/replace all severe or moderately severe regurgitant valves (3-4+).
- The threshold for intervening on moderate aortic valve stenosis may be lowered in the setting of an MVR.

- Moderate aortic regurgitation (2+) does not necessarily require repair in the setting of an MVR but requires evaluation by intraoperative TEE and possibly direct inspection.
- Moderate mitral regurge (2+) does not necessarily require repair but requires evaluation by intraoperative TEE and possibly direct inspection depending on the TEE.
- Moderate mitral stenosis should be carefully evaluated with right heart catheterization and TEE. Replace the mitral in the setting of an AVR if there is evidence that it is contributing to the clinical picture (elevated PAP, NYHA III-IV, afib).
- Bioprosthetic valves are generally acceptable if patient > 65 years old.
- Remember that the order of replacement/repair is imperative: open aorta, excise leaflets, and debride annulus *prior* to performing mitral replacement/repair.
- Size the aortic valve *after* replacing the mitral valve.
- Take care not to oversize the mitral valve. This can lead to effective downsizing of the aortic valve and the possibility of having to use too small of an aortic valve (patient prosthesis mismatch).
- As in any mitral repair or replacement, take care when placing sutures in the mitral annulus around P1 and A1—do not want to compromise the circumflex artery.
- After performing mitral valve replacement, avoid lifting the heart (see below).
- Bright red blood coming from behind the heart after coming off bypass—think AV dissociation. Do not lift the heart to examine. Go back on bypass, then determine where blood is coming from and repair as appropriate.
- See pearls/pitfalls in Chapters 34, 38, 41, on Aortic stenosis, Ischemic mitral regurgitation, and Mitral stenosis.

Suggested readings
- Bonow B. Tricuspid, Pulmonic and Multivalvular Disease. Braunwald's Heart Disease—A textbook of Cardiovascular Medicine, 9th ed. 2011.
- Gillinov AM, Blackstone EH, Cosgrove DM, et al. Mitral valve repair with aortic valve replacement is superior to double valve replacement. J Thorac Cardiovasc Surg 2003;125:1372-87.
- Carpentier A, Adams D, Filsoufi F. Carpentier's Reconstructive Valve Surgery. Section II, IV, V. 2010.
- Nishimura R, Grantham JA, Connolly HM, et al. Low-Output, Low-Gradient Aortic Stenosis in Patients With Depressed Left Ventricular Systolic Function: The Clinical Utility of the Dobutamine Challenge in the Catheterization Laboratory.

Circulation. 2002;106:809-813.

Notes

44. Combined coronary and carotid procedures
Gabriel Loor, MD, and Douglas R. Johnston, MD

Concept
- Identification of patients with carotid disease undergoing CABG
- Justify the sequence of interventions
- Perioperative strategies for stroke reduction

Chief complaint
"A 70 yo man presents with a 2 month h/o chest pain to his local cardiologist. He recommends a stress test which is positive for myocardial ischemia. Cardiac catheterization shows the following lesions: 70% mid RCA, 80% mid circumflex and 60% proximal LAD. The patient had a transient ischemic attack (TIA) 1 month ago with no residual deficits. How would you proceed with evaluation and treatment?"

Differential
The patient has coronary disease for certain. The neurologic disease may be accounted for by embolic disease from arrhythmias or atherosclerotic disease in small or large vessels.

History and physical
The history for any patient undergoing open heart surgery should include a search for risk factors of carotid disease including prior strokes, peripheral vascular disease, coronary artery disease, age, prior carotid endarterectomy (CEA), smoking, diabetes or hypertension. The physical exam should assess for any gross neurologic deficits and carotid bruits.

Tests
The patient in this scenario has risk factors for carotid disease (age, CAD and prior TIA) and should undergo a carotid duplex as well as a computed tomography (CT) scan of the head to evaluate for and characterize any new or old strokes. An MRA or angiography may be considered for equivocal carotid lesions. It is important to document a complete preop neurologic exam in the event there are deficits postoperatively.

Index scenario (additional information)
"He has a history of hypertension and non-insulin dependent diabetes mellitus. He has a right carotid bruit and a duplex shows 70% right ICA stenosis. CT of the head showed no evidence of a prior stroke."

Treatment/management

The options for this man with symptomatic carotid disease (prior TIA) and multivessel symptomatic coronary disease include staged repair (CEA and then CABG in either order) or a combined approach under one anesthetic. Meta-analysis has shown that the mortality and stroke rate are higher with a combined approach (death - 5% versus 3%; stroke - 6% versus 3%). Thus a combined approach should be avoided when possible and used only when absolutely necessary. The risk of a myocardial infarction (MI) is higher with CEA followed by a CABG and the risk of stroke is higher for CABG followed by CEA. In general the most symptomatic territories should be addressed first and in combination if both are equally severe. This patient has symptomatic carotid disease and symptomatic coronary disease thus he is at high risk of an MI with a CEA and a stroke with a CABG. The most prudent option would be a combined procedure.

If the carotid disease was symptomatic and his coronary disease was not as burdensome (no recent symptoms, chronic stable plaques,mostly < 70%) then it would be reasonable to proceed with the CEA followed in 4-6 weeks by CABG. MI is more common in this situation. If the carotid lesion was asymptomatic with no prior TIA or stroke then he should undergo a CABG followed by a CEA in 4-6 weeks. A severe carotid lesion (> 60% by angio or > 80% by duplex) that is asymptomatic is still grounds for a CEA either first or in combination depending on the severity and symptomatology of the coronary disease. The same goes for a 60-80% stenosis and contralateral occlusion.

Operative steps

- Supine position, arterial line, ETT, swan, cerebral oximetry.
- Prep and drape for both a CEA and CABG.
- Begin with the CEA while the leg vein is being harvested.
- Decide ahead of time what conduits to use and determine if an adequate length of vein is available for both the bypass and CEA. Otherwise use a hemashield patch.
- Oblique incision along the anterior border of the sternocleidomastoid muscle (SCM). Divide the facial vein.
- Dissect down to the carotid artery and expose the common, internal and external carotid. Take care not to injure the vagus during this dissection.
- Get proximal and distal control (external and internal) with vessel loops.

- Give 10,000 units of heparin,clamp. Consider a shunt if the cerebral oximetry drops excessively. Open the artery from the proximal common carotid up to the internal carotid beyond the area of gross intimal disease.
- Dissect the plaque with a blunt dissector. Close with a vein patch or hemashield patch.
- Flush all vessels beginning with the external then the internal and finally the common carotid.
- Obtain hemostasis and pack the wound.
- Complete the vein harvest, median sternotomy, and mammary takedown. Carefully palpate the aorta given the risk for ascending calcification which may require axillary cannulation.
- General measures to reduce stroke risk would include keeping MAPs greater than 70 mmHg during bypass, avoiding excessive manipulation of the aorta and limiting cross clamp time. After heparin has been reversed, ensure hemostasis in the neck and close over a drain.

Potential questions/alternative scenarios

"Postoperatively the patient has evidence of left sided upper extremity weakness."

A neuro exam should be performed as soon as possible following the combined approach. Any abnormalities warrant a head CT, neuro consultation and carotid duplex. Maintain a low threshold for returning to the operating room to explore the patch if there is any hint that the neurologic impairment is due to a structural issue with the patch.

"Postoperatively the patient develops a large neck hematoma with tracheal deviation."

If a neck hematoma develops and compromises the airway it should be opened immediately at the bedside or in the operating room if time permits. Always protect the airway with an endotracheal tube if the patient has already been extubated. After draining the hematoma, ensure hemostasis, irrigate and close over a drain.

Pearls/pitfalls

- Symptomatic coronary artery disease (worsening angina, NSTEMI, STEMI) requires coronary intervention urgently. If the patient has symptomatic carotid disease with at least moderate grade carotid stenosis (50% by duplex) then perform a CEA in the same setting.
- CEA should also be considered in the same setting if a patient who needs an urgent CABG has an asymptomatic carotid lesion > 60% by angio or > 80% by duplex. Same goes for a patient with 60-80% stenosis but contralateral occlusion.

- CEA can be safely delayed in patients undergoing CABG with mild or moderate grade lesions (< 80% duplex) who have not had a prior stroke or TIA.
- If the carotid disease is symptomatic and his coronary disease is not as burdensome (no recent symptoms, chronic stable plaques, mostly < 70%) then it would be reasonable to proceed with the CEA followed in 4-6 weeks by CABG.

Suggested readings

- Burger MA et al. Coronary bypass and carotid endarterectomy: does a combined approach increase risk of stroke? A metaanalysis. *Ann Thor Surg* 1999;68;14-20.
- Barbour JR and Ikonomidis JS. Chapter 28 Concomitant carotid endarterectomy and coronary artery bypass. Yuh D, Vricella LA, Baumgartner WA (eds). *Manual of Cardiothoracic Surgery* 2007.
- Gewertz B. Chapter 12 Carotid endarterectomy. Fischer JE (ed). *Mastery of Surgery 5th ed.* 2009.

Notes

45. Endocarditis

Katherine B. Harrington, MD, and Bruce A. Reitz, MD

Concept
- Indications for surgical management of infective endocarditis
- Timing of surgical intervention
- Valve repair or replacement options
- Options for complicated reconstruction

Chief complaint
"A 72 yo man with diabetes presents with 2-3 days of low grade fevers, weight loss, lethargy, and shortness of breath. About a week ago he completed treatment for a right knee infection with antibiotics. Preliminary blood cultures are growing gram positive cocci in 4 of 4 bottles. TTE shows moderate-severe aortic insufficiency (AI). How would you proceed with management?"

Differential
Endocarditis, bacteremia, structural valve disease, coronary disease, CHF

Definition and pathophysiology
- Infective endocarditis (IE) is infection of the endocardial surface of the heart, with the heart valves most commonly affected (mitral > aortic > tricuspid > pulmonary), and also frequently, prosthetic valves. IE may also involve congenital heart lesions such as septal defects, patent ductus arteriosis, and coarctation of the aorta.
- The endocardial or valvular surface is damaged by turbulence, providing the substrate for the infective agent and a platelet/fibrin matrix to initiate colonization and persistence.

History and physical
The H&P should help establish the diagnosis, source, any adverse sequelae and stratify the patient for surgery if needed. *Establishing the diagnosis* - history of murmurs, structural heart disease, or immunosuppression. Social history focused on IV drug usage. Timing and duration of symptoms as well as any recent treatment. *Source* - inquire about infection (dental procedures, GI illnesses, recent invasive procedures). Inquire about recent skin/soft tissue infections or joint infections suggestive of septic arthritis. *Sequelae* - Evaluate for signs and symptoms of congestive heart failure, distal embolic phenomena, stroke/TIA. *Risk stratify* - other significant comorbidities, renal dysfunction, dialysis, diabetes, cardiopulmonary disease. Focused physical exam including vital signs, sequelae of possible neurologic emboli, murmurs, pulmonary congestion/edema, and endocarditis

stigmata: Osler's nodes-painful nodules on hands and feet, Janeway lesions- small, flat, non-painful erythematous lesions on palms and soles, Roth's spots- pale retinal hemorrhages, and splinter hemorrhages in nails. Investigate all possible sources and whether source control has been achieved.

Tests

- *Blood cultures.* Follow-up speciation and full sensitivities. *Streptococcus viridans* is most frequently identified. *Staphylococcus aureus* and fungal endocarditis are now more frequently seen, especially in medical settings. If *strep. bovis* is the causative organism, should get colonoscopy to rule out GI malignancy. If fungal infection, an ophthalmologic evaluation is required.

- Frequent EKG, to follow PR interval and look for the development of heart block, or evolving bundle branch block. This would indicate the development of annular abscess near the conduction system.

- *TEE.* Recommended as the first line study for all prosthetic valve endocarditis. Recommended in all cases of suspected endocarditis when the transthoracic echo is non-diagnostic or to further assess the severity of known endocarditis (i.e., annular abscess).

- Cardiac catheterization may be indicated pre-op for all females over 50 and all males over 40. Consider CT coronary angiography instead, especially if patient has no risk factors and left heart catheterization may cause embolization of known aortic valve vegetations.

- CT head if any neurologic deficits to evaluate possible embolic phenomena, and identify site and size of ischemic versus hemorrhagic lesions.

- *Chest CT/CXR*: pulmonary infarcts or abscesses.

Criteria for diagnosis of IE

- If there is no explicit clinical diagnosis of endocarditis, then the Modified Duke criteria can be used. Modified Duke criteria requires 2 major criteria, or 1 major and 3 minor, or 5 minor criteria for a "definite" diagnosis of IE.

Table 45-1. Modified Duke criteria for diagnosis of infective endocarditis.

Major criteria

Microbiologic evidence of endocarditis
   - Typical organisms in 2 cultures
   - Atypical organisms in 2 cultures drawn at
     least 12 hours apart or in 3 of 4 cultures
     drawn at least an hour apart
Evidence of endocardial involvement on echo:
   - New valvular regurgitation
   - Abscess
   - Oscillating cardiac mass
Partial dehiscence of a prosthetic valve

Minor criteria

Predisposition to endocarditis
   - Intravenous drug use
   - Prior prosthetic valve
   - Structural heart disease

Fever > 38° C

Vascular phenomenon.
   - Systemic embolism
   - Mycotic aneurysm
   - Janeway's lesions

Immunologic phenomenon
   - Osler's nodes
   - Roth's spots
   - Glomerulonephritis

Microbiology finding not meeting major criteria

Index scenario (additional information)
"The TEE confirms moderate-severe AI and also shows a 0.8 cm vegetation on the posterior leaflet of his mitral valve. Blood cultures are positive for methicillin sensitive staphylococcus aureus. He is otherwise hemodynamically stable."

Treatment/management
The decisions regarding surgical management of the patient with IE should be individualized, and requires consultation with the infectious disease physician, the cardiologist, and the cardiac surgeon. Appropriate antibiotic therapy based on blood culture data is the mainstay of IE therapy. If the patient is hemodynamically stable, serial blood cultures demonstrating blood sterilization after 48 hours of antibiotics is optimal (3 cultures drawn at least 24 hours apart), and may indicate effective treatment.

The patient in this scenario has two major criteria for endocarditis with septic arthritis as the most likely inciting event. He appears to have source control and with the severe AI he meets criteria for surgical intervention.

The following generalities can be made regarding timing of intervention for endocarditis:

Emergency (24 hrs)
- Acute AI with early closure of the mitral valve or hemodynamic instability.
- Rupture or any sudden deterioration in hemodynamics.

Urgent (48 hours)
- Severe AI/MR with evidence of heart failure (NYHA 3-4).
- Annular abscess, fistula.
- New conduction deficit.
- Unstable prosthesis, mobile vegetation > 1-1.5 mm.

Elective (earlier the better)
- Staph prosthetic valve endocarditis (PVE).
- PVE within 2 months (early).
- Worsening regurge.
- Increasing size of vegetation despite antibiotics.
- Fungal endocarditis.
- Persistent infection after 10 days despite antibiotics.

Late PVE can be treated like native valve endocarditis with regards to indications and timing.

Valve replacement or repair considerations
If replacement is needed, valve choice can be discussed based on individual patient characteristics and preference. However, it is not until the valve is excised, debrided and inspected in the OR that the final decision regarding conduits can be made. There is no difference in reinfection risks between mechanical and bioprosthetic valves, so long as the annulus is not involved with extensive infection. In the presence of more extensive annular involvement, abscess formation, or septal perforation, a tissue valve option such as a homograft or autologous valve has been demonstrated to be a superior alternative. After surgical correction, at least six weeks of appropriate antibiotic therapy is recommended.

Operative steps

- The most important operative goal for endocarditis is to *debride ALL infected tissue.*
- The conduct of the operation is similar as that in standard aortic valve replacement and mitral valve replacement. See those chapters for detailed steps. The exception is that you really have to be prepared to tackle anything from a simple valve replacement to a valve and patch, double valve, root and even reconstruction of the fibrous skeleton of the heart.
- Aortic cannulation, bicaval cannulation, retrograde and antegrade cardioplegia access.
- Begin with the aortotomy above the STJ and inspect the leaflets, annulus, membranous septum and anterior leaflet of the mitral valve. Resect the aortic leaflets along with all infected tissue.
- Do the mitral valve first, then the aortic valve (presence of the aortic valve prosthesis will make mitral valve visualization difficult).
- Left atriotomy of choice, but make sure the exposure is perfect. With acute endocarditis the left atrium may be small and an extended transeptal may give the best exposure. Send tissue for gram stain and culture.
- An attempt to repair the mitral valve should be made if at all possible. This includes resection of the vegetation, and use of standard valve repair techniques, with or without autologous pericardium. Avoid prosthetic bands or rings unless absolutely needed.
- Repair of the aortic valve is much less frequent, and is usually limited to pericardial patch repair of a leaflet with a perforation. More often the valve is replaced with a tissue valve, mechanical valve or homograft root replacement. All fistulae and abscesses should be completely unroofed. Repair perforations with autologous pericardium.

Potential questions/alternative scenarios

"There is an annular abscess at the right-noncoronary commissure."
If there is an abscess, it must be completely unroofed and all grossly infected tissue debrided. The defect is then patched with autologous or bovine pericardium. The valve stitches are then anchored through the patch at that site in the annulus. For a small abscess this patch will suffice. The right-non commissure is the site of the membranous septum, so there is high risk for VSD creation with aggressive debridement. This patient also has a high risk for conduction disturbance and pacemaker need. If the abscess is even more extensive and debridement of a large part of the annulus is needed, a homograft root replacement may be the best option. The muscular annulus of the homograft helps fill any tissue

defects after extensive debridement. The homograft is affixed to the annulus with multiple simple interrupted sutures or several running prolene sutures. The coronaries are reimplanted to the homograft. The homograft must be trimmed to the appropriate height from the donor RCA. Leave a cuff of mitral leaflet for orientation. The mitral leaflet is aligned along the posterior aspect of the annulus to line up the donor and recipient coronaries.

Another option for extensive infection involving both the aortic and mitral valve with infection of the common annular area, is to use autologous or bovine pericardium to reconstruct the aorto-mitral curtain and create a neo-annulus for the aortic and mitral valve sutures. If conduction block is expected consider placing 2 sets of ventricular pacing wires and an early consult to electrophysiology.

"Upon visualization the endocarditis appears to be confined to the P2 segment of his mitral valve."
Repair mitral when possible. The infected segment can be removed with a triangular or quadrangular excision. Avoiding placement of a prosthetic valve in the mitral location is preferable in an infected setting, provided you can confidently excise all infected tissue. Any small focal holes in the mitral or aortic valves can be debrided and patched with autologous or bovine pericardium.

"The lesion is not on the posterior leaflet, but on the underside of the anterior leaflet."
This is known as a "drop lesion" and can be resected and patched with autologous or bovine pericardium through the aortotomy. If using a homograft, the mitral skirt of the homograft can be used to reconstruct the base of the leaflet at the aortomitral curtain.

"The patient is persistently hypotensive weaning off pump."
Assure through TEE and measuring cardiac output that it is not primarily cardiogenic. Endocarditis patients with active infection or large inflammatory response can be quite vasoplegic after bypass. Start neosynephrine and vasopressin infusions. If non-responsive, can give methylene blue.

"His initial blood cultures are negative."
If the clinical suspicion of endocarditis is high, empiric antibiotics should be started and continued. The HACEK (*Haemophilus, Actinobacillus, Cardiobacterium, Eikenella,* and *Kingella*) organisms are difficult to isolate and are a likely cause of culture negative endocarditis. These organisms are also likely to cause large vegetations. Fungal organisms may also be slow or difficult to isolate, and a patient who is not

improving on empiric antibiotics should have an antifungal added.

"Patient is found to have multiple embolic lesions on preoperative head CT."

The operative timing of patients with cerebral embolic lesions is controversial. Systemic embolic phenomena alone can be an indication for operation, but only if they are recurrent after appropriate antibiotics have been started. However once cerebral emboli have happened, there is some worry that the lesions will convert to a hemorrhagic infarct and expand while fully heparinized for bypass. On the basis of the head CT, determine the size and type of lesion. Some studies suggest that patients with ischemic infarcts of less than 1 cm, can be operated on safely after 5-7 days. For hemorrhagic lesions less than 1 cm or ischemic lesions of 2 cms or greater, a delay of 2 weeks is recommended. Attempt to wait four weeks after a large ischemic stroke and > 2 cm hemorrhagic stroke, prior to placing on CPB. The risk of embolization usually decreases after the second week of antibiotics. Of course, if the patient requires operation for progressive congestive heart failure, or other life threatening indication, the increased operative risk in the presence of a cerebral infarct might be justified, and an earlier operation performed.

"A 50 yo IV drug abuser is diagnosed with 3+TR and a 1 cm vegetation on the tricuspid valve. He also complains of worsening shortness of breath and lower extremity edema."

Early initiation of antibiotics and prompt surgical treatment is key as these patients can rapidly spiral into right sided heart failure and respiratory insufficiency. This patient needs a careful TEE and right heart catheterization to evaluate right sided function and pressures. Usually medical management with antibiotics is sufficient. Surgical indications include sepsis/bacteremia/worsening TR unresponsive to antibiotics, RV failure from TR, and recurrent pulmonary emboli with respiratory compromise. Surgical options include:

- Simple vegectomy.
- *Valve repair*: procedure of choice. Repair of perforations, sliding commissural plasty, and triangular/quadrangular resections with local annuloplasty or annular plication with pericardial pledgets. Annular plication or devegas annuloplasty can be used for reinforcement of most repairs without adding prosthetic material. Prosthetic bands decrease recurrence of TR but at the potential expense of recurrent infection.
- *Valve replacement*: mechanical versus bioprosthetic - no real survival advantage. Mechanical - keep INR > 3.0, risk of bleeding, more durable; bioprosthetics - theoretically less risk of reinfection.

- *Valve excision without replacement*: need good RV and LV function, normal pulmonary vascular resistance and no left sided endocarditis to withstand the stress on the RV. Roughly 10-15% will require replacement.

"A 68 yo male undergoes a mini AVR for aortic stenosis and returns one month later with leaflet vegetations, fevers and chills."
Early PVE < 2 months is often aggressive and most often requires intervention within 1-2 weeks of treatment. Any high risk features such as an unstable prosthesis requires earlier intervention (24-48 hours). The principles of the operation are similar to those listed above. The prosthesis and all pledgets are removed and all infected tissue is debrided. Usually a homograft is required. For late PVE > 2 months the indications for operation are similar to those for native valve endocarditis.

Pearls/pitfalls
- Surgical treatment of endocarditis is indicated with valvular lesions causing heart failure, conduction disturbance, annular or sub-annular abscess, fungal
  endocarditis, recurrent embolic phenomenon, or progressive prosthetic valve regurgitation.
- Debride all infected tissue, repair mitral and tricuspid valves when possible, replace aortic valves.
- Be prepared for anything with these procedures. Range of procedures can include simple AVR, homograft, mitral repair/replacement, double valve, double valve with reconstruction of the fibrous skeleton, and tricuspid repair/replacement.
- Prepare for postoperative heart block and vasoplegia.
- The patient will need at least six weeks of antibiotics postoperatively.

Suggested readings
- Bonow RO et al. Focused update incorporated into the ACC/AHA 2006 guidelines for the management of patients with valvular heart disease: a report of the American College of Cardiology/American Heart Association Task Force on Practice Guidelines. J Am Coll Cardiol. 2008 Sep 23;52(13):e1-142.
- David TE. Surgical treatment of Aortic Valve Endocarditis. Cohn LH. Cardiac Surgery in the Adult. 2008.
- Stamou SC, Gosta P, Gillinov AM. Surgical Treatment of Mitral Valve Endocarditis. Cohn LH. Cardiac Surgery in the Adult. 2008.

- Moon MR, Miller DC, Moore KA, Oyer PE, Mitchell RS, Robbins RC, Stinson EB, Shumway NE, Reitz BA. Treatment of endocarditis with valve replacement: the question of tissue versus mechanical prosthesis. Ann Thorac Surg. 2001 Apr;71(4):1164-71.

Notes

46. Cardiac trauma

Mark Joseph, MD, and Andy C. Kiser, MD

Concept
- Management of penetrating cardiac trauma
- Preoperative considerations
- Operative strategies and choice of incision
- Pitfalls and alternative solutions

Chief complaint
"A 24 yo man presents with a gunshot wound (GSW) to the chest. The patient is talking but confused, bedside sonography shows evidence of a pericardial effusion. The patient becomes increasingly agitated and hypotensive. What is the next step in management?"

Differential
Injury to the great vessels or heart.

History and physical
Proceed with standard ATLS workup and primary survey (ABCD's - secure airway, ventilation, IV access, fluid/blood resuscitation). Secondary survey - define the pattern of chest injury (anterior box - mid clavicular, notch to xiphoid = cardiac injury until proven otherwise; posterior box - between scapula = esophagus, aorta, airway; chest or thoracoabdominal = pulmonary, aortic, cardiac if transmediastinal, abdominal organs if thoracoabdominal). Quickly assess for other associated life threatening injuries (head trauma, GCS), order chest x ray, auscultate for breath sounds, prepare for a thoracostomy tube insertion on the side of the injury, review the echo, and send labs. CT scans should be performed on hemodynamically stable patients only and is warranted if the CXR shows a widened mediastinum. Sonography can determine the presence of pericardial fluid, physical examination may reveal Beck's triad (muffled heart sounds, jugular venous distention, and hypotension) or Kussmaul's sign (jugular venous distention with inspiration) indicating pericardial tamponade. Should the patient decompensate and lose their pulse, an emergency left anterolateral thoracotomy becomes part of the primary survey (see below).

Tests
- *CXR*: evaluate widened mediastinum.
- *FAST (focused assessment with sonography for trauma)*: evaluate pericardial fluid and other potential injuries.

- *Echocardiography (the gold standard)*: can be used to further delineate valves, pericardial effusions, RV compression, tamponade physiology and foreign bodies/missiles within the myocardium or cardiac chambers.
- *CT scan*: may be helpful to identify additional injuries (abdominal) if patient is stable, but in general not helpful unless a vascular injury is suspected.

Index scenario (additional information)

"FAST revealed pericardial fluid with a wide mediastinum on CXR. The patient became pulseless. You performed an antero-lateral thoracotomy and found a hole in the left ventricle."

Treatment/management

On arrival, nearly half of patients with cardiac injury may are hemodynamically stable and then suddenly deteriorate. Unstable patients may respond to fluid resuscitation but arrest is always eminent. Establishing an airway with appropriate ventilation and large bore IV access are critical. If the patient responds to fluids, its usually transient but does provide the clinician time to formulate a plan. The main branch point in the treatment algorithm is to discern whether a patient is stable (or nearly stable) or unstable (or pulseless). Stable patients can get a CXR, echo, labs, access, and chest tube if warranted. If a pericardial effusion is present assume a cardiac injury has occurred and plan to get to the OR immediately. A subxiphoid pericardiocentesis may help buy time if the patient needs other critical preoperative information (i.e., a head CT in the setting of severe head trauma). But in general penetrating and isolated chest trauma with an effusion requires a trip to the OR for a median sternotomy. If the patient with penetrating trauma arrests in transit to the ED (within 20 minutes) or in the trauma bay then an ED thoracotomy (left anterior thoracotomy) is warranted to evacuate the tamponade, open cardiac massage and identify/control the injury if possible. If the patient is in the OR, a median sternotomy is acceptable for penetrating wounds. As with all trauma patients, be sure to prep from the patient's chin to ankles in the event there's a need to harvest the saphenous vein for a coronary artery injury. Otherwise a bilateral trans-sternal anterolateral thoracotomy ("clam shell") provides excellent exposure to the mediastinum and pleural spaces (see below).

Operative steps

ED thoracotomy

- Have airway secured, NG tube in place (helps to locate the esophagus), IV access.
- Small towel roll under the left chest, prep and drape expeditiously.

- Perform left anterior thoracotomy in approximately the 5th intercostal space (below the nipple) down to the bone (anterolateral exposure).
- Chest retractor.
- Open the pericardium longitudinally. Stay above the phrenic nerve.
- Identify, bluntly dissect and clamp the descending aorta to optimize perfusion to the heart.
- During the left anterior thoracotomy if the source of bleeding is not immediately identified and left ventricular injury suspected, inflow may be reduced by manually occluding the left hilum. Left ventricular injuries can be temporarily managed with a finger or occlusion using a foley catheter balloon.
- If the patient is stabilized then proceed to the operating room for definitive management. The types of injuries that may be encountered and the operation required may be highly variable. Epicardial lacerations may undergo simple closure with prolene sutures. Coronary artery injuries may require ligation and distal bypass with vein. An intraop TEE will reveal valvular injuries that may require debridement and repair/replacement. Aortic injuries are treated like ruptures and may require anything from simple suture ligation to circulatory arrest and aortic graft placement.
- In stable patients with a pericardial effusion and suspected cardiac injury, skip the ED thoracotomy and proceed to the OR for median sternotomy +/- CPB.

Potential questions/alternative scenarios
"You wean off bypass and the echo shows new localized anterolateral wall motion abnormalities and the patient is started on high dose inotropic support."
Strongly consider a coronary artery injury in the region of your repair and bypass the appropriate vessel.

"You open the chest, and identify a right atrial injury."
Right atrial injuries can usually be controlled with a clamp and do not necessitate the need for CPB. A series of clamps can be used to approximate long injuries. Suture closure can be performed under the clamps. The repair can usually be performed with pledgeted suture. Caution should be given to avoid tearing the atrium with traction. Similarly, superior caval injuries can sometimes be repaired without institution of bypass. The benefit of avoiding CPB is the avoidance of heparin in a patient with multisystem trauma (i.e., heparin would not be ideal in the setting of a GSW to the abdomen, head or extremity). On the other hand, if you are reasonably certain you have an isolated chest trauma involving vascular structures and or lung parenchyma then CPB

and arresting the heart gives you the best chance of a successful and hemostatic repair.

"You notice both right atrial and ventricular injury?"

Injuries from gunshot wounds can damage all chambers of the heart. The friability of the tissue, injury location, and hemodynamic instability may necessitate CPB. Injuries that involve multiple chambers require thorough investigation to rule out valvular or septal injury. Direct visualization of the bullets path and intraoperative echo are invaluable. Trans cardiac injuries imply a path from one chamber to the next and the potential for an intracardiac injury. CPB and cardiac arrest with cardiotomy are necessary. If the injury is small, use horizontal pledgeted mattress sutures. Larger defects, however, require reconstruction using pericardium. Posterior cardiac injuries can be visualized by elevating the heart out of the pericardium while on CPB. Injuries to the coronary sinus should be ligated as a patch repair is very difficult in a heart that is already friable. Still, a patch can be considered for reinforcement. If reasonable hemostasis is achieved but the patient is spiraling into a coagulopathy then you can always pack and leave the chest open until coags normalize.

"A stab wound has caused a laceration to the distal LAD?"

Coronary artery injuries require CPB and may require coronary bypass using a conduit. Vein conduit is most appropriate in an emergency situation. Distal coronary artery injuries, especially beyond the distal third of the vessel, may only require ligation. However, if there is salvageable ventricular dysfunction, then the vessel should be bypassed. Cardiac injuries in proximity but without direct injury to the coronary artery may require repair without compromising coronary flow. Passing the pledgeted sutures through the myocardium behind the coronary allows repair without compromising coronary patency.

Pearls/pitfalls

- In a patient with penetrating trauma who is pulseless within 20 min of arriving to the ED or in the ED, an anterolateral thoracotomy with release of tamponade, open cardiac massage and cross clamping the aorta is the procedure of choice.
- Cardiac injuries in proximity to coronary arteries can be managed with horizontal mattress sutures going under the vessel as to avoid occlusion or injury to the artery. If artery is injured then bypass should be considered.
- Complex injuries to the heart and other blood vessels should be treated in order of most life-threatening first followed by other injuries such as intracardiac or valvular injuries.

Suggested readings

- Asensio JA, Stewart BM, Murray JA, et al: Penetrating cardiac injuries. *Surg Clin North Am* 1996;76:685.
- Thourani VH, Feliciano DV, Cooper WA, et al: Penetrating cardiac trauma at an urban trauma center: a 22-year perspective. *Am Surg* 1999;65:811.
- Ivatury RR, Rohman M, Steichen FM, et al: Penetrating cardiac injuries: twenty year experience. *Am J Surg* 1987;53:310.
- Wall Jr. MJ, Mattox KL, Chen C, et al: Acute management of complex cardiac injuries. *J Trauma* 1997;42:905.

Notes

47. Iatrogenic aortic dissection

Vakhtang Tchantchaleishvili, MD, and Peter A. Knight, MD

Concept
- Predisposing risks
- Timely recognition of iatrogenic aortic dissection
- Delayed iatrogenic aortic dissection
- Critical operative steps
- Complications of iatrogenic aortic dissection
- Pearls/pitfalls

Chief complaint
"A 68 yo man is brought to the OR for a CABG. Shortly after placement of the arterial cannula in the ascending aorta, the perfusionist notes a high line pressure with the test transfusion and a purple colored hematoma begins to form."

Differential
Iatrogenic aortic dissection from cannulation should always remain high on the differential in this scenario because early recognition and therapy can be life saving. Adventitial hematoma is another possibility but would not explain the high line pressure and you are entitled to check a TEE immediately either way. Non-functioning or misplaced aortic cannula is possible but should be a diagnosis of exclusion.

History and physical
Prompt evaluation of cannula site, look for adventitial discoloration. Check systemic blood pressure.

Tests
Immediate transesophageal echocardiography is needed even if you suspect a simple hematoma. TEE is able to demonstrate an intimal tear in the ascending aorta at the cannulation site with a dissection flap that may extend proximally and or distally

Index scenario (additional information)
"The patient has three-vessel disease for which he is undergoing a CABG. Preoperative CT scan showed a normal aorta with no aneurysm. You just placed an arterial cannula in the ascending aorta. Shortly afterwards there was an increase in arterial line pressure and the purple hematoma has now involved the entire ascending aorta. The patient is hypotensive with MAPs at 50. There are no ST changes and the pericardium appears unchanged. The TEE demonstrates a flap in the ascending aorta. How do you proceed?"

Treatment/management

The patient has an iatrogenic aortic dissection from arterial cannulation. Aortic dissection occurs in 0.01-0.09% of all ascending aortic cannulations. The following factors seem to be associated with iatrogenic aortic dissection: dilated ascending aorta, atherosclerosis, older age and high blood pressure at the time of dissection. In the majority of cases, aortic dissection occurs at the start of the procedure, however it may occur hours or even days after the cardiac procedure. When recognized early, survival ranges 66-85%. When discovered in a delayed fashion the survival drops to 50%. Prompt action is needed to maintain perfusion and limit the dissection. This includes pharmacologic control of hypotension and operative repair of the dissection. Step #1 is to stop perfusing through the cannula, and treat hypotension as you normally would with volume and pressors as needed using the central line. Remember that in this scenario you discovered the dissection very early. You have time. You will not tamponade because the pericardium is opened. You are unlikely to rupture. The most likely "serious" thing that could be giving you severe hypotension is myocardial ischemia from a dissected coronary or potentially acute AI. You need to secure an alternative cannulation site relatively quickly and hopefully you have time to make it the axillary. The femoral is the second option. Finally you have the ascending aorta with a percutaneous and TEE guided approach to ensure cannulation of the true lumen (learn your cannulas and have a sense of how you would do this). After/during the initial resuscitation, the first option is the best but you may be forced down an alternative pathway if the patient is crashing despite best medical therapy.

Operative steps

- Remove the cannula and tie down purse string sutures.
- Obtain right axillary access with a graft or alternative access as discussed above.
- Have the anesthesiologist assess the degree of dissection as well as the presence of AI and LV dysfunction. (LV distention is a sign of retrograde dissection and new onset AI.)
- If the dissection was appreciated once you started flowing on CPB then stop flowing, remove the arterial cannula and use the venous line as a volume line as needed.
- Otherwise, obtain venous access; institution specific - single RA cannula versus bicaval depending on your mode of brain protection (i.e., antegrade brain versus retrograde brain).
- Place your retrograde coronary sinus catheter and make space in the AP window for a cross-clamp.
- Begin cooling to 18° C.
- Be prepared to clamp and arrest if the heart distends and fibrillates.

- The benefit of an LV vent for treating distention and fibrillation would be in a situation where you could not physically clamp the aorta as in a porcelain aorta or extremely distended aorta which is rarely the case.
- Do not place a root vent.
- Arrest the heart with retrograde and vent the root by making your aortotomy above the STJ. Antegrade coronary perfusion can be used if needed only if the integrity of the coronaries is not at all in question. If they are and the retro is inadequate, place bicaval snares, open the atrium and place the retrograde direct.
- Refer to Chpater 48, standard aortic dissection repair, but in short, do your proximal work on the valve as needed (resuspension versus replacement), circ arrest, brain perfusion of choice, hemiarch repair (some might consider an ascending depending on how clearly localized the tear is and how aneurysmal the distal ascending is), deair and resume full flow, perform the proximal and place a root vent.
- Once the graft is constructed, perform your distal anastomoses followed by the proximals off the graft as usual. The one caveat is that if the coronary was dissected then you should suspect that your distal coronary anatomy may have been altered. For instance if the left main is dissected then make sure you graft the distal LAD and OM, if the right was dissected graft the PDA. Dissected coronaries can be difficult to reimplant and distal perfusion will be uncertain unless an angio is done.

Potential questions/alternative scenarios

"During cooling the heart begins to over distend."

This is not uncommon and reflects valve incompetence. You have to prepare for this prior to initiating bypass so be sure to have room to clamp and access to arrest. The easiest venting strategy is an aortotomy but an LV vent is used as safe practice in many institutions. The main benefit of the LV vent is in improving exposure during the proximal valve work (see above).

"Dissection diagnosed at the end of operation by routine transesophageal echocardiography evaluation."

This can occur from removal of the cross clamp under pressure, the proximal anastomosis or an unrecognized tear from the antegrade or proximal cannulation. Re-heparinize, axillary cannulation and follow the steps addressed above.

"In addition to dissection at the cannula site, TEE demonstrates 3+ AI but the leaflets appear intact. The patient had only trivial AI preoperatively. How do you proceed?"

Repair aortic dissection as outlined in the operative steps above. Resuspend the aortic valve as long as the leaflets are clearly preserved and the anatomy is such that the resuspension will realign you with the center of coaptation. Reevaluate the valve function with the TEE postoperatively. 1-2+ may be acceptable in most situations but be prepared for the possibility of 3-4+.

"You complete a CABG. In the CVICU, shortly after the operation, the patient develops signs of myocardial ischemia and unexplained hemodynamic instability. What is your next step?"

Differential diagnoses include graft dysfunction and thrombosis, reperfusion injury, coronary artery embolus, iatrogenic aortic dissection. Obtain STAT chest X-ray, EKG, and transthoracic echocardiography; if non diagnostic get TEE. If a dissection is present return to the OR for a dissection repair as outlined above.

"Your patient is three years status post CABG. He had a chest CT done for workup of a cough, and was found to have an ascending aortic dissection. What is the most likely explanation?"

Chronic dissection that developed as a result of the prior cardiac operation. While this patient is asymptomatic and the aorta is non-aneurysmal, a chronic ascending dissection has the potential to cause valvular incompetence, chest pain, dilation of the aorta or even rupture, all of which are indications for surgery. Careful follow up with echo and CT imaging is needed but surgery is not warranted unless any of the indications are met.

"During an mini-thoracotomy for mitral valve surgery, resistance is noted while threading the wire for antegrade arterial access. You remove the wire and do an angio through the sheath and discover a dissection that appears to extend up towards the infrarenal aorta."

Abort the procedure. Check a TEE to rule out an ascending component. Check a post op CT. Treat the patient medically for a Type B dissection for as long as possible (> 4-6 weeks) prior to returning to the OR and performing the mitral repair with central cannulation.

"You complete a CABG on a patient with an EF of 20% with a balloon pump that was placed preoperatively. In the ICU he loses his RLE pulse. The patient is on minimal inotropic support."

The differential includes embolic disease, localized thrombosis/dissection/mechanical occlusion from the sheath, or a descending aortic dissection from the IABP. Assuming the patient does not need the IABP the best initial therapy is to remove it and follow the vascular exam. Vascular duplex maybe helpful. If ischemia persists, check a CTA of the chest abdomen and pelvis with lower extremity runoff. If a Type B dissection is discovered with persistent evidence of limb ischemia then go the OR urgently for a Fem-Fem bypass using inflow from the non-dissected limb.

Pearls/pitfalls

- Ascending aortic dilatation, known atherosclerosis, older age, and high blood pressure are risk factors for iatrogenic aortic dissection.
- Mostly common they present at the beginning of the operation, although they may present in a delayed fashion after cardiac surgery.
- Immediately discontinue use of the offending cannula. Let anesthesia resuscitate while you switch to axillary cannulation.
- Know alternative cannulating strategies if needed and know the conduct of a dissection repair as this may come up in a number of different cardiac surgical scenarios.

Suggested readings

- Januzzi JL, Sabatine MS, Eagle KA, et al. Iatrogenic aortic dissection. Am J Cardiol. 2002 Mar 1;89(5):623-6.
- Fleck T et al. Intraoperative iatrogenic Type A aortic dissection and perioperative outcome. Interact Cardiovasc Thorac Surg. 2006 Feb;5(1):11-4.

Notes

48. Type A aortic dissection

Armin Kiankhooy, MD, and Ravi Ghanta, MD

Concept

- Clinical presentation
- Diagnostics
- Surgical strategy
- Postoperative management

Chief complaint

"A pale 63 yo man presents to the emergency room with severe tearing anterior chest and mid-scapular back pain."

Differential

This presentation calls for a high index of suspicion for acute aortic dissection. Up to 30% of patients with with acute dissection are initially thought to have another diagnosis. Differential includes acute aortic dissection, acute myocardial infarction, pulmonary embolism, and pericarditis.

History and physical

A focused history to elicit the quality, location (mid-sternum or interscapular) and timing of the pain (acute vs. chronic > 14 days) and presence of malperfusion, i.e., stroke, paraplegia, abdominal pain, anuria/oliguria, and claudication. Physical exam concordantly should focus on discerning the level and propagation of the dissection. Retrograde propagation involving the aortic root and aortic valve can lead to severe aortic regurgitation with a murmur (blowing, diastolic, decrescendo at the left 3rd intercostal space). Aortic rupture will lead to tamponade with characteristic JVD, pulsus paradoxus, and pericardial friction rub. Neurologic exam is key to evaluate for CVA from arch vessel involvement as well as lower extremity neurological deficit. This should be clearly document
prior to surgery. Bilateral blood pressure measurement and pulse exam will also help identify patients with distal aortic branch and peripheral vessel involvement.

Pathophysiology

Cystic medial necrosis, intramural hematoma, penetrating atherosclerotic ulcers, and connective tissue disorders have all been associated with development of aortic dissection. Hypertension is now thought to be the most likely mechanical force associated with dissection. The tear is typically > 50% of the circumference and usually occurs along the right anterior aspect of the ascending aorta and circumferentially spirals around the arch and into the descending thoracic and abdominal aorta on the left and posteriorly. Approximately 10% of the time the dissection propagates in a retrograde fashion to involve the coronary ostia. MI and rupture into the pericardium are the most common (80%) causes of death. 1% per hour risk of mortality in the first 48 hours, 50% mortality in the first 48 hours, and 90% mortality at 72 hours if untreated. If rupture does not occur, weakening of the outer media and adventitia over time will result in aneurysm formation with resultant root dilation. Patients with Type A Dissections ultimately die from 5 causes: 1) hemorrhage; 2) heart failure from acute AI; 3) myocardial infarction from dissection into coronary; 4) acute tamponade; and/or 5) brain malperfusion.

Risk factors
Hypertension, connective tissue disease, aneurysms, pregnancy, iatrogenic trauma (catheterization, CPB, cross-clamping, IABP), prior aneurysm)

Tests
- *Labs*: establish baseline lab values (CMP, CBC, Coags).
- *EKG*: EKG may show evidence of myocardial ischemia.
- *CXR*: widening of the mediastinal silhouette (50%) and pleural effusion.
- *CT angiography*. Diagnostic study of choice due to widespread availability and high sensitivity/specificity. Identify proximal and distal flap extent (sensitivity 82-100%; specificity 90-100%). Also helps identify aortic root and arch aneurysms or presence of pericardial effusion. If high suspicion for dissection CT down to level of femoral vessels is ideal.
- *TEE*: confirmatory but invasive study that may exacerbate the tear or rupture. Identifies proximal intimal tear (distinguishing Type A from B), true and false lumens, aortic valve characteristics, presence of AI, proximal coronary involvement, and pericardial effusion. Some of these features can be picked up with the less invasive TTE. It is safest to perform the TEE in the operating room. Intraoperative TEE is the diagnostic study of choice in an unstable patient with high suspicion of Type A dissection.
- *Any imaging study revealing pericardial effusion or pleural effusion may signify imminent rupture requiring emergency surgery!*

Index scenario (additional information)
"This patient has < 24 hours of pain and CT angiography reveals a Type A dissection involving the ascending aorta. There is no aortic root or arch involvement. How would you like to proceed?"

Treatment/management

This patient meets the criteria for acute Type A aortic dissection *without arch or root involvement*. Surgery is warranted to prevent life-threatening complications of aortic rupture. The goal is to prevent death and irreversible end-organ damage. Pre-operative anti-impulse (dp/dt) treatment with beta-blockade (esmolol) and sodium nitroprusside, with goal heart rate (60 to 80 bpm), systolic pressure (90-110 mmHg) and mean arterial pressure (60-75 mmHg) is critical. Calcium channel blockers may be used in patients who are unable to tolerate beta-blockade. Pain control is important. The presence of Type A is an indication for immediate repair. Only minor delays for CT imaging of a stable patient can be justified. Hemodynamic instability demands immediate surgery. Focal neurologic deficits mandate a head CT. Major neurologic insult (stroke or hemorrhage) is at least a relative contraindication. Age over 80 years old and significant comorbidities or sepsis are also relative contraindications. For the most part Type A dissections will be operative without delay.

Operative steps

Acute Type A dissection repair

Goals – The primary goal is to save the patient's life by eliminating the possibility of tamponade, coronary malperfusion, brain malperfusion, acute aortic regurgitation, or hemorrhage. The extent of aorta requiring replacement depends on the location and extent of the tear and aneurysm. The most common operation is a supra-coronary tube graft to the level of the hemi-arch. In all cases, an open distal anastomosis is performed and thus deep hypothermic circulatory arrest is utilized. Many variations on surgical approach exist (axillary vs. femoral cannulation; antegrade vs. retrograde brain perfusion), so stick with the one that works for you and be able to describe it well.

- Anesthesia & monitoring
    - Single lumen endotracheal intubation, central venous access, PA catheter, radial (single or bilateral) and femoral arterial lines, TEE, bladder and esophageal temperature probes. Prep wide for possible axillary and femoral cannulation. Neurologic and spinal perfusion monitoring with EEG, transcranial Doppler, somatosensory evoked potentials or near-infrared spectroscopy.
    - Cell saver should be utilized. PRBCs and FFP available at the start of the case.
- Cannulation and cardiopulmonary bypass
    - Arterial cannulation is a critical step in the management of aortic dissection. In general there are 4 major options: 1) Right Axillary, 2) Femoral, 3) Ascending Aorta, and

4) LV Apex. The choice of cannulation site is dependent on patient stability and extent of dissection. The critical factor in arterial cannulation is that the true lumen is cannulated. In general right axillary and femoral are the preferred cannulation sites. Right axillary allows for antegrade flow and antegrade brain perfusion during circulatory arrest. Femoral cannulation is the most rapid and easiest cannulation to perform. Left axillary is another option. Direct aortic cannulation can be performed using a wire guided cannula with TEE guidance to cannulate the true lumen. LV apex cannulation can be performed as a last ditch "bailout" as it allows for successful cannulation of the true lumen when the cannula is introduced into the apex and then passed through the aortic valve.

- If high line pressures are encountered, you may have cannulated the false lumen with resultant high pressures. Come off bypass and readdress your arterial cannulation. Likely will need to choose a different site.
- *Venous cannulation*: depends on whether you want retrograde brain perfusion or not. The safest approach is to do bicaval so you have the option. Otherwise right atrium using a two-stage venous cannula will suffice for a short circulatory arrest time.
- Left ventricular vent via right superior pulmonary vein may be helpful.
- *Cardioplegia*: Retrograde cardioplegia cannulation is required. If it can not be placed correctly, then the aorta must be opened following cross-clamp and direct coronary ostial cardiplegia should be given. One may then switch to direct retrograde insertion for intermittent cardioplegia throughout the case.

- *Incision*: median sternotomy with possible extension along the left SCM.
- Cannulation (see above).
- Initiate CPB and begin systemic cooling. Slow cool with a maximal temperature gradient of 10° C between the patient and perfusate. Measure brain temperature with nasopharyngeal and tympanic thermometers. Cool to 18-20° C and place ice-bags around the head.
- During cooling, perform proximal dissection. Cross clamp the mid-ascending aorta and divide the aorta. Inspect aortic root and aortic valve. Perform as much proximal work (see below) while cooling.
- Once cooled to at least 20° C and electrocerebral silence is achieved (EEG monitoring), give a dose of cardioplegia, place the patient in Trendelenburg and initiate circulatory arrest. Utilize the brain

protection method of your choice. Selective antegrade can be administered via the right axillary (10 cc/kg/min) with occlusion of the innominate artery but remember that you are unlikely to know the status of the patient's circle of willis circulation. Retrograde brain may be more predictable in these acute scenarios and can be administered via the SVC cannula (flow rate of 500-800 mL/min to achieve a pressure (CVP) of 15-25 mmHg, but not exceeding 25-30 mmHg). Following circulatory arrest, some centers use furosemide and mannitol to promote diuresis and free radical scavenging.

- Up to 40 minutes of circulatory arrest with deep hypothermia is acceptable, there is a 60% peri-operative TIA risk at 60 minutes.
- Perform an open distal anastomosis between the tube graft and aorta. The distal flap is usually not fenestrated in the setting of an acute dissection as this would promote perfusion of the false lumen (different than chronic where you may need to maintain patency of both). The true lumen is usually clearly evident. The walls of the false lumen are re-approximated with the suture line. A variety of suture reinforcement techniques can be used including felt or pericardial strips on the outside and sometimes a felt sandwich technique. If the tear extends into the arch and is within your capacity to fix it with a simple or pledgeted suture or a pericardial patch then it may be worth doing so. You should try to extend your resection of the ascending aorta to involve the tear. The problem is what to do if the tear is beyond your anastamosis at the mid to distal arch and cannot be repaired with a patch or suture. A total arch or elephant trunk would work but adds significant time to the operation. It is reasonable to do the ascending as planned, leave the tear and follow the patient for downstream events clinically and radiologically.
- After confirming good hemostasis, resume cardiopulmonary bypass. Deair and clamp the graft. Consider relocation (particularly if femoral) of the arterial cannula to the graft. A number of grafts have side-arms for cannulation. The beauty of the axillary is you can simply resume flow.
- Complete proximal work. In this scenario, the root is ok without a tear. However, just as you considered the implications of a tear in the distal arch also consider what you might do if the tear were below the coronaries. In this case your options are root replacement, patch or other local repair (particularly if located in the noncoronary sinus).
- Perform proximal anastomosis.
  - If the sinotubular ridge is involved, reapproximate the dissected layers with a teflon felt sandwich technique using 4-0 Prolene. (Biological glues have also been used but are

associated with toxicity and redissection).
- Perform the proximal anastomosis to the Dacron tube graft using 4-0 prolene in a simple running fashion with teflon felt buttress.
• Wean bypass/deair/decannulate.

Potential questions/alternative scenarios
"This patient's CT angiography demonstrates a Type A aortic dissection with arch vessel involvement. How would you like to proceed?"
In almost all scenarios of arch involvement, a hemiarch will be sufficient to exclude the false lumen and re-establish arch vessel perfusion. Rarely, a total arch is needed with reimplantation of the arch vessels individually or as a Carrel patch. The only real indication is an aneurysmal arch at risk of rupture (> 5.5 cm) (please refer to arch aneurysms). Note that a tear in the arch is not sufficient indication to perform a total arch (see above operative discussion under distal anastamosis).

There are a variety of ways to intervene on the arch during a dissection if intervention is warranted. If the vessels are dissected their proximal portions should be resected and replaced with a separate tube graft in an end to end fashion. If they are not dissected then the arch vessels may be sewn to the graft as a patch. If the isthmus is aneurysmal than an elephant trunk may be used. As the procedure becomes more involved, greater thought should be given to antegrade brain perfusion.

"This patient has an unknown connective tissue disorder (possible Marfan's, annulo-aortic ectasia) and CT angiography reveals the aforementioned findings as well as a widened aortic root. TEE demonstrates additional findings of retrograde propagation involving the aortic root and severe aortic regurgitation). How would you like to proceed?"
If the regurgitation is secondary to commissural detachment (*without the presence of connective tissue disorder*), an appropriate resuspension with pledgeted teflon and closure of the proximal false lumen will provide a competent aortic valve and repair in most of these specific cases and allows preservation of the sinuses.

If the valve is regurgitant secondary to root dissection and the patient *has* a connective tissue disorder replacing the aortic valve and root with a composite valve-graft and coronary reimplantation is likely your best option (modified Bentall). A valve-sparing aortic root replacement (David procedure) is not unreasonable in stable patients with normal leaflets and without evidence of end-organ damage but is not necessary, as this typically will require more time.

"Upon opening the aorta you are surprised to find that this patient has dissection of both coronary ostia. How would you specifically address the coronary dissections?"

This is challenging and the approach depends on the extent of the coronary dissection. Local repair techniques have been described including mobilization of coronary buttons and reapproximating the dissected layers (mainly if the coronary itself is not torn but the dissection does reach the coronary). If the coronary itself is dissected then either patch repair of the coronary or complete transection with saphenous interposition have been described. If you are familiar with these techniques then you can use them as options. Otherwise, a saphenous vein graft is a perfectly acceptable alternative.

"The patient demonstrates a decrease in the femoral pressure after initiation of bypass."

Distal malperfusion is caused in most cases by false lumen compression on the true lumen. Either your femoral arterial line is in the false lumen or your arterial cannula is in the false lumen. To clarify the later check the radial pressure reading. If it is normal then the femoral line is unreliable or a regional malperfusion event has occurred due to a distal re-entry tear. If the radial line is dampened then stop the pump and switch your cannulation. Due to re-entry tears in the dissection flap and changes in distal flow dynamics it is possible to have malperfusion events during initiation of CPB, cross clamping or after circulatory arrest. In these cases you are essentially dealing with a Type B situation and can clarify and address the distal perfusion issues once the ascending repair is completed (i.e., angio, fenestration vs. bypass - please see Type B dissection section for more information).

"A 52 yo african american man presents with an acute Type A dissection. He complains of severe abdominal pain and a CTA demonstrates occlusion of the SMA by the false lumen. How would you proceed?"

Most distal complications associated with a Type A dissection will resolve by re-establishing flow to the true lumen. If there is a question of the integrity of the bowel then a laparotomy should be done in the same setting after the dissection repair. For prolonged preoperative limb ischemia consider four quadrant fasciotomies. After the operation, distal complications can be monitored through clinical examination, CT scan and duplex as needed.

"A 63 yo male patient undergoes a CT chest for evaluation of a solitary lung nodule. Incidentally a 5.6 cm ascending aortic aneurysm is noticed with signs of chronic dissection. How would you like to proceed?"

Treatment/management

Chronic Type A dissection

Uncommon (4-31%) as most patients do not spontaneously heal acute Type A dissections, but when they present in the chronic phase they usually present asymptomatically and incidentally discovered on imaging. Most commonly intervene for new symptoms, increasing associated ascending aneurysm (5.5 cm or 5 cm if associated connective tissue disorder), eccentric expansion, rapid expansion (> 1 cm per year) or aortic insufficiency. Annual imaging follow-up with CT or MRI is recommended.

Operative considerations
- Generally the surgery is similar to acute Type A dissection however the rate of native aortic valve preservation (50%) is considerable less due to the chronicity of the disease. The distal chronic dissection flap should be resected and the distal anastomosis should be made to the outer wall of the aorta. A staged elephant trunk procedure is required in rare instances when the chronic Type A dissection with aneurysm dilation extends from the ascending aorta through the arch and into the descending thoracic aorta.

Outcomes
- Operative mortality for chronic Type A dissection: 4-17%
- Stroke: 4%
- Reoperation rate if native aortic valve preserved: 20%

Long-term management
- Despite Type A dissection surgical repair, most patients on follow-up reveal distal false lumen perfusion. This places patients at risk for aneurysmal dilatation and potential rupture. Therefore blood pressure control (< 120 mmHg) is critical to prevent late death from rupture and chronic dissection.
- A vast majority (80-90%) of patients are free from reoperation at 10 years, however routine echocardiographic monitoring of the aortic valve and diagnostic imaging of the aortic diameter are still warranted.

Pearls/pitfalls
- High index of suspicion
- Diagnosis with CT angiography
- Be comfortable describing alternative cannulation
- Circulatory arrest with cooling to 18-20° C
- Hemiarch most common repair (full arch rarely needed)
- Resuspend commissures if possible to preserve the native valve

- Replace the root if known connective tissue disorder
- Strict dp/dt control pre/post-op with esmolol and nitroprusside
- Monitor for malperfusion pre/intra-/post-op

Suggested readings

- Reece B, et al. Aortic Dissection. Cardiac Surgery in the Adult. Cohn LH. *Cardiac Surgery in the Adult* 2008;Ch 51.
- Coselli JS et al. *Operative Techniques in Thoracic and Cardiovascular Surgery: A Comparative Atlas.* 1999;(4):13-32.
- Bolman RM. *Operative Techniques in Thoracic and Cardiovascular Surgery: A Comparative Atlas.* 2009;14:124-135.

Notes

49. Type B aortic dissection

Katherine B. Harrington, MD, and Michael P. Fischbein, MD, PhD

Concept
- Presentation and classification of aortic dissections
- Initial treatment
- Medical versus surgical therapy
- Operative steps for repair

Chief complaint
"A 56 yo man presents to the ED with sharp, tearing back pain. CT scan shows an aortic dissection extending from just distal to the left subclavian artery to the aortic bifurcation."

Differential
The diagnosis, aortic dissection, is already known. The dissection must be classified into Type A vs. Type B, acute vs. chronic, and complicated vs. uncomplicated. Dissections are considered "acute" in the first 14 days after development of symptoms. After 14 days dissections are considered "chronic" as patients typically stabilize after this time and are managed under a different algorithm.

There are several anatomic classification schemes for describing aortic dissections. The Stanford system considers all dissections which involve the ascending aorta, i.e., the aorta proximal to the right innominate artery, to be Type A, and those which involve only the descending aorta, i.e., everything distal to the left subclavian, to be Type B dissections. The Debakey classification classifies dissections into three groups. Type I and II include the ascending aorta. In Type I it propagates at least to the aortic arch and often further distally, while Type II is confined to the ascending aorta. Type III originates in the descending aorta is further broken down into Type IIIa (descending thoracic aorta only) and Type IIIb (extending into abdominal aorta).

"Complicated" dissections are those with persistent pain, thoracoabdominal malperfusion (spinal, visceral, and extremity), impending rupture, or other life-threatening complications. The majority of Type B dissections are "uncomplicated."

History and physical
The most common presenting symptom is abrupt onset, sharp, severe, chest or back pain. Patients tend to be significantly hypertensive when they present. Most patients have a history of long standing hypertension.

Social history should query amphetamine or cocaine use, both risk factors for dissection. A brief skeletal exam should assess for connective tissue disorders, especially in younger patients. A very thorough vascular exam should be documented. Pulse deficits are present in approximately 10% of patients.

Tests

- *Initial CXR*: mediastinal widening or abnormal aortic contour in 56% of patients.
- *Laboratory*: serum creatinine, liver function tests, and lactate (evaluate for renal or visercal malperfusion).
- *Diagnostic procedures*: computed tomographic angiographic scanning (CTA), transesophageal echocardiography, and magnetic resonance angiography. Study interpretation should include dissection classification, extent, primary intimal tear (PIT) location, and presence/absence organ malperfusion. Further information can also be acquired for possible endovascular stent graft insertion including the dimensions of descending aorta, size of true and false lumen, arch branch vessel anatomy, potential landing zones, and femoral/iliac dimensions for access.

Index scenario (additional information)

"Upon further questioning the patient's pain started this morning. He continues to have severe pain even after his blood pressure is brought to appropriate levels and is requiring a large amount of narcotics."

Treatment/management

As soon as acute aortic dissection is suspected, emergency medical therapy should be initiated and continued while the diagnostic procedures are performed. Medical treatment includes reduction of mean, peak, and rate of rise in arterial pressure (*dP/dt*) with both an intravenous (a) B-Blocker (esmolol, labetolol) and (b) vasodilator (nipride). Parenteral calcium channel antagonists, like diltiazem or nifedipine, that lower arterial blood pressure and left ventricular dP/dt can also be used.

For Type B dissections medical treatment results in equal if not better results than surgical repair. Current registry studies show medical management carries a 30-day mortality between 9-16% while surgical management yields an operative mortality of 27-32%, biased by the more complicated patients receiving intervention. Comparative retrospective studies which attempted to match risk adjusted cohorts have shown that long-term survival, as well as freedom from late aortic reintervention, is similar for both medically and surgically treated patients.

Currently, a "complication-specific" approach is recommended, reserving surgical or endovascular intervention on the descending aorta for those with complicated dissections. Other conditions that should prompt consideration of early intervention include extensive aortic arch involvement, expectations of poor medical compliance, and underlying connective tissue disorders.

After determining that an intervention is required, the surgeon must decide between an open versus endovascular approach. Endovascular stent grafts should be considered in patients who are older, poor operative risks (renal failure, COPD, poor cardiac function, acidotic from malperfusion), and have favorable anatomy. Younger patients, good surgical candidates, patients with connective tissue diseases, and patients with unfavorable endovascular stent graft anatomy receive a central aortic operation.

Operative steps

Goals – patients with acute Type B aortic dissection is graft replacement of a limited segment of the descending thoracic aorta, hopefully including the site of the PIT, to restore flow to the true lumen and obliterate flow to the false lumen.

- After insertion of a double-lumen endobronchial tube, and often a lumbar intrathecal catheter for cerebrospinal fluid drainage, patients with acute Type B dissections are explored through a left posterolateral thoracotomy through the third or fourth intercostal space, providing access to the transverse arch and proximal descending aorta. Alternatively, a second entry point into the 7th intercostal space may provide access to the distal thoracic aorta.
- Full cardiopulmonary bypass with antegrade perfusion is preferred. Arterial cannulation strategies include the following: perfusion into the arch, left subclavian artery, left common carotid artery, right subclavian artery, left ventricular apex and across the aortic valve, or femoral artery (perfuse true lumen). Venous return can be accomplished with central venous cannulation via the femoral vein or retrograde cannulation through the main pulmonary artery.
- Hypothermic circulatory arrest is utilized to perform an open proximal anastomosis. Most Type B dissection tears originate at the origin of the subclavian artery; clamping between the left common carotid and left subclavian arteries may be utilized, but frequently results in insufficient length for a proximal anastomosis. If left ventricular distension occurs during systemic cooling and subsequent ventricular fibrillation, the left heart may need to be decompressed with a vent via the left superior pulmonary vein or left ventricular apex. During hypothermic circulatory arrest, myocardial protection is from systemic hypothermia only.

- The phrenic and vagus nerves are identified and dissected free from the transverse arch, with special attention paid to the recurrent laryngeal nerve near the ligamentum and along the posterior proximal aortic neck. The transverse arch, proximal descending thoracic aorta, left subclavian artery, and distal aortic anastomotic site are circumferentially dissected.
- The primary goal is to replace only a short segment of aorta to redirect flow into the true lumen. This strategy allows one to stay above T7 and therefore prevents the need to re-implant intercostal arteries.
- When the goal hypothermic temperature is achieved (18-22° C core temperature), the pump is turned off, and the proximal descending aorta opened. An appropriately sized woven double velour Dacron graft is selected and sewn proximally to undissected aorta with an open technique taking care to excise the entire PIT. If the dissection extends into the arch (retrograde from the PIT), incorporate both the aortic intima and adventitia while performing the anastomosis to obliterate the false lumen. The left subclavian artery may need to be individually reimplanted if the PIT is very close or proximal to the left subclavian artery. Carefully identify the recurrent laryngeal nerve along the proximal aortic neck, especially while transecting the aorta along the posterior wall (common site of nerve injury while performing proximal anatomosis).
- Resume arterial flow to the head and heart slowly (about 500-700 mL/hr) either through the axillary or a perfusion cannula inserted directly into the graft. Replace the cross clamp on the graft after taking care to evacuate any air trapped in the heart or ascending aorta.
- Proximal intercostals arteries (above T7) are oversewn to eliminate steal of blood from the spinal cord.
- The distal anastomosis is also performed with an open technique under circulatory arrest, taking care to incorporate both aortic layers and obliterate the false lumen. Distally, intima and adventitia may occasionally be reapproximated with a Teflon felt media or adventitial bolster. Proximal cross-clamp is released, air is evacuated both proximally and distally prior to tying the sutures, and both anastomoses checked for hemostasis. Systemic rewarming is commenced approximately 10 minutes after reperfusion to allow oxygen debt reversal. After warming to 35-36° C, CPB is discontinued. Transesophageal echo should be used to assure perfusion of the true lumen at the level of the diaphragm.

Potential questions/alternative scenarios

"Post-operatively the patient has a rising lactate and creatinine…"
Visceral malperfusion postoperatively should be monitored with urine output and serial lactates/ABGs. Malperfusion results when a dissection compromises blood flow to end-organs, and occurs in approximately 21% of dissections. Two pathophysiological mechanisms of malperfusion are commonly described: dynamic and static branch malperfusion. Dynamic branch compromise is the more common mechanism of malperfusion (80%), and occurs when the true lumen is narrowed or compressed due to the majority of flow occurring in the false lumen- this should be alleviated by open repair. Static branch malperfusion occurs when the dissection flap or intimal tear extends into a branch vessel ostium, leading to mechanical obstruction of flow from the intimal intussusception. This may be treated percutaneously with balloon septal fenestration and uncovered stenting in collaboration with an interventional radiologist.

"The patient wakes up and is not able to move his/her legs."
Paraplegia is a significant risk of any descending thoracic aortic repair (both open and endovascular). Dissection patients have an increased risk, although short segment replacement mitigates this somewhat. Patients with prexisting AAA repair have a higher risk. Pre-operative lumbar drain placement is commonly done, but not required. If it was not done pre-operatively in this patient, it needs to be placed now. If pre-existing, the amount of drainage should be increased and every effort should be made to get the ICP to less than 10, if not as low as possible. However, caution should be used in draining more than 20 mL per hour due to the risk of subdural hemorrhage. MAP should be increased to > 80-90 mmHg with neosynephrine or vasopressin to increase spinal cord perfusion pressure. Several adjunct strategies, such as a naloxone drip may be used, but no data support its benefit. There is no benefit to high dose steroid treatment.

"A similar patient presents but there is no visible flap, just hematoma within the wall of descending thoracic aorta."
Intramural hematomas (IMH) and penetrating aortic ulcers (PAU) are pathological variants of the classic aortic dissection. Importantly, in contrast to the dissection, neither IMH nor PAU has blood flow down a false lumen. IMH likely results following aortic vasa vasorum rupture, causing hemorrhage into the aortic media. PAU originates from an intimal lesion (ruptured atherosclerotic plaque) that penetrates into the aortic media and results in a variable amount of IMH. IMH is treated similarly to a dissection. Emergency anti-impulse therapy should be initiated.

"A patient with a previously uncomplicated Type B dissection several years ago returns with pain and a descending thoracic aorta that has now grown to 7 cm."

All patients with acute Type B dissections should have serial CT scans at 3 months, 6 months, and then yearly to monitor for aneursymal development of the dissection. Surgical intervention for chronic Type B dissections may be considered for both symptomatic patients (pain, mesenteric ischemia) and asymptomatic patients (rapidly expanding or > 6 cm aneurysmal aortic dissections). The techniques utilized are identical to those for an acute Type B dissection, although the extent of resection is usually greater (remove all enlarged aorta) (Refer to descending aneurysm section). Importantly, prior to performing the distal anastomosis, a "tongue" of chronic dissection flap is excised from the aorta- a "flap septectomy," allowing blood flow into both true and false lumens distally (visceral or iliac arteries may originate from either true or false lumens). Surgical resections distal to T-7 may require reimplantation of large intercostal arteries to avoid spinal cord ischemia.

Pearls/pitfalls

- Type B dissections involve the descending aorta. Current management for acute dissections involves aggressive anti-impulse blood pressure therapy with a beta blocker and vasodilator.
- Surgical or endovascular management is generally reserved for "complicated" dissections: those with persistent pain, refractory hypertension, thoracoabdominal malperfusion (spinal, visceral, and extremity), impending rupture, or other life-threatening complications.
- Endovascular stent grafting is reserved for elderly or non-operative candidates. Younger patients or those with connective tissue disorder should reccieve an open central aortic operation, if indicated.
- The goal of surgical treatment is graft replacement of a *short segment* of the descending thoracic aorta, including the site of the PIT, to restore flow to the true lumen and obliterate flow to the false lumen.
- Circulatory arrest with axillary cannulation is the simplest way to deal with the proximal and distal anastamosis.

Suggested readings

- Hagan PG, Nienaber CA, Isselbacher EM et al. The International Registry of Acute Aortic Dissection (IRAD): new insights into an old disease. JAMA 2000 February 16;283(7):897-903.

- Umana JP, Lai DT, Mitchell RS et al. Is medical therapy still the optimal treatment strategy for patients with acute Type B aortic dissections? J Thorac Cardiovasc Surg 2002 November;124(5):896-910.
- Suzuki T, Mehta RH, Ince H et al. Clinical profiles and outcomes of acute Type B aortic dissection in the current era: lessons from the International Registry of Aortic Dissection (IRAD). Circulation 2003 September 9;108 Suppl 1:II312-II317.
- Ehrlich MP, Dumfarth J, Schoder M et al. Midterm results after endovascular treatment of acute, complicated Type B aortic dissection. Ann Thorac Surg 2010 November;90(5):
- 1444-8.

Notes

50. Aortic root aneurysm

Muhammad Aftab, MD, Ismael de Armas, MD, and Faisal G. Bakaeen, MD, FACS

Concept

- Clinical Presentation of aortic root aneurysms
- Diagnostic modalities
- Indications for surgery and choice of conduit
- Technique of aortic root replacement
- Complications
- Follow up

Chief complaint

"A 44 yo man is referred to you by his cardiologist for the evaluation of severe aortic regurgitation and enlarged aortic root after presenting with a 1 month history of increasing shortness of breath and cough. How would you proceed with work up and management?"

Differential

Usually patients with aortic root aneurysm are asymptomatic and the condition is diagnosed during the workup of other disease processes or it could cause symptoms such as pulmonary congestion that can masquerade as respiratory in origin. Symptoms such as shortness of breath and chest pain should also raise concern for pneumonia, dissection, aneurysmal disease, pulmonary embolism, or MI.

History and physical

A focused history should attempt to elicit any symptoms relevant to the aneurysm or aortic regurgitation such as chest pain, back pain or shortness of breath. Significant history of bleeding diathesis or significant dental pathology e.g., caries, infection is also important in preparation and planning for surgery. Ask for history/family history of Marfan disease, other connective tissue disorders or aneurysms. Evaluate for the risk factors of aneurysm formation and progression such as hypertension, atherosclerosis, and smoking. Physical examination of patient with un-ruptured aortic root aneurysms is often unremarkable. Nonetheless, check lungs for evidence of pulmonary edema, listen for murmurs and evaluate distal pulses. One may discover findings such as a water-hammer pulse with wide pulse pressure and low diastolic pressure and a decrescendo diastolic murmur. AAA is present in 10-20% of patients with atherosclerotic ascending aortic aneurysm. Patients with Marfan syndrome have characteristic features including thin, tall stature, lax joints, ectopia lentis and high arched palate. Also evaluate for the phenotypic features of Loeys-Dietz syndrome such as blue sclera, hypotelorism, bifid uvula, malar flattening, retrognathia, translucent skin with visible veins and arachnodactyly.

Tests

- *CXR*: prominent right mediastinal border. Aortic valve and aortic root calcifications (lateral projection).
- *EKG*. Usually there will be no EKG abnormality specific to aortic root aneurysm. However left ventricular volume overload from aortic regurgitation is supported by increased QRS complex voltage (best seen in the chest leads) and prominent septal depolarization reflected by Q waves in leads V4 to V6.
- *Echocardiogram*. TEE is the imaging modality of choice. Accurate visualization of aortic root and ascending aorta is imperative. It is also important to determine if the aortic valve is bileaflet, since this may influence when to surgically intervene. Carefully evaluate valve anatomy to determine whether the valve repair is feasible. For aortic root measurements, the widest diameter, typically at the mid-sinus level should be used.
- *Computed tomography angiography (CTA)*. Most common imaging to study the aorta. Ability to image the entire aorta including lumen, wall, branch vessels, arch, periaortic regions and distal aorta with 3-dimensional data. EKG gated imaging helps to eliminate motion artifact at the aortic root and helps assess coronary arteries, aortic valve morphology and function. While the widest diameter is typically at the mid sinus level, measurements should be taken at all four levels including annulus, sinotubular junction, mid sinus and ascending aorta. Limitation includes risk of contrast-induced nephropathy.
- *Magnetic resonance imaging (MRI)*. A valuable imaging modality for diagnosis of thoracic aortic diseases in stable patients with sensitivities and specificities comparable to CT and TEE. A preferred imaging modality for patients requiring repeat imaging for the follow-up of aortic pathology without exposing them to radiation and iodinated contrast agents.
- *Cardiac catheterization*. Considerations should be given to perform cardiac catheterization to rule out presence of coronary artery disease in patients greater than 40. Make sure to define the ostial anatomy and look for anomalies such as a left from the right, right from left, or separate circumflex and LAD orifices.

Index scenario (additional information)

"He is a 6 foot tall, thin gentleman with a significant smoking history and worsening dyspnea on exertion. He is noted to have a holo diastolic murmur radiating towards the apex. His CXR revealed a

prominent right mediastinal border. On echocardiogram he is noticed to have gross aortic root dilatation, a trileaflet non-stenotic aortic valve with severe aortic valve regurgitation, mild mitral regurgitation and moderately dilated LV. His aortic root diameter is 7.2 cm (mid sinus) on CT scan and tapers down to normal size at the mid ascending."

Treatment/management

Criteria for surgical intervention of an ascending aortic aneurysm includes:

- Sporadic (5.5 to 6.0 cm)
- Connective tissue disorder (4.5 to 5.0 cm)
- Bicuspid aortic valve (5.0 to 5.5 cm)

The surgical procedure to be performed on an aortic root aneurysm will be dictated by the status of the aortic valve and the condition of the patient. If the aortic valve is structurally normal a valve sparing procedure is becoming a popular treatment choice at experienced centers. When choosing the valved conduit consideration should be given to the patients' age, life expectancy, underlying disease condition, comorbidities, lifestyle, preference, risk of bleeding from anticoagulation, risk of possible reoperation and finally surgeons experience. Aortic root replacement using a graft and mechanical valve (composite or separate) is recommended for younger patients (age < 60 years) with no contraindication to anticoagulation or patients of any age requiring anticoagulation for other indication such as pulmonary thromboembolism, atrial fibrillation or mechanical valve in other valvular position. Advantages include long term durability and relatively ease of implantation compared to other root replacement options. Complications are related to thromboembolic events and anticoagulation.

When tissue valve is desired during aortic root replacement, a stented bovine or porcine bioprosthetic valve is hand sewn to a tube graft to make a composite biological valve graft conduit. Bioprosthetic grafts are recommended in patients older than 65 years of age with the benefit of freedom from anticoagulation as well as better durability in elderly patients. Bioprosthetic valved graft conduit may also be used in patients of any age with medical or personal contraindication to anticoagulation.

For the David procedure (valve sparing root replacement) the aortic valve is preserved by reimplanting it inside the Dacron tube graft. This is possible in almost 30% of patients requiring aortic root replacement. This is ideal in patients with root dilatation, AI and structurally normal valves.

The stentless composite porcine aortic root grafts such as Freestyle (Medtronic, Inc., Minneapolis, MN), Prima plus (Edwards Life Sciences,

Irvine, CA) and Toronto Root (St. Jude, Minneapolis, MN) are alternate options for biological root replacement. The most commonly used graft is Freestyle porcine root. This option is recommended in patients older than 65 years with no risk factor for thromboembolic conditions, thus offering them freedom from anticoagulation. Benefits over the tissue valve may include enhanced durability, superior hemodynamics, and less patient prosthesis mismatch. Homografts may be considered for endocarditis and a Ross is an option for very young patients < 40 yo who do not want anticoagulation.

Operative steps

Aortic root replacement

- Wide prep and drape in case the femoral vessels and or right axillary artery are necessary for cannulation. Median sternotomy and pericardial dissection, carefully palpate the aorta for calcifications. The distal ascending aorta at the location free of disease is the preferred access for arterial cannulation. Other option is the axillary or femoral artery. In general a dual stage atriocaval cannula through the right atrial appendage is the preferred method for venous drainage, unless the aortic aneurysm is large enough to preclude the access of the right atrium for cannula placement. In this case the right femoral vein becomes an option for venous cannulation.
- A large aortic aneurysm abutting the sternum, redo aneurysm or evidence of contained rupture are situations where one may consider being on pump through the axillary and femoral vein prior to the sternotomy. A surgeon should be prepared to go on emergency cardiopulmonary bypass by femoral arterial and venous cannulation in a patient who becomes hemodynamically unstable (due to rupture or tamponade).
- Prior to initiating CPB, have the necessary exposure and access for retrograde cardioplegia and cross clamping since a patient with severe AI may very well fibrillate with CPB. Initiate CPB with moderate hypothermia, +/- LV vent through right superior pulmonary vein (RSPV). Cardioplegia is delivered in an antegrade fashion into aortic root if there is no aortic regurgitation or directly into each coronary ostium as well as retrograde cardioplegia into the coronary sinus.
- Ascending aorta is transected 3 to 4 cm above the sinotubular junction. Aortic valve is inspected for possible preservation otherwise leaflets are excised and annulus is debrided if necessary.
- Orientation of right and left coronary arteries and their height above the annulus is noted for coronary reimplantation. The coronary arteries are dissected free from the root with few millimeters of aortic wall as coronaries buttons, and are adequately but carefully

mobilized to allow for tension free implantation into the root graft.

Mechanical composite valve graft (CVG) conduit
- After excising the aortic leaflets and debridement of aortic annulus, mechanical valve sizers are used to choose appropriate CVG. The valve and conduit can also be sewn as separate entities if desired. Pledgeted horizontal mattress non-absorbable sutures are used to implant the valved conduit with the rigid sewing cuff in an intra-annular position. These sutures are placed across the annulus from the aorta to LVOT and then across the sewing ring of CVG. CVG is seated and sutures are tied. Coronary arteries are then reimplanted. A round opening is made in the tube graft using an ophthalmic cautery device. Coronary artery buttons are sutured to the opening with continuous 5-0 prolene sutures starting with the left and finishing with the right coronary implantation without tension or kinking. If the aortic tissue is friable a ring of felt may be used to reinforce the anastomosis.

Bioprosthetic stented composite valved graft (CVG) conduit
- Bioprosthetic valve sizers are used to select the valve required. Usually a tube graft of size 3 to 5 mm larger than the valve is chosen. The hand sewn composite valve graft conduit is then sewn to the annulus using the same technique as described for mechanical CVG conduit implantation.

Valve sparing aortic root replacement
- Aorta is transected just beyond the aneurysmal dilatation. Aortic root is first dissected circumferentially down to the lowest point of aortic annulus. All three aortic sinuses of valsalva are excised, leaving a 5 mm aortic wall rim around the valve leaflets. Multiple interrupted horizontal mattress 2-0 Ticron sutures are placed from inside to outside the LVOT just below the aortic valve. Sutures are placed in a single horizontal plane along the fibrous portion of LVOT and below the nadir of the valve leaflets and commissural structures. Care should be taken to avoid injury to the conduction system in the membranous septum and the number of sutures in this area could be minimized because this is not the haemostatic suture line. A Dacron tube graft with diameter equal to double the average leaflet height is selected. This is typically 26-28 mm for women and 28-30 mm for men. Previously placed sutures through LVOT are passed through the graft and tied on outside of the graft. Sutures are spaced symmetrically along the muscular interventricular septum and correspondingly closer on the Dacron graft in the fibrous portion of LVOT thus correcting the annular dilatation. Fibrous portion of LOVT is the location where dilatation occurs in patients

with connective tissue syndromes. The Dacron graft is trimmed 2-3 cm above the commissures, which are then pulled vertically and suspended to the graft using 4-0 pledgeted mattress prolene sutures. Now the valve, which sits entirely inside the graft, is re-implanted to the graft using 4-0 prolene sutures in running fashion along the residual sinus tissue. Coronary buttons are then reimplanted to their respective sinuses. Aortic cusps are inspected for coaptation and any leaflet prolapse is corrected if necessary. Neoaortic sinuses are created by plicating 2-3 mm of graft material in each sinus at the level of commissure by placing figure of eight 5-0 prolene suture. Alternatively a commercially available graft with the sinuses of valsalva can also be used. Intraoperative aortic valve competence can be evaluated by clamping the distal end of graft and injecting cardioplegia under pressure. Absence of ventricular distension suggests no more than trace aortic insufficiency. Distal anastomosis is then performed to distal ascending aorta.

Stentless aortic root xenograft

- The implantation technique of aortic root xenograft is similar to that described for CVG replacement with few technical considerations. After excising the aortic valve leaflets the size of aortic annulus is measured. The bioprosthesis selected may be of the same size or 2 mm larger than aortic annulus. The coronary anatomy of porcine aortic root differs from the human root as the coronary ostia of porcine root are relatively closer to each other (90-110° apart) compared to humans (120-140° apart). To place the prosthesis in an anatomical position relative to the coronaries it is usually rotated 120° such that the porcine non-coronary sinus will be used for reimplantation of either right or left coronary artery. It is also very critical to attach the left coronary artery perfectly to its corresponding sinus, avoiding any kinking which may result into postoperative coronary insufficiency. The inflow suture cuff of the bioprosthesis is attached to the aortic valve annulus using either continuous or interrupted horizontal mattress sutures. The suture line can be further reinforced with either Teflon felt or strip of autologous pericardium.

- After completion of aortic root replacement using your procedure of choice systemic rewarming is started. The heart is deaired with TEE guidance and a warm shot of cardioplegia is typically given before removing the cross clamp. That final shot of cardioplegia can help detect significant bleeding along suture lines and test for valve competence. The cross clamp is removed, an aortic vent is placed. Temporary pacing wires are placed and the LV vent could be removed if there is no ventricular distension and the cardiac contractility is resumed. Lung ventilation is started.

"You just finished replacing the aortic root and while deairing, you notice > 1 mm ST elevation in the inferior leads (II, III, and AVF). How would you manage that?"

Postoperative coronary insufficiency is the most dreaded complication. Although it is not a common complication after aortic root replacement, it is often caused by the kinking and changes in the orientation of the proximal RCA. This can be prevented by careful sizing with the heart engorged, meticulous technique of coronary implantation and ensuring that coronary ostia are properly aligned. It is suspected in the situation of difficulty in coming off cardiopulmonary bypass, new regional wall motion abnormality, arrhythmias, new EKG changes and unexplained right ventricular failure in the presence of non-obstructed coronaries. This can also be caused by inadequate myocardial protection, coronary air embolism, and protamine or transfusion related reaction. An early decision to bypass the involved artery with the saphenous vein graft is crucial.

"You complete a valve sparing root replacement and discover 3+ AI."

If this occurs you have to be prepared to go back on CPB, arrest the heart, resect the valve and replace with a mechanical or bioprosthetic valve.

"When coming off CPB you notice persistent blood coming from behind the proximal anastomosis."

This can be a serious condition that is difficult to fix. One should anticipate that the etiology is bleeding from the root. The other possibility is bleeding from the LCA suture line. Manipulating the graft and placing sutures posteriorly in a blinded fashion is not advisable. The most prudent course of action is to pack the root with sponges or mild topical agents and wait. Do not give protamine until you have reasonable hemostasis. Eventually remove the packing and check. If it is persistent and the source is not clear then go back on CPB and address. One may even have to re-arrest to adequately achieve hemostasis and potentially replace the root. An alternative in a patient who will not withstand a second cross clamp at that point in time is to pack, give heparin and, if needed, leave the chest open with a planned second look after reversing all coagulation factors. If you need to replace the root, you might consider a homograft or xenograft which may offer better hemostasis for friable tissues.

"How do you follow these patients?"

Blood pressure control and anticoagulation management requires a close postoperative follow up. Scheduling of post-operative CT or MRI is required to assess the growth of non-resected aorta and to evaluate for possible aneurysm formation. CT scan or MRI of the aorta is reasonable at 1, 3, 6, and 12 months and, if stable, annually thereafter so that any threatening enlargement can be detected in a timely fashion.

"How would you manage this patient if he is asymptomatic and aortic root diameter is 3.5 cm?"
There is no medical therapy which will treat the underlying condition resulting into aortic root dilatation or aneurysm. Guidelines for the medical treatment of patients with aortic aneurysms include strict control of hypertension, optimization of lipid profile, smoking cessation, and risk factor modifications for the atherosclerosis.

"What are the Genetic syndromes and familial conditions associated with aortic root aneurysms and how do they affect treatment and management?"
The genetic syndromes associated with aortic root aneurysms are Marfan syndrome, Loeys-Dietz Syndrome, Ehlers-Danlos Syndrome and familial thoracic aortic aneurysm and dissection syndrome. Bicuspid aortic valve patients are also known to have associated aneurysmal disease. Patients with these conditions should undergo elective operation at smaller diameters (4.0 to 5.0 cm depending on the condition) to avoid acute dissection or rupture.

- *Marfan syndrome* – Symptomatic aneurysm, asymptomatic with of diameter > 5.0 cm, Asymptomatic with diameter < 5.0 cm with family history of aortic dissection at < 5.0 cm, rapidly expanding > 0.5 cm/year, Aortic diameter > 4.0 cm in Marfan women desiring pregnancy (Class IIA, Level of evidence C).

- *Loeys-Dietz syndrome* - Aortic diameter ≥ 4.2 cm by transesophageal echocardiogram (internal diameter) or 4.4 to 4.6 cm or greater by computed tomographic imaging and/or magnetic resonance imaging (external diameter), Class IIA, *Level of Evidence: C.*

- *Bicuspid Aortic Valve* - Symptomatic aneurysm, Asymptomatic aneurysm with diameter > 5.0 cm or diameter > 4.5 cm in patients undergoing aortic valve repair or replacement (Class I, level of evidence C).

"You are doing a redo aortic root replacement and you find it very difficult to dissect the tissue around the aortic root especially posteriorly. What are its implications and your options?"
This implies that mobilization of coronary arteries will be difficult or even dangerous. One option is the Cabrol technique which involves coronary reimplantation by placement of 8-10 mm interposition tube graft to each coronary ostium and then side to side anastomosis to the main aortic graft.

Alternate option includes the direct implantation of right coronary button, which is usually easier to mobilize, and reimplantation of left coronary artery using an interposition graft between left coronary ostium and aortic graft (Hemi-Cabrol).

Pearls/pitfalls

- Criteria for surgical intervention includes: sporadic (5.5 to 6.0 cm), connective tissue disorder (4.5 to 5.0 cm), bicuspid aortic valve (5.0 to 5.5 cm).
- When presented with an aortic root aneurysm decide whether it needs to be resected or not.
- Decide what type of root replacement technique is ideal and which one you are the most comfortable describing.
- Make sure the preoperative workup is complete including risk assessment distal aortic imaging and cardiac catheterization.
- Recognize potential complications and solutions of root replacement.

Suggested readings

- Yuh DD, Vricella LA, Baumgartner VA (eds). *The Johns Hopkins Manual of Cardiothoracic Surgery*. 1st ed. New York, NY: McGraw Hill; 2007:585-606.
- Khonsari S, Sintek CF. *Cardiac Surgery: Safeguards and Pitfalls in Operative Technique*. 4th ed.Philadelphia, PA: Lippincott Williams & Wilkins; 2008.
- Franco KL and Thorani VH (eds). *Cardiothoracic Surgery Review*. 1st ed. Philadelphia, PA: Lippincott Williams & Wilkins;2012:315-327.
- Hiratzka LF, Bakris GL, Beckman JA, et al. 2010. ACCF/AHA/AATS/ACR/ASA/SCA/SCAI/SIR/STS/SVM Guidelines for the Diagnosis and Management of Patients with Thoracic Aortic Disease. *J Am Coll Cardiol*. 2010;55:e27-e129.
- Bonow RO, Carabello BA, Chatterjee K, et al. ACC/AHA 2006 Guidelines for the Management of Patients with Valvular Heart Disease: a Report of the American College of Cardiology/American Heart Association Task Force on Practice Guidelines (writing committee to revise the 1998 Guidelines for the Management of Patients With Valvular Heart Disease). *Circulation*. 2006;114:e84-231.

Notes

51. Ascending aortic aneurysm
Leora Yarboro, MD, and John A. Kern, MD

Concept
- Pathophysiology of aortic aneurysms
- Associated genetic syndromes
- Indications for operation
- Preoperative evaluation
- Imaging
- Operative strategy
- Conduit
- Distal anastomosis
- Bicuspid aortic valve disease

Chief complaint
"A 58 yo man presents to clinic for evaluation of incidentally noted ascending aortic aneurysm (5.8 cm) and aortic stenosis."

Differential
In this case there is little else in the differential. However, it is important to personally review the films to confirm the measurements of the aorta as well as the extent of involvement (i.e., root–transverse arch). Obtain any previous studies to determine rate of growth. Rule out chronic dissection.

History and physical
Many patients with ascending aortic aneurysms are asymptomatic. However, in your history be sure to ask about any chest pain, dyspnea, embolic events and ask about commonly associated conditions including: atherosclerosis, bicuspid aortic valve, family history, connective tissue disorders (Marfan's syndrome, Loeys-Dietz, Ehlers-Danlos) and inflammatory conditions. Perform complete cardiovascular, pulmonary, and neurologic exams.

Pathophysiology
Aortic aneurysms can arise in the setting of connective tissue disorders, bicuspid valve disease or in an otherwise normal tri-leaflet valve (degenerative). The natural history of aortic aneurysms is to continue to dilate over time due to forces imposed in accordance with the Law of Laplace Tension = Pressure x Radius. Although some aneurysms stay remarkably stable over time. Risk of rupture and dissection are directly related to the diameter of the aneurysm with significant increase in mortality for ascending aneurysms > 6 cm.

Connective tissue disorders
Recommendations are covered under Chapter 50, Aortic root aneurysm, but here are a few additional details:

Patients with connective tissue disorders typically present at a younger age and have higher risk of rupture at smaller diameters. Most centers recommend surgical intervention for ascending aortic aneurysm associated with connective tissue disorders at 4.5-5.0 cm.

- *Marfan's syndrome*
    - Autosomal dominant, prevalence 1/5000, mutation in gene on chromosome 15 encodes fibrillin-1. Phenotype is highly variable. Major diagnostic criteria include: positive family history of Marfan's, pectus excavatum and/or arm span - height ratio > 1.05. Mitral insufficiency can also be associated with Marfan's syndrome. Without surgery most patients with Marfan's die in their third decade from complications of aortic root aneurysm. There is data to suggest that patients with Marfan's syndrome should be on beta-blockers and angiotensin receptor blockers to reduce the rate of growth of aneurysms.
- *Loeys-Dietz*
    - Mutation in TGF-B receptor. Patients may have hypertelorism, bifid uvula, and arterial tortuosity. Dissection can occur in children. May consider surgery for adults if aortic root > 4.4 cm (by CT) or descending thoracic aorta > 5 cm. For children, consider surgery when aortic root z-score is > 3 or expansion greater than 0.5 cm/yr.
- *Ehlers-Danlos syndrome*
    - Autosomal inherited disorder of connective tissue COL3a1 gene encodes Type III collagen. Present with arterial or visceral rupture. Any surgery in this population carries increased risk—as such no formal guidelines exist for operative intervention.

Degenerative (sporadic) ascending aortic aneurysms
Occur in the setting of tri-leaflet aortic valve in patients without connective tissue disorders. May be associated with family history, hypertension, smoking and/or atherosclerosis. Aneurysms tend to grow at a rate of 0.1 cm/yr. Serial imaging is important in this population either with echo or CT scan. Growth rate > 1 cm/year or diameter > 5.5 cm in a patient with acceptable surgical risk is an indication for surgery.

Infectious/inflammatory aortic aneurysms
Syphilis destroys muscular and elastic fibers of media. Once commonly associated with ascending aneurysms, now less prevalent since improved antibiotic therapy.

Aneurysms associated with aortic dissection
Patients with previous dissection may have continued dilation of the ascending aorta. There is a faster growth rate and associated rate of rupture when compared to degenerative aneurysms.

Tests
- *Contrasted CT scan or MRA*: to evaluate the extent of the aneurysm including the carotids. You should know preoperatively whether a root or arch replacement is necessary. The CT scan should include abdomen and pelvis if femoral cannulation is considered. Carefully evaluate CT or MRA to see if aneurysm is abutting the sternum. This may increase risk of rupture during sternotomy.
- *Echocardiogram*: is also important in preoperative evaluation with special attention to valve disease and overall cardiac function. This study is limited and may be used to follow root aneurysms but should not be the sole study for operative planning for an ascending aneurysm.
- *Cardiac catheterization*: to evaluate coronary vessel disease .
- *Pulmonary function tests (PFTs)*. Aneurysmal disease is more common in smokers with COPD. PFTs are not always essential but may help to determine perioperative risk.
- *Labs*: CBC, CHEM, Coagulations studies, Type and cross.

Index scenario (additional information)
"The patient has no family history of aneurysmal disease. He has no symptoms. His CT shows an isolated mid ascending aneurysm with no effacement of the sinotubular junction. The aneurysm tapers down to 4 cm proximal to the innominate artery. The AV mean gradient is 45 mmHg."

Treatment/management
If the patient meets criteria for intervention, a thorough preoperative assessment is warranted. This patient needs an aortic valve replacement and ascending repair above the sinotubular junction. Imaging and preoperative assessment should proceed as discussed above. The patients systolic blood pressure should be kept between 90 and 110 mmHg.

Operative steps

The procedural steps will vary depending on the extent of the aneurysm and whether or not the aortic valve needs to be replaced.

Normal aortic valve, no root or arch involvement

- *Perioperative monitors.* PA catheter, cerebral oximetry, Foley catheter with temperature probe, transesophageal echo, and arterial line.
- *Cannulation.* Central cannulation can be used for an isolated ascending aortic aneurysm as long as there is enough room to cannulate and clamp beyond the dilated portion. This is usually accomplished with a high cannulation in the arch. These purse strings need to be very secure. Consider pledgeted purse strings. An alternative is to axillary cannulate.
- *Cardioprotection.* Antegrade and retrograde cardioplegia lines are placed as well as a left ventricular vent. A left ventricular vent can be omitted if there is no significant aortic insufficiency (be able to describe alternate methods of decompressing the left ventricle in the case of fibrillation). Cool to 34° C.
- *Dissection.* Transect ascending aortic aneurysm at midpoint. Extend proximally leaving enough room to safely do the anastomosis above the coronary ostia. Distally leave a rim of aorta to sew to before the clamp.
- *Graft.* Impregnated Dacron graft and 4-0 prolene suture to perform anastomosis. Felt may be used to reinforce aorta if tissue is felt to be of poor quality or connective tissue disorder. Remember not to leave the graft too long as it may kink when the heart fills. Perform the distal anastomosis first with running 4-0 prolene suture. Then you may clamp the graft and check the back side for hemostasis. Then pack and perform the proximal anastomosis in a running fashion. Place root vent in the graft prior to cross clamp removal and turn off vents while performing the distal anastomosis to aid in deairing.
- Postoperatively maintain tight blood pressure control. Discharge on beta-blocker, ARB and statin.

Expected outcomes

- Known complications from aortic surgery include bleeding (2.4-11% requiring reoperation) neurologic injury (1.9-5%). Reports of perioperative mortality range from 1.7%-17.1%.

Potential questions/alternative scenarios

"Not enough room to cannulate and cross clamp distally."
Plan for axillary or femoral cannulation. If still not able to clamp with adequate sewing cuff then may need circulatory arrest (see Chapter 52, Arch aneurysms).

"Graft is kinked when heart fills."
It can be easy to overestimate the amount of graft necessary. You can try to plicate the graft along the lesser curve. You may need to cross clamp and arrest the heart in order to remove a portion of the graft and sew graft to graft.

"Aortic dissection occurs with cannulation."
Potential complication of untreated aneurysms and can occur during cannulation of the aneurysm. Be prepared to discuss alternate cannulation strategies, cooling protocols and repair (see Chapter 47, Iatrogenic aortic dissection).

"Patient has left ventricular distension once commencing bypass."
Significant aortic insufficiency may be present. You should have a sense that this may happen preoperatively. Be prepared to clamp and arrest the heart with retrograde. In the acute setting if you do not yet have an antegrade vent in place, you can decompress the heart by transecting the aorta. You can then deliver direct coronary cardioplegia. You can also decompress the heart via an LV vent if you have one in place. If the valve is not competent it should be replaced.

"Patient has a bicuspid aortic valve with mean gradient of 48 mmHg, shortness of breath and a 4.7 cm ascending aneurysm."
Bicuspid aortic valve disease occurs in 1-2% of the population. Males 4:1. Most have 3 sinuses and 2 cusps (fusion of the right and left cusps). Dominant circumflex circulation with small right coronary. At risk for premature degenerative changes in the media of aortic root and ascending aorta. Consider ascending aorta replacement if performing aortic valve replacement in bicuspid aortic valve and ascending aorta > 4.5 cm.

"The aorta ruptures during the median sternotomy."
For a presumed rupture you need to ensure you have sufficient help available in the room. Place towel clamps to close the sternum. Ask anesthesia to get PRBC in the room. Let perfusion know of impending need for cannulation. Do not try and fix or dissect out the rupture at this time since this will only make the tear worse. For the most part, towel clamps on the sternum can provide reasonable tamponade. Dissect out the femoral artery, give heparin, place your retractor attempt to tamponade the ruptured area if possible with manual compression while

you gain venous access by direct puncture and cannulation of the right atrium. Place a basket sucker in the field for drainage into the CPB reservoir. Start cooling in the event you need circulatory arrest. Once you are stable on bypass try to clamp the aorta above the rupture and arrest the heart. Now continue with your resection and repair. Place your retrograde coronary sinus cannula and LV vent if needed. Note that for aneurysms that are at risk of rupture or closely abutting the sternum it may be best to perform your sternotomy with the heart on bypass through the axillary and groin. If there is a very high chance of entering the vessel you might even cool to 18° C for circulatory arrest if needed prior to sternotomy.

Pearls/pitfalls
- Surgical intervention for ascending aneurysm > 5.5 cm diameter.
- Consider surgery for ascending aneurysm > 5 cm in patients with bicuspid aortic valve or 4.5 cm for connective tissue disorder.
- Aneurysms tend to grow at a rate of 0.1 cm/year. Growth rate > 0.5 cm/year or diameter > 5.5 cm in a patient with acceptable surgical risk is an indication for surgery.
- Make sure to look for root or arch involvement prior to surgery.

Suggested readings
- Elefteriades JA. Natural history of thoracic aortic aneurysms: indications for surgery, and surgical versus nonsurgical risks. *Ann Thorac Surg.* 2002 Nov;74(5):S1877-80.

Notes

52. Aortic arch aneurysm

John F. Lazar, MD, and Peter A. Knight, MD

Concept
- Indications
- Preoperative assessment
- Operative management (hemiarch/total arch/elephant trunk)
- Circulatory arrest
- Brain protection options
- Chronic dissection

Chief complaint
"A 57 yo man with known aortic diastolic murmur presents to your clinic after complaining to his PCP that he has increased shortness of breath. After a full work up, including chest CT and an echo he is found to have moderate aortic insufficiency and an ascending aortic aneurysm extending to the proximal arch of 5.5 cm in size."

Differential
Aortic insufficiency with ascending/arch aneurysm, aortic dissection, coronary artery disease.

History and physical
Most patients with aortic aneurysms are asymptomatic and are discovered incidentally. Of those who present with symptoms, 25-75% present with chest pain (usually anterior chest). Acute pain generally implies impending rupture or dissection. Hoarseness of the voice implies stretching or damage to the recurrent laryngeal nerve. Risk factors include smoking, hypertension, atherosclerosis, personal history of chronic aneurysms or previous repair, bicuspid aortic valves, trauma, and genetic disorders such as Marfan and Ehlers-Danlos syndromes. The physical exam is often unremarkable. A diastolic murmur will be heard if dilation of aortic annulus results in AI.

If a thoracic aneurysm is diagnosed, a thorough vascular examination should follow looking for any peripheral vascular disease, carotid disease, and sequelae of distal embolization. It is also important to document a thorough neurologic exam to establish baseline clinical status in the event of changes postoperatively. Abdominal aortic aneurysms are present in 10 to 20% of patients with atherosclerotic involvement of an ascending aortic aneurysm.

Tests

- *EKG*: may be completely normal; if AI is present may have LV enlargement; assess for ischemic coronary changes.
- *CXR*: may be the first test to detect a silent aneurysm. An enlarged ascending aorta produces a convex contour of right superior mediastinum.
- *CTA*: is the test of choice for assessing the aortic aneurysm and provides rapid and precise evaluation of the root, ascending and arch. CT scanning detects areas of calcification, and accurately identifies dissections and mural thrombus. Axial measurements should be taken perpendicular to the line of flow. The entire thoracic and abdominal aorta should be scanned. The main disadvantage of CT scans is the need for contrast solution for optimal resolution, which may be contraindicated in those patients with renal insufficiency or a history of a dye allergy.
- *MRI/MRA*: effective means of assessing the aorta but is more suitable for those who cannot tolerate CTA dye and in a non-urgent setting.
- *ECHO*. TTE is good for evaluating the valves and ascending aorta but gives little information on the arch. Echo can also be used to corroborate aortic dimensions found by either CTA or MRI/MRA. TEE is done in the operating room and can help rule out Type A dissections.
- *Cardiac catheterization*. Rule out coronary artery disease in patients undergoing aneurysm repair prior to surgery. May be omitted safely in females of age < 35 and males < 40 with no cardiac risk factors.

Index scenario (additional information)

"Patient has no past medical or surgical history. He takes no medications. He used to smoke a pack a day for 20 years but quit 7 years ago. His father died suddenly in his 50's from a ruptured aneurysm but the rest of his family is still alive and well. Other than being overweight and having a 3/6 diastolic murmur in the right parasternal position his physical exam is completely benign. The aneurysm extends into the proximal arch but tapers to normal size by mid-distal arch. The root is not dilated. The echo shows normal function, 3+ AI and a normal root. How would you like to proceed?"

Treatment/management

This patient has symptomatic AI which requires intervention as well as a 5.5 cm uncomplicated ascending/arch aneurysm that requires repair. In general, 5.5 cm is a safe cutoff for interventions on the arch. 5 cm is the threshold for Marfans, Ehlers-Danlos or bicuspid aortic valve, while even lower thresholds may be used for Loeys-Dietz (4.5 cm). Symptomatic aneurysms of any size require surgical intervention. Asymptomatic aneurysms should be addressed at the time of surgery for aortic valve procedures if the size is at least 4.5 cm and the patient is a reasonably good candidate. Finally, a growth rate of > 0.5 cm/yr justifies repair in asymptomatic patients with aneurysms less than 5.5 cm.

Additional preoperative testing
- Patients with poor pulmonary function should have spirometry and room air arterial blood gases.
- Smoking cessation, antibiotic treatment of chronic bronchitis, and chest physiotherapy may prove beneficial in elective situations.
- Severe carotid disease is a risk factor for stroke during aortic operations. Patients > 65 should have duplex imaging of their carotids pre-operatively or any patient with h/o TIA or bruits.
- Abdominal aortic aneurysms occur in 10 to 20% of patients with ascending aortic aneurysms and should be investigated.
- Head CT to ensure an intact Circle of Willis.

Operative steps
There are a few different ways to approach aortic arch aneurysm repairs. The main decision is whether to perform a hemiarch, total arch or elephant trunk. This decision depends almost exclusively on the distal extent of the aneurysm. Usually you can be well prepared for either intervention ahead of time based on the CT scan but things may get altered in the OR. All of these cases require circulatory arrest. Right axillary cannulation is safe for all of these. Retrograde brain perfusion through the SVC is reasonable for an uncomplicated hemiarch but the more advanced the procedure becomes the more likely that antegrade brain protection will be needed. The operative details that follow all assume axillary artery cannulation with antegrade brain perfusion (see below for details of circulatory arrest).
- Left brachial IV, arterial line in left arm and leg, general endotracheal anesthesia, pulmonary artery catheter, foley.
- Temp probe in the bladder, nasopharynx and venous perfusate.
- *Brain monitoring*: EEG, Bispectral index (BIS).
- Check the intraoperative TEE for AI and aortic dimensions.
- Dissect right axillary artery (or right femoral artery for arterial cannulation).
- Median sternotomy, pericardial stay sutures, inspect aorta.
- Heparin 400 mg/kg, arterial cannulation, 2 stage venous cannula or bicaval if retrograde brain perfusion, retrograde coronary cannula; once ACT is 480 initiate CPB, +/-LV vent through right superior pulmonary vein.

- Commence cooling while you mobilize the distal ascending aorta and proximal arch and dissect out the great vessels.
- Clamp and arrest with antegrade/retro/direct coronary.
- Once the patient is at 18-20° C and the EEG is silent, give a dose of cardioplegia, position the patient in Trendelenburg and pack the head in ice. +/- pentobarbital and mannitol given.
- CPB is turned off.

Hemiarch

- The aorta is transected longitudinally along the ascending aneurysm and inspected proximally and distally.
- Ascending aorta is transected along the lesser curve to create a cuff extending from the base of the innominate artery on the right to approximately mid arch or 1 cm proximal to the ligamentum arteriosum and the recurrent laryngeal nerve. The further you transect the more difficult the anastomosis becomes.
- Clamp the right innominate and initiate antegrade brain perfusion at 500 mL/min (or 10-15 cc/kg) with a mean pressure of 40-60 mmHg. Check for backflow through the LCCA. If not then place a coronary perfusion catheter up the LCCA and Y it into the antegrade perfusion circuit at a similar flow rate.
- Size the aorta with freestyle sizers to determine the aortic graft diameter required.
- The distal graft is beveled and anastomosed to the aorta with a continuous 3-0 or 4-0 polypropylene suture (a cuff of Teflon felt or strip of pericardium can be used outside the aorta for friable tissue).
- Once the anastomosis is complete, remove the clamp on the right innominate, gradually resume systemic flow while deairing the graft, clamp the graft and check the back wall carefully for hemostasis.
- Begin rewarming at approximately 1° C/5 min until 36° C.
- This completes the hemiarch—the remainder of the procedure is dictated by the proximal pathology.

Total arch

- Indicated when the aneurysm extends into the mid arch. Need to decide if head vessels are aneurysmal and need reconstruction. If not, the head vessels can be fashioned to the graft as an island.
- While cooling dissect out the arch and head vessels (may need an expanding incision into the neck). Prepare the appropriate graft. The limbs to the innominate and head vessels/LSCA are typically 12 and 8 mm respectively. Trifurcated grafts are available, or any combination of bifurcated or single limb grafts can be sewn individually to the respective vessels.

- Once the circulation is arrested, transect the proximal arch vessels and the aorta along the lesser curve up to the level of the distal arch which is often beyond the LSCA. Clamp the LCCA if too much blood return obscures your view. Note that if the LSCA is too deep in the chest for a feasible anastomosis it can be ligated. The distal anastomosis can then be done proximal to the LSCA which can be bypassed at a future date or off pump at the end of the case, prior to protamine.
- Usually a bifurcated graft to the R innominate and the LCCA is sewn first and then clamped to allow antegrade brain flow through both head vessels. If reimplanting the LSCA it is sewn next. Then the distal anastomosis and finally the appropriate graft to graft anastomoses. Trifurcated grafts may decrease the number of anastomoses. Whatever the method, stick to what you know best.
- Note that if the proximal arch vessels can be preserved then you may be able to sew them into the graft collectively as an island.
- Deair, clamp the graft, resume systemic flow and complete your proximal work or proximal anastomosis. A graft extension may be required to avoid kinking if an ascending is being performed as well.

Elephant trunk
- Indicated for distal arch or isthmus involvement.
- Follow the same steps as in the total arch except instead of an end-to-end anastomosis between the distal aorta and distal graft the distal 5-10 cm of the graft needs to be invaginated within the aorta and then sutured into place.
- On completion of the suture line, the graft is everted, and the head vessels are sewn into the graft with a running prolene as an island.
- The graft is de-aired, clamped and hemostasis is assessed. The proximal work is completed.
- The trunk can later be incorporated into the reconstruction of the descending aorta either by open or endovascular techniques.

Circulatory arrest
- At 18° C cerebral metabolism and oxygen consumption are 17 to 40% of normothermia. Measure temperatures at the bladder, nasopharyngeal and venous perfusate. Monitor brain with EEG or BIS. Most investigators report increased mortality and adverse neurologic outcomes after 40 to 65 minutes of circulatory arrest. Most surgeons try to keep the period of arrest at less than 40 minutes if the operation allows. Consider antegrade brain perfusion for procedures lasting > 30 minute.

Brain protection options
- Antegrade brain perfusion: Line pressure is monitored. The head vessels are collectively perfused with cold blood between 10-18° C and at approximate flows of 10-15 mL/kg/min. Perfusion pressures are restricted to 40 to 60 mmHg which can be difficult to monitor unless you have a left radial arterial line. Most go off of either weight based flows or a flat rate of 500 mL/min.
- Retrograde brain perfusion (RBP): During RBP the SVC is snared and perfused at blood pressures not exceeding 25-30 mmHg that is monitored via CVP, temperatures between 8 and 18°C, and flows between 250 and 400 mL/min. In theory RBP has the added benefit of flushing atherosclerotic material and air from the brachiocephalic vessels while keeping the brain cool.

Potential questions/alternative scenarios

"A stable patient with occasional chest pain is referred to you for evaluation of a chronic Type I dissection with a 5.7 cm aneurysm involving the ascending and proximal arch."

This patient has a symptomatic dissection and aneurysmal disease both of which require treatment. The operation proceeds very much like that of a Type A dissection with circulatory arrest and an open distal anastomosis. In this case the aneurysm involves the proximal arch and thus requires a hemiarch configuration as described above. If the aneurysm proceeded more distally, a total arch or even elephant trunk may be necessary. The only technical difference in the setting of dissected head vessels is that these vessels must be anastomosed directly in an end-end fashion to the tube graft limbs rather than an island for a total arch or elephant trunk. Also the chronic dissection flaps should be fenestrated or resected as far as possible.

"On the preoperative imaging you notice an aberrant left vertebral artery on a patient who was being worked up for a total arch replacement due to an isolated arch aneurysm."

On occasion the left vertebral artery (LVA) will exit the arch directly. This requires duplex US evaluation of the right vertebral artery (RVA) to ensure patency and antegrade flow. With a patent normal RVA, the LVA can be temporarily occluded during selective brain perfusion and reimplanted during patient rewarming. Three options have been used: 1) direct reimplantation of the LVA into the left common carotid artery 2) attachment of a portion of reverse saphenous vein to the vertebral artery 3) anastomosis to the arch graft or the left subclavian limb of the trifurcated graft. A very small LVA (< 2 mm) with a patent RVA may be ligated.

"You are called to evaluate a patient with a known arch and descending aneurysm who is complaining of excruciating chest pain. Workup for MI is negative and there is no evidence of dissection. However, there is some periaortic density concerning for a contained early rupture."

The issue here is that an elephant trunk would normally be the ideal procedure for this patient but it does not allow for a distal seal until the completion elephant trunk is performed. This patient is in need of a complete procedure involving the arch and descending thoracic aorta. A hemi-clamshell incision or "thoracosternotomy" extended into left 4th ICS allows adequate exposure for both the standard cannulation techniques and the distal repair. An elephant trunk-like strategy can still be used with the graft invaginated through the isthmus and anastomosed distally to the descending aorta. The head vessels would be sewn as an island unless they were aneurysmal.

"You are presented with an 86 yo relatively healthy female with a 6.5 cm ascending aneurysm which tapers to 4.5 cm at the proximal arch. She has no familial genetic syndromes."

Elderly patients do not tolerate circulatory arrest as well as their younger counterparts. They have a higher risk of stroke and heart failure. The 4.5 cm proximal arch does not necessarily have to be addressed in this setting. The arterial cannula can be placed high on the arch with carefully placed pledgeted cannulation sutures and the clamp can be beveled proximal to the cannula and along the lesser curve. Alternatively, the axillary can be cannulated if it proves too hazardous to cannulate high on the arch. An isolated ascending replacement can then be performed without circulatory arrest.

Pearls/pitfalls

- Clarify whether the patient does or does not have an indication for repair of the aneurysm.
- Clarify the location and extent and decide whether it needs a hemiarch, total arch, or elephant trunk.
- Consider whether a hemiclamshell is needed to definitively address the arch and descending in a single setting (usually only in the case of rupture).
- Decide on your cannulation strategy and brain protection strategy.
- Know the sequence of arch anastomosis depending the type of graft you are using. Also know the sequence of de-airing and removal of clamps.

Suggested readings

- Brinster DR, Rizzo RJ, and Bolman RM. Ascending aortic aneurysms. Cohn LH (ed). Cardiac Surgery in the Adult. New York: McGraw-Hill Medical. 2008:1223-1250.
- Spielvogel D, Mathur MN, and Griepp RB. Aneurysms of the aortic arch. Cohn LH (ed). Cardiac Surgery in the Adult. New York: McGraw-Hill Medical. 2008:1251-1276.
- Caffarelli AD, Van der Starre PJ, and Mitchell RS. Ascending and arch aneurysms of the aorta. Yu DD et al. (eds). The Johns Hopkins Manual of Cardiothoracic Surgery. New York: McGraw-Hill Medical Pub. 2007:663-700.

Notes

53. Descending aortic aneurysm

David Griffin, MD, and Stephen Bailey, MD

Concept
- Pathophysiology/classification (isolated descending vs. thoracoabdominal)
- Indications for repair
- Open versus endovascular approaches
- Considerations for thoracoabdominal aneurysms
- Outcomes
- Pitfalls

Chief complaint

"A 75 yo woman with a history of hypertension, Chronic Obstructive Pulmonary Disease (COPD) and Marfan's disease is referred to you after her primary care physician obtained a CXR during a recent COPD exacerbation and found a enlarged descending aorta. After recovering from her COPD exacerbation, she is referred to you for evaluation and further management if warranted."

Differential

Type I or B Dissection (acute/chronic) with associated aneurysm, thoracic or thoracoabdominal aortic aneurysm, mediastinal mass

History and physical

Approximately 50% of descending aortic aneurysms (DAA) are found incidentally. Most common symptoms attributed to DAA are pain from expansion or erosion into the spine. Pain is described as sharp or stabbing usually between the scapulae. Acute severe pain may signal dissection or rupture. Enlargement may cause compression of the mediastinal structures causing hoarseness (recurrent laryngeal nerve impingement), dyspnea (airway obstruction) or dysphagia (esophageal compression). Occasionally, evidence of distal embolization such as trash foot may be present. Pathophysiology is generally related to degenerative disease of the media or prior Type B dissection. Less commonly, infections or connective tissue disorders (particularly in young patients or those with a family history of Marfan's, Ehlers-Danlos or Loeys-Dietz syndromes) may also result in aneurysmal degeneration of the descending aorta.

Always perform a complete history and physical exam focusing on potential symptoms such as pain or evidence of malperfusion, risk factors including hypertension, tobacco abuse, steroid use as well as personal history of aortic dissection or family history of connective tissue disease or aortic problems. Evaluation should also include an ocular exam of the

413

sclera and lens as well as arachnodactyly or other stigmata of Marfan's, particularly in young patients as well as a detailed neurologic exam in the event there are postoperative neurologic complications. It is also important to perform a complete examination of radial and femoral pulses for symmetry. Also assess operative risk (history of diabetes, renal disease, pulmonary and cardiac complications, heart and lung exam, extremities).

Tests

The justification for these imaging modalities are discussed under other chapters devoted to aneurysmal disease. Essentially you are clarifying the anatomical features of the aneurysm, determining other cardiovascular problems that may be surgical (valves, coronaries) and risk stratifying.

- CTA chest/abdomen/pelvis
- Labs
- Carotid duplex
- EKG/echocardiography/left heart catheterization
- PFTs

Index scenario (additional information)

"A careful history and physical reveals no evidence of pain, malperfusion or distal embolization. She is not on oxygen or steroids currently for her COPD. She has not smoked for several years but has a 60 pack year history. Her PFTs show a mild obstructive defect but her DLCO is preserved. She has no symptoms to suggest myocardial ischemia. She is on a low dose ACE inhibitor for her hypertension. You obtained a CTA which demonstrates a 6.5 cm fusiform descending aneurysm. It begins 3 cm distal to the left subclavian artery (LSCA) and tapers down to normal size by about 4 cm above the aortic hiatus. How would you proceed with managing this patient?"

Treatment/management

Isolated DAAs occur between the takeoff of the LSCA and the aortic hiatus/suprarenal aorta. This is different than a thoracoabdominal aneurysm (TAA) which by definition extends to the abdominal aorta at least to or near the level of the celiac artery. Management for both entities depends on whether the aneurysm is symptomatic, rapidly enlarging or meets established size criteria for intervention. Symptomatic aneurysms require urgent or emergency repair by endovascular means if possible or open repair.

Asymptomatic aneurysms should undergo elective open repair when the size is > 5.5 cm in the setting of chronic dissections or connective tissue disorders. Endovascular repair is recommended for patients with comorbidities and an isolated descending > 5.5 cm (class IIa - AHA/ACC). Endovascular repair is given a class IIb recommendation in the setting of a descending aneurysm > 5.5 cm without comorbidities. Thus, do the procedure you are most comfortable with in these patients. Asymptomatic DAA or TAA should be stented or repaired if the growth is more than 0.5-1 cm/year. Note that the threshold for intervening on asymptomatic TAA is slightly higher than DAA (6.0 cm - stent if possible, open repair if not). This threshold may be lower for connective tissue disorders, dissections, saccular aneurysms, contained ruptures etc. Expectant management includes blood pressure control and smoking cessation which may slow progression. Patients not yet undergoing repair should be followed with serial imaging. Initially, every 3-6 months and then yearly to document stability or progression.

Elective repair in appropriate candidates should be undertaken following evaluation of cardiopulmonary function and operative risk. In this patient COPD exacerbations place her at increased risk of respiratory complications and should be discussed with the patient. Either operative or endovascular repairs are reasonable options here but given her pulmonary issues a stent graft would be ideal. In general, DAA are treated with open repair if the anatomy is not favorable for stenting, in the setting of connective tissue disease, and in chronic dissections.

Operative steps
Open repair of isolated DAA
- Spinal drainage is placed by anesthesia usually the day prior to surgery. The patient is positioned in a well padded right lateral decubitus with the hips flexed back to expose the femorals.
- Single lung ventilation of the right lung is established.
- radial and femoral a-lines. The radial tells you the pressure generated by the heart's contraction on partial bypass while the femorals tell you the pressure generated by the pump. You want to keep similar pressures or slightly higher on the upper extremities. This governs how much you can empty with the left atrial cannula.
- Left posterolateral thoracotomy through the 4th, 5th, or 6th interspace is made. The exact interspace for entry is determined by the location of the aneurysm. A rib below or above may be partially resected to improve exposure to the aneurysm.
- The inferior pulmonary ligament is divided and the lung retracted medially.
- *Proximal control.* The distal arch and left subclavian are identified and dissected proximally. The vagus, recurrent and phrenic nerves are identified and preserved. Tacking sutures on the soft tissue can help to reflect the nerves gently out of the operative field. The

ductus remnant is divided if needed. The vagus nerve may be ligated distally to prevent traction injuries to the recurrent branch if absolutely needed.

- *Distal control.* The distal extent is identified. The descending aorta is dissected free taking care to avoid the thoracic duct and esophagus.
- It is most convenient to cannulate the left inferior pulmonary vein for inflow (i.e., venous drainage) and the descending aorta below the aneurysm for distal perfusion (i.e., outflow). The left atrial appendage and the left femoral artery are also acceptable for cannulation. Left heart bypass (LHB) with moderate hypothermia (32° C) is begun after systemic heparinization (150 U/kg Heparin).
- *Proximal anastomosis.* Ideally the cross clamp is placed distal to the takeoff of the left subclavian artery. A second clamp is placed a few centimeters distal to the first. The aorta is opened between the clamps and the proximal anastamosis is fashioned with a running prolene suture and properly sized graft. Teflon reinforcement can be used if needed. The proximal clamp is moved onto the graft and hemostasis of the suture line is achieved.
- *Intercostal ligation/reimplantation (30-60 min).* Clamp the distal descending aorta. Resect the throacic aneurysm longitudinally. Any upper thoracic intercostal branches (above T8) are suture ligated from within the aorta (this can be done after the graft is completed). More distal branches are incorporated into the proximal graft as a patch with running prolene to improve spinal cord protection. The proximal clamp is now replaced on the graft distal to the patch to check for hemostasis.
- *Distal anastomosis.* The distal anastomosis is fashioned with a running prolene, clamps are removed and hemostasis is ensured. Chest tubes are placed, cannulas are removed and heparin is reversed.
- *Alternative sequence.* There are different ways to do this procedure and do what is most comfortable. An alternative and efficient method is to clamp proximally and distally, make the longitudinal cut along the aneurysmal aorta but bevel the distal end of the aorta proximal to the distal clamp in such a way as to preserve the intercostal arteries below T8. Bevel the distal graft accordingly and perform the distal anastomosis such that it incorporates the distal lumen and all the distal intercostals in one beveled anastomosis. Now clamp the graft, reperfusing the intercostals, check hemostasis and sew the proximal.

"A 75 yo woman with a history of COPD, diabetes and malnutrition presents with an isolated asymptomatic descending aortic aneurysm 6.0 cm in diameter. She has no history of dissection or connective tissue disorder."

Endovascular repair

- Appropriate candidates are screened with a CTA to evaluate potential access sites, the tortuosity and calcification of the vascular system and the relationship of the aneurysm to the arch vessels.
- A lumbar drain is placed and then vascular access is obtained either through the groin or a retroperitoneal approach (you need at least an 8 mm femoral vessel).
- Otherwise, a chimney graft may be required for safe access. A guidewire is advanced into the distal arch using fluoroscopy.
- The aneurysm is measured using fluoroscopy and then one of several commercially available stent grafts is deployed according to manufacturer instructions.
- A landing zone of at least 20 mm of uninvolved and healthy aorta is needed on either end of the graft to reduce the risk of a Type I endoleak.
- The left subclavian artery may be covered in the proximal landing zone (zone 2) and may require revascularization with a carotid to subclavian bypass should collateral flow be inadequate.
- The graft is typically oversized by 10-20% to ensure a tight seal.
- A completion angiogram is then obtained.
- Balloon aortoplasty or extension grafts are applied as needed.

"A 68 yo male with h/o HTN and an MI in the past presents with a 7 cm aneurysm beginning distal to the LSCA and extending to the infrarenal abdominal aorta."

This represents a Crawford Type II thoracoabdominal aneurysm (I - proximal descending to proximal abdominal, II - proximal descending to distal abdominal, III - distal descending to proximal abdominal, IV - distal descending to distal abdominal). These almost always require surgical intervention as described above with a few modifications:

- *Incision*: posterolateral thoracotomy exposure extending inferiorly towards the umbilicus. The 4th ICS is entered, the 5th rib is removed and the 6th rib can be shingled. Again, the exact incision is adjusted to the proximal and distal extent of the aneurysm. The retroperitoneum is entered through the abdominal incision and the costal margin is divided. The diaphragm is incised circumferentially leaving a 2 cm cuff along the chest wall. Now the retroperitoneum and left chest are one cavity. An Omni or Bookwalter retractor stabilizes the exposure. The aorta and involved visceral and intercostal branches are identified and dissected carefully. Do not dissect behind the aorta if you can avoid it until you have proximal and distal control and are ready to initiate bypass.

- LHB is initiated, proximal and intercostal reimplantation proceeds as described above.
- *Visceral reimplantation*: the distal aortic clamp is moved to just above the renals and the celiac is reimplanted to the proximal graft. After deairing, the graft is clamped distal to the new anastomosis and hemostasis is addressed. The distal clamp is then placed below the SMA and renal arteries, which are reimplanted to the graft. There are a variety of ways to reimplant the visceral vessels as well as a variety of grafts that can be used. Be prepared to describe the method that works best for you.
- *Distal anastomosis.* Now replace the clamp on the infrarenal aorta and perform the final anastomosis.

"A similar patient with a Type II thoracoabdominal aorta presents with a ruptured aneurysm."

Aggressive up front resuscitation. Unlikely to have time for spinal drain (can be placed postoperatively). Simplest and most versatile bypass strategy will be femoral venous and arterial (fem-fem). All steps as discussed above with an emphasis on gaining immediate proximal and distal control with cross clamps. In this emergency scenario you do not have to replace the entire distal aorta if there is a reasonably normal appearing distal to sew to. The patient can return for a followup operation if they survive. If the rupture is in the abdominal aorta then it may suffice to start with the abdominal exposure as you would for a AAA and clamp the supraceliac aorta. If the aorta is too aneurysmal in this area then extend the exposure to the left chest through the costal margin.

"Postoperatively the patient is unable to move his legs."

Differential includes ischemic injury from the clamp period, embolic disease, spinal hematoma, or central stroke. Ischemic injury - Need to optimize spinal cord perfusion. Check to make sure the spinal drain is working well and is draining to keep the CSF pressure no greater than 8 mmHg. Improve the systemic MAP to > 80 mmHg. Avoid hypotensive episodes. Risk of paralysis is greatest after 30 minutes of cross clamping during "cut and sew procedures" using moderate hypothermia. LHB reduces the risk of spinal cord ischemia. Reimplantation of intercostal arteries below T8 seems to reduce the risk of paraplegia but still a safe window for ischemic time is 30-60 minutes. Spinal hematoma/central stroke - check head CT and MRI of the spinal cord if feasible. To rule out embolic disease as a culprit check the distal pulses. If they are full then emboli is unlikely to account for this amount of paresis.

"Postoperatively the patient has a bloody bowel movement."
Differential includes ischemia reperfusion injury to the bowel after mesenteric vessels were reimplanted. 30-60 min window is a safe time frame for clamping and re-implanting the visceral vessels. Prior to this the visceral circulation is supported by LHB and distal femoral perfusion. Embolic disease - showering to the mesenteric vessels may also result in ischemia. Obtain an emergency general surgery consult. Antibiotics and optimize forward flow. Colonoscopy and possibly exploratory laparotomy if transmural necrosis is suspected.

"Postoperatively the patient stops making urine and her creatinine triples."
If the renal vessels are reimplanted then a 30-60 min ischemic time frame with LHB support is reasonable. You should make an attempt to clamp above the renals when reimplanting the celiac if possible although it may be necessary to implant them collectively as a patch. Individual renal perfusion catheters can be used as well. Optimize the patients forward flow in the ICU. If the CVP is optimized and the patient is still oliguric it may ultimately be necessary to challenge the patient with diuretics and consider renal replacement therapy since fluid overload can be devastating to the patient's pulmonary recovery.

"Following a technically successful repair, her left hemidiaphragm is persistently elevated and she remains ventilated on the third postoperative day. What is the suspected problem and work up?"
A left phrenic nerve injury is suspected. Vent weaning proceeds as able. Fluoroscopy (Sniff Test) can confirm paradoxical motion of the affected diaphragm. Early enteral nutrition should be initiated. Surgical plication, either open or by thoracoscopic means is considered if unable to wean from the ventilator. A tracheostomy may be considered as well.

"She is extubated on the first postoperative day and is noted to have a hoarse voice."
A recurrent laryngeal nerve injury is suspected. ENT evaluation and direct laryngoscopy is warranted. A trial of conservative measures including vocal exercises, regulated diet and aspiration precautions is tried first. As long as there is no aspiration, there is a chance that this represents paresis rather than paralysis and conservative measures may suffice. Medialization of the paralyzed cord can improve voice quality and is often done after demonstrating no improvement with voice therapy after 6 months.

"You placed a covered stent in the descending aneurysm and partially occluded the origin of the left subclavian artery to obtain fixation. Postoperatively, the ipsilateral hand is cold and she reports paresthesias."
Unfortunately, there is inadequate collateral circulation to the left subclavian system that was not apparent on preoperative evaluation. The extremity should be revascularized either with a carotid to subclavian bypass or subclavian transposition immediately.

"The patient has high output milky secretion from the left chest tube on POD 2."
See Chapter 14, Chylothorax.

"Preoperatively the patient is found to have a 6.5 cm aneurysm of the arch extending down to the celiac vessels. The patient notes both chest and abdominal pain that wakes her up from sleep."
This discussion assumes that you need to address both the arch and descending component in the same setting. Indications for this include evidence of contained rupture or severe symptoms where waiting for a staged repair is not ideal. If a staged repair is reasonable then it is by far the best option. Elephant trunk through a median sternotomy followed by descending or thoracoabdominal repair after 2-3 months. This may also decrease the risk of paraplegia. If you are called upon to address the proximal and distal components in a single stage and the aneurysm is too far proximal to clamp between the LCCA and LSCA then circulatory arrest is required. This poses challenges to the usual LHB setup and you need to have a more versatile cannulation strategy. Hopefully this was anticipated preoperatively based on imaging. Considerations include achieving full flow and drainage for cooling (axillary and femoral arterial plus femoral venous cannulation), circulatory arrest with brain protection (axillary artery cannulation), and resumption of full flow to the upper and lower body after circulatory arrest with partial heart bypass while the descending repair is completed (axillary and femoral arterial cannulation with femoral venous). In the standard right lateral decubitus and thoracoabdominal exposure, right axillary artery with left femoral venous and arterial cannulation can achieve most of these objectives. An alternative for aneurysms contained within the chest is a clamshell incision. This allows complete control of the pericardial arterial and venous structures as well as axillary cannulation.

"The patient has a chronic Type B dissection with a 7 cm Crawford Type I aneurysm."
The repair proceeds just like the thoracoabdominal repairs described above with a few exceptions. You need to be careful about distal perfusion and make sure you sew a graft to the non dissected femoral

artery. Also make sure that flow is being directed to the appropriate lumen (i.e., the lumen that is supplying the visceral segments). The proximal anastomosis should be reinforced with felt or pericardium within and around the dissected intima/media. The distal flap should be fenestrated with whatever method you are most comfortable with to ensure perfusion to both lumens. Note Chapter 49, Type B aortic dissection, which suggests axillary cannulation, circulatory arrest and a short segment graft interposition to address the tear. The difference in this scenario with an aneurysm is that you need a longer tube graft that requires reimplantation of the distal intercostals. The circulatory arrest period would be too long for all this work. Partial left heart bypass strategies as described above gives you more flexibility but at the expense of potential problems with the femoral cannulation. Note that axillary artery cannulation with a brief circ arrest may be warranted for the proximal anastamosis. Dissected aortic tissue may be flimsy and sewing to this just distal to a clamp near the arch could result in a retrograde dissection or other disaster.

Pearls/pitfalls

- Asymptomatic TAA > 6.0 cm should be surgically addressed.
- Endografting is appropriate for patients with isolated thoracic DAAs with 20 mm landing zones proximally and distally especially with comorbidities. Thoracic endografts should be oversized by 15-20%.
- Thoracic and thoracoabdominal repairs require a thoracotomy dictated by the proximal extent of disease. Distal retroperitoneal exposure is needed for abdominal involvement.
- *Alternative cannulation strategies.* In general LHB through the left atrial appendage or left inferior pulmonary vein with descending or femoral artery cannulation. Axillary artery and femoral venous should be considered if circulatory arrest is required. Femoral-fem AV cannulation is the most expeditious if a rupture is present.
- *Principles of thoracic or thoracoabdominal repairs include*: appropriate exposure, LHB, proximal anastomosis, ligation/ reimplantation of intercostals, sequential distal anastomosis with reimplantation of visceral segments.
- In the setting of diffuse aortic enlargement such as in Marfan's disease, repair is generally staged with the symptomatic segment treated first. If asymptomatic, the proximal segment is addressed first. An elephant trunk or hybrid repair may be needed.

Suggested readings
- Descending and Thoracoabdominal Aneurysms. Cohn LH. *Cardiac Surgery in the Adult*, 3rd Edition. 2008.
- Descending Thoracic and Thoracoabdominal Aortic Surgery. *Sabiston and Spencer - Surgery of the Chest 8th Edition*. 2010.
- Coady et al. "Surgical Management of descending thoracic aortic disease: Open and endovascular approaches: A scientific statement from the American Heart Association." *Circulation*. 2010; 121:2780-2804.

Notes

54. Arrhythmia surgery

Muhammad Habib Zubair, MD, and Yoshiya Toyoda, MD, PhD

Concept
- Indications for invasive intervention
- Primary procedure
- Medical/cath options
- Concomitant valve or coronary procedure (indication, operative strategy, devices)

Chief complaint
"A 57 yo woman with a history of obesity and atrial fibrillation (AF) was treated initially with antiarrhythmic medications and was not compliant due to the side effects. She underwent 2 catheter ablations for persistent afib with a short period of relief but now returns with recurrent palpitations, generalized weakness and dizziness for more than a week. It has been 4 months after catheter ablation and the cardiology refers her to you for a surgical alternative?"

Differential
The diagnosis was established initially by the cardiologist. Recognizing other associated diseases will be important for planning surgical interventions. Also, review the EKG carefully to ensure that the rhythm is labelled correctly.

History and physical
Attempt to determine the pattern of afib (paroxysmal - spontaneous conversion, recurrent - requires ECV/antiarrythmics or persistent), medications (anticoagulation, antiarrhythmics), and complications of afib (stroke, peripheral emboli). Identify signs and symptoms of diseases that predispose to a high recurrence rate after catheter ablation: hypertension, hypercholesterolemia, persistent AF, or obstructive sleep apnea. Predisposing factors include age, male sex (because of the tall stature), hypertension, hyperthyroidism, chronic kidney disease, alcohol, PE, obesity (BMI > 30 kg/m2) and family history. Ask about any known ischemic or valvular issues.

Tests
- *Labs*: CBC, BMP, Coags.
- 12 lead EKG to establish the rate and rhythm.
- 24 Holter monitoring especially if the patient is currently in sinus rhythm.

- *CT scan or MRI*: pulmonary vein protocol in patients with a failed catheter ablation (to rule out pulmonary stenosis).
- *Echo*: complete valvular assessment, septal anatomy, right and left function, and left atrial size. Severely dilated left atrium decreases the likelihood of achieving sustained sinus rhythm.
- *Left heart catheterization*: for IHD and for establishing coronary anatomy (left dominant patients are at slightly increased risk of injury to their coronary arteries while ablating close to the coronary sinus).
- *Electrophysiological mapping*: which utilizes the combination of pace/anatomic/activation mapping to identify potential sites for ablation.

Index scenario (additional information)
"The patient has normal electrolytes, no valve abnormalities and evidence of persistent afib on 24 hour holter monitoring with a rate between 70 and 90. Her cardiac catheterization is normal."

Treatment/management
- Indications for catheter or surgical ablation include paroxysmal (PAF), persistent or recurrent AF in patients who do not tolerate or have failed antiarrhythmics. Catheter ablation is usually attempted first once or even twice prior to referral for surgery unless the patient is undergoing surgery for a concomitant lesion.
- This patient has failed medical and catheter based interventions and is thus a candidate for stand alone surgical ablation. Options include pulmonary vein isolation (works well for PAF), or Cox MAZE IV (cut and sew or the modified ablation protocol). For this patient Cox MAZE IV will give her the greatest chance of sinus rhythm control.

Operative steps
Goals – establishing atrioventricular synchrony, return and preservation of atrial mechanical function to enhance ventricular diastolic filling and abolish electrophysiologic substrates propagating the arrhythmia.

Cox maze IV
- Many different ways to do this but here we describe the critical lesion sets using a single cryoablation catheter (nitric oxide).
- Standard median sternotomy, aortic and bicaval cannulation, antegrade cardioplegia.
- Initiate CPB, clamp, antegrade arrest, snares around the IVC/SVC, right atriotomy, place the retrograde coronary sinus catheter in directly and administer cardioplegia (although may also do the case entirely with antegrade).

- Left atrial incision through Sondergaards groove. Alternative is transeptal incision through the fossa ovalis.
- *Left sided lesions*: the unipolar cryoablation (nitric oxide), can be used for all the lesions in the Cox Maze IV and may be more cost effective than using both bipolar radiofrequency (RF) and cryoablation. 1) Start with a box lesion around the four pulmonary veins. Success may be documented by demonstrating exit block from each PV. Note that this lesion can also be done with the bipolar ablation device. If using the cryoprobe you need to have the TEE probe pulled up towards the upper mediastinum and lift anteriorly on the backwall of the atrium during freezing so as to avoid esophageal injury. 2) Excise the LAA and make a lesion from here to the left superior pulmonary vein. Close the left atrial appendage incision. 3) Lesion from the atrial incision to the posterior mitral annulus (P3) - this is the circumflex lesion and should be performed both inside and outside of the atrium for transmural ablation. De-air and close the septal incision. Care with the phrenic nerves while doing left sided lesions. A moist lap pad to insulate the nerve maybe helpful.
- *Right sided lesions (can be done with the heart beating)*. 1) Right transverse atriotomy. 2) Epicardial surface of the SVC to the IVC (can use bipolar here, watch for the SA node). 3) Right atrial appendage (RAA) incision with a free wall lesion down the anterior RA wall with a cut or ablation (be sure to keep a 2 cm uninvolved atrial bridge between this lesion and the transverse atriotomy). 4) RAA lesion to the 10'oclock position on the tricuspid annulus. 5) Atriotomy to the 2 o'oclock position on the tricuspid valve.
- Close the right atriotomy, and release your snares.

Potential questions/alternative scenarios

"A 65 yo female with a history of PAF is undergoing an AVR and is noted to have PAF."

This is an excellent indication for pulmonary vein isolation (PVI). PVI can be used as a stand alone procedure for PAF especially in patients with comorbidities who need a limited operation. However, it is not as complete as the Cox Maze IV and is not as successful for persistent or recurrent AF. PVI is very often used for PAF in patients undergoing valve surgery with good results.

Pulmonary venous isolation (PVI)

- Median sternotomy, aortic and single stage venous cannulation. Initiate CPB and perform the right sided lesions first.
- *Right sided lesions*: carefully get around the right superior pulmonary vein (RSPV) and right inferior pulmonary vein (RIPV) with blunt and sharp dissection. Stay away from the phrenic nerve.

The bipolar RF jaws are inserted around the right sided pulmonary veins and then clamped on the atrial tissue to avoid pulmonary vein stenosis.

- *Left sided lesions*: now arrest the heart and get around the left sided pulmonary veins in a similar fashion. Identify and divide the ligament of Marshall. Here you have to make sure that you are away from the circumflex artery on the AV groove when clamping on the left atrial tissue.
- *Excise/ligate LAA*: excise and suture or occlude the LAAL with a variety of commercially available devices.
- Perform the AVR.

"A 58 yo male is undergoing a mitral valve repair and has a history of PAF."

For this patient the PVI is best performed when the left atrium is opened with a single cryoablation catheter. BIpolar devices can be used for the inferior and superior connecting lesions to prevent injury to the esophagus. But remember to excise or exclude the LAA prior to repairing or replacing the mitral valve. You do not want to lift up on the heart after the mitral is completed due to the potential for AV groove disruption.

"The same patient has a history of persistent afib."

There are a few different ways to do this. It is reasonable to plan for left and right sided lesions (Cox Maze IV) as well as LAAL as described above. Make the left atriotomy through Sondergaard's groove, address the left sided lesions, LAAL, repair/replace the valve and make a separate right atriotomy for the right sided lesions. Alternatively, perform the mitral through a transseptal incision. The one risk with the transseptal is that if the mitral exposure is not great and you need an extended transseptal then you risk injury to the artery supplying the SA node.

"A 59 yo diabetic, hypertensive male patient with chronic kidney disease is suffering from persistent atrial fibrillation. She had an intracranial bleed while on warfarin and other class 1 and 3 anti arrhythmics. How would you proceed?"

This patient is at increased risk of intracranial hemorrhage with CPB. Thus catheter ablation with best medical management may be her best option.

"On electrophysiologic mapping a patient is a suitable candidate for minimally invasive PVI, but a thrombus is discovered intraoperatively on TEE, how will you proceed?"

The minimally invasive PVI will be converted to an open procedure.

"A 57 yo obese, female who is a known case of atrial fibrillation (AF) was treated initially with antiarrhythmic drugs and she was non compliant due to the side effects, this was followed by a catheter ablation procedure but she is still having occasional palpitations 2 months after catheter ablation?"

If she is highly symptomatic and antiarrhythmics are not effective or tolerated a second attempt at catheter ablation after careful electrophysiologic mapping can be attempted. If this fails wait for three months and proceed with surgical management.

Pearls/pitfalls

- There could be potential overlap in the type of AF, therefore patients should be classified according to the most dominant AF pattern in the last six months.
- PVI is good for PAF and Cox Maze is preferred for persistent or recurrent afib.
- For PAF in the setting of valvular or coronary surgery, PVI using RF ablation and LAAL are sufficient. If already in the LA for MVR then do the PVI box lesions with cryoablation/bipolar.

Suggested readings

- http://www.ctsnet.org/sections/videosection/giants/2011Giants_DamianoRalph.html
- Calkins H et al. Heart Rhythm Society Task Force on Catheter and Surgical Ablation of Atrial Fibrillation. 2012 HRS/EHRA/ECAS expert consensus statement on catheter and surgical ablation of atrial fibrillation...Heart Rhythm. 2012;9(4):632-696.e21.
- Melby SJ, Damiano, Jr. RJ. Surgery for atrial fibrillation. Cohn LH (ed). Cardiac Surgery in the Adult. New York: McGraw-Hill. 2008.

Notes

55. Hypertrophic obstructive cardiomyopathy

Muhammad F. Masood, MD, and Vinay Badhwar, MD

Concept
- Establishing the diagnosis as primary entity or in conjunction with aortic stenosis
- Indications for operation and preoperative planning
- Anatomic landmarks and extent of myomectomy
- Role of surgical treatment of the mitral valve in the setting of left ventricular outflow tract obstruction (LVOTO)

Chief complaint
"A 30 yo previously healthy man has presented to you with a complaint of 6 months of progressive worsening shortness of breath and left sided chest pain that is exacerbated with exercise and relieved by rest. He usually runs 5 miles twice a week but now can only run 1 mile. His symptoms however are relieved by rest. He states his older brother died suddenly at age 35. Patient is apprehensive about what is going on?"

Differential
Hypertrophic obstructive cardiomyopathy (HOCM), arrhythmogenic right ventricular dysplasia (ARVD), Wolff-Parkinson-White (WPW) syndrome, long QT syndrome, and Brugada syndrome are the most common causes of sudden cardiac death in young healthy/athletic individuals. The progressive nature of this patient's symptoms without syncope is suggestive of HOCM.

History and physical
Focused history to elicit symptoms of angina, dizziness, or dyspnea, which are often exacerbated with exercise. Diuretic or vasodilator therapy, used to treat presumed congestive heart failure, will often exacerbate symptoms. Family history of sudden cardiac death in young first degree relative is important. Focused examination to elicit a systolic ejection murmur and premature ventricular contractions (PVC) is essential. Increased murmur intensity with valsalva and notation of a brisk bisferens pulse can often hint towards HOCM instead of aortic stenosis.

Tests
- *EKG.* Left ventricular strain pattern, large T-waves in pre cordial leads, frequent PVCs.

- *Echocardiogram*: to evaluate level and degree of left ventricular outflow obstruction (LVOTO), degree of systolic anterior motion of mitral valve (SAM), and determine if cavitary hypertrophy is diffuse as in HOCM or asymmetric and focal as can be associated with aortic stenosis or hypertension.
- *Gradients*: diagnosis defined by peak instantaneous LV outflow tract gradient (not mean gradient).
  a. Basal (resting) gradient: > 30 mmHg
  b. Provocative gradients: with stress valsalva or amyl nitrite > 30 mmHg
  c. Intervention is considered when gradient is > 50 mmHg
- *Septum*. Septal hypertrophy of > 15 mm is helpful in identifying HOCM. Other abnormalities causing ventricular and septal hypertrophy must be ruled out, e.g., HTN, aortic stenosis. Asymmetric septal hypertrophy is noted when the hypertrophy is focused and limited to the outflow tract septum. Wall thickness of > 30 mm in HOCM patients has a strong correlation with sudden cardiac death (SCD).
- *Mitral Valve*. Systolic anterior motion of mitral valve (SAM) – due to the Venturi effect of blood ejecting from LV, resulting in outflow obstruction by the anterior mitral leaflet which may often be associated with secondary mitral regurgitation. SAM may often involve the body of the anterior leaflet. In some cases this may be limited to just the subvalvular structures, which may be referred to as chordal SAM.
- *Chamber size and function*. Athletic hearts can have 13-15 mm LV thickness with normal relaxation and chamber dilation. In HOCM, ejection fraction is supra-normal and if LV dilation occurs it often represents advanced heart failure.
- Exercise echo is performed in asymptomatic patients with gradients of < 50 mmHg.
  - *Angiography*. Brockenbrough–Braunwald–Morrow sign occurs following a PVC in HOCM where the LV pressure on the aortic tracing is much greater than prior to the PVC due to more time for LV filling.
  - *Cardiac MRI*: can be adjunctive to echocardiography if available. In many experienced centers it can be the diagnostic and primary tool for following HOCM patients.

Index scenario (additional information)
"This young patient does not have CHF. He does have apical heave and a systolic murmur. EKG demonstrates paroxsysmal atrial flutter. Echo reveals peak instantaneous LVOT gradient of 60 mmHg with septal thickness of 27 mm and left ventricular

outflow tract obstruction due to SAM. His coronary angiogram was normal. What are his treatment options?"

Treatment/management

This patient meets criteria for treatment. His options are medical, interventional, or surgical. His symptoms of angina and dyspnea are caused by outflow obstruction, subendocardial ischemia and SAM with potential MR. His atrial dysrhythmia is further decreasing his LV filling and cardiac output thus making his symptoms worse. Medical therapy may be used to relieve symptoms. Initial pharmacotherapy is with beta blockers for rate control to optimize LV filling. For patients that cannot tolerate beta blockade, non-dihydropiridine calcium channel blockers such as verapamil may be used. In this case, attempts at medical or electrical cardioversion of atrial fibrillation should be considered to optimize LV filling and relieve symptoms. Disopyramide can be used if symptoms persist. Diuretic use should be very judicious and only in setting of marked volume overload as they could worsen the LVOTO.

"Patient was started on a low dose beta blocker but was not able to tolerate it due to bradycardia."
"Treatment with disopyramide was started, however, 4 months later he developed dry mouth, blurred vision and constipation."
Although utilization of medications for symptomatic control is often attempted first, adverse side-effects or persistent symptoms would prompt options to mechanically relieve the LVOTO. While surgical myectomy is often considered first line for symptomatic patients who fail medical therapy, other options include alcohol septal ablation, ventricular pacing, or even cardiac transplantation.

Septal myectomy is indicated in symptomatic patients who fail conservative medical therapy. Patients with septal thickness of > 30 mm have an increased risk of SCD and long standing LVOT obstruction leads to heart failure. Excellent 5 year and 10 year survival of 96% and 83% has been demonstrated with < 1% peri operative mortality. Care should be taken with the anterior mitral leaflet and degree of SAM as this may influence the degree of myectomy. If MR is present it is often improved with myectomy alone although sometimes you may need to address the valve.

Trans-aortic septal myectomy
Goals – relieve LVOTO, improve hemodynamics and symptoms.

- Establish invasive monitoring. Arterial line, central venous catheter, PA catheter, foley.
- *Intra operative TEE*: re-evaluate septal thickness, gradients, mitral valve pathology to include degree of anterior leaflet involvement (body of leaflet vs. chordal SAM only), degree of MR severity, presence of anterior leaflet calcification or posterior leaflet excess. The concomitant presence of myxomatous mitral disease or excess posterior mitral leaflet tissue may point to the necessity to address the mitral valve or highlight a potential pitfall in isolated septal myomectomy. The intraoperative TEE interpretation will be a key point for planning the operative approach.
- Sternotomy and pericardial marsupialization. Administer heparin. Standard aortic cannulation, but bicaval venous cannulation is recommended. If mitral valve pathology is identified or if after septal myectomy any need arises to address the mitral or septum, it will be easier to address with bicaval cannulation and this will show important foresight in your operative planning.
- Myocardial protection is critical. Antegrade and retrograde recommended (thick ventricle may need both routes for myocardial protection). LV vent through right superior pulmonary vein (RSPV). Myocardial septal temperature probe can be considered.
- A low transverse aortotomy with extension into the non-coronary sinus is performed. Exposure of the aortic valve and sub-aortic septum can be performed with sutures if needed (careful not to damage leaflets), or a Ross retractor in certain cases. Sub-aortic septum may be transiently exposed additionally by a gentle push on the free wall of right ventricle.
- *Extended myectomy*. Using #11 scalpel on long handle, an incision is made below the nadir of right coronary sinus and a parallel incision below the left coronary commissure is made and connected 3 mm below the aortic annulus. The area between the two incisions is cut as a trough, towards the base of the anterior papillary muscle. This incision provides a myectomy length of 7 cm. Extreme care is taken not to allow muscle tissue to drop in the ventricle; one way is to place a traction suture (a pledgetted 4-0 prolene for example) prior to commencing your resection. The landmarks of importance are the anterior leaflet of the mitral valve, the membranous ventricular septum and the aortic leaflets; all of which could be damaged as part of the myectomy.
- Close aortotomy and re-animate. Ventricular ectopy is common and one should be prepared for chemical or electrical defibrillation. Wean bypass, fill the heart (restrict venous drainage and stop RSPV

vent). Evaluate using TEE: LVOT velocity, gradient, presence/absence of VSD, SAM or MR. If an obstructive concern is raised, come off bypass but remain cannulated and volume load. Repeat myectomy is recommended if the gradient is > 10-15 mmHg. You can challenge the patient intraoperatively with a vasodilator to look for SAM when tachycardic.

- Once successful myomectomy is performed, decannulate and close in the standard fashion.
- Postoperatively avoid tachycardia and keep volume loaded.

Potential questions/alternative scenarios
"Patient is apprehensive about surgical intervention and would like to consider catheter based therapies."
Ventricular pacing has been used in some patients to activate the septum before the LV free wall in an asynchronous manner in an attempt to reduce the LV outflow tract gradient. The benefit of pacing remains controversial with perceived benefits being limited.

Alcohol septal ablation involves injecting alcohol into septal perforators of the left anterior descending coronary artery to create what amounts to a controlled myocardial infarction of the outflow tract septum. It has been shown to improve symptoms in experienced hands but the outcome can be highly variable based on center experience. It is associated with relatively higher incidence of mortality (1.5% as opposed to 1%). Morbidity can be significant: 11% pacemaker rate due to permanent heart block, 1.8% risk of coronary artery dissection, 2.2% rate of ventricular fibrillation, 1.1% risk of stroke, with 6% patients requiring repeat ablation and 2% requiring surgical myectomy. Patients with multiple co-morbidities with high or prohibitive surgical risk may be offered this therapy. In addition, catheter-based septal ablation does not address the potential need for concomitant treatment of mitral valve or coronary pathology and therefore cannot be offered to this group of patients.

"Before incision is made, on table TEE demonstrates presence of mild to moderate mitral regurgitation."
Evaluation of the mitral valve is of paramount importance. The principle mechanism of symptomatic LVOTO is from SAM so it is expected that the mitral valve will be involved and that in many cases MR will exist. Deciding how much of the MR is from SAM and how much may be related to primary mitral pathology is the key question here. Ask about the relationship between the posterior mitral leaflet (PML) and anterior mitral leaflet (AML) in terms of length or excess leaflet tissue or the presence of primary mitral pathology such as ruptured chordae, clear myxomatous degeneration or annular dilation. If you have excess PML height, anticipate the

potential need to add an adjunctive PML treatment to decrease PML height. This may require concomitant repair (sliding valvuloplasty) or low-profile mitral replacement based on the comfort of the surgeon and the discussion with the patient preoperatively.

Presuming mild to moderate MR as stated in the question it is likely that there is not major valvular pathology and that the SAM (likely chordal SAM) will likely resolve with therapeutic septal myomectomy. If no significant primary valve pathology exists that predisposes to SAM, over 85% of cases will demonstrate resolution of regurgitation and will not require additional mitral valve interventions.

"Patient post-operative day 2 after septal myectomy is having increasing oxygen requirements. A new harsh holosystolic systolic murmur is heard. PA systolic pressures have increased from 35 to 55 mmHg."

The importance of this question is to ascertain if these findings are due to SAM or a more rare complication of post myectomy, VSD. Evaluate if the patient had received diuretics or vasodilators or if the patient was in atrial fibrillation, all of which could decrease LV preload, recurrence of SAM and MR that could explain the above symptoms. These would be readily treatable with volume loading, restoration of sinus rhythm and medical therapy. However, as the question specifically notes a "new harsh holosystolic murmur" this is likely due to a postoperative VSD. Focused physical exam should demonstrate the above mentioned murmur, precordial heave and elevated CVP manifested by jugular venous distension. Diagnostic confirmation may be obtained by transthoracic or transesophageal echocardiography or by a PA catheter to document a step-up in oxygen saturation between the proximal and distal ports. Imaging to establish the location and size of the VSD will be imperative to determine treatment and surgical therapy. Once confirming the diagnosis and location, plan return to OR with TEE to re-evaluate VSD, septum, mitral valve and presence or absence of a new wall motion abnormality. Following sternal re-entry and bicaval cannulation, a right atriotomy is then performed and the tricuspid valve exposed. The membranous septum is exposed below the septal leaflet of the triscupid valve. Repair is then performed using autologous pericardium or a GoreTex patch. Avoid primary suture repair in these cases due to tissue friability. It is important to identify that there is not a mid-ventricular defect by preoperative imaging as your operative approach will need to be tailored to assure coverage and repair appropriately.

- Septal myectomy in HOCM is the best, most effective and proven approach to change the course of heart failure by relieving obstruction at LVOT.
- *Classic Morrow's technique for myectomy.* Using #11 blade, incision is made below the nadir of right coronary and resection of 3 cm of sub aortic muscle is performed. Extended myectomy is a long 7 cm resection up to the LV apex and often the treatment of choice of true HOCM.
- Vasoconstrictors (i.e., phenylephrine or vasopressin) are used for acute hypotension. Positive inotropy, vasodilators and diuretics should be avoided.
- Mitral valve replacement is no longer commonly performed as the first line surgical therapy of HOCM. Septal myectomy usually corrects the MR and SAM when there is no major concomitant mitral pathology. Mitral valve repair is performed with the goal of reduction of PML height when clear myxomatous degeneration exists or ruptured chordae is revealed. If repair is contemplated, be sure to place a large ring following repair and consider concomitant septal myomectomy. In the setting of severe mitral pathology, a low profile prosthetic replacement with/without myomectomy is a safe strategy.
- Aggressive treatment of pre or post-operative atrial fibrillation is of key importance.
- Routine septal myectomy for sub-valvular hypertrophy at time of aortic valve replacement for severe aortic stenosis is not yet a universally accepted treatment recommendation. The diagnosis of asymmetric septal hypertrophy is made by preoperative TEE or catheterization to document non-valvular LVOT sub-valvular gradients. The scenario may be one of a diagnosis of aortic stenosis but normal aortic leaflets are noted. If asymmetric septal hypertrophy is identified in the absence of HOCM, septal myectomy can be performed to improve symptoms of heart failure.
- Genetic testing (GT) is not used for establishing a diagnosis of HOCM, but rather for screening potential family members once a diagnosis is made. It may also be useful in predicting the progression or complications of HOCM.

Suggested readings

- Gersh BJ, et al. 2011 ACCF/AHA guideline for the diagnosis and treatment of hypertrophic cardiomyopathy. A report of the American College of Cardiology Foundation/American Heart Association Task Force on Practice Guidelines. *J Thorac Cardiovasc Surg* 2011;142;e153-e203.

- Brown ML and Schaff HV. Surgical management of obstructive hypertrophic cardiomyopathy: the gold standard. *Expert Review of Cardiovascular Therapy* June 2008 p715-725.
- Di Tommaso L, Stassano P, Mannacio V, et al. Asymmetric septal hypertrophy in patients with severe aortic stenosis: The usefulness of associated septal myectomy. *J Thorac Cardiovasc Surg* 2012 Feb epub p1-5.
- Bonde P, Yuh D. Surgical management of hypertrophic obstructive cardiomopathy. Yuh D, Vricella LA, and Baumgartner WA (eds). *Johns Hopkins manual of cardiothoracic surgery* 2007.

Notes

56. Cardiac tumors

Muhammad F. Masood, MD, and Vinay Badhwar, MD

Concept

- Identification of cardiac tumor as a differential diagnosis
- Knowledge of sub-types of cardiac tumors, their prognosis and treatment
- Operative strategy: cannulation, tumor handling and reconstruction of chamber walls

Chief complaint

"You are evaluating a 45 yo woman who presents with a 3 week history of fatigue and feeling unwell. She reports a syncopal episode 2 weeks ago. Over last week she has experienced progressive worsening shortness of breath (SOB), both during exertion and lying down. She is admitted to the hospital due to SOB and currently is on 4 liters of oxygen via nasal cannula."

Differential

Endocarditis with mitral or multi-valvular involvement, cardiomyopathy with arrhythmias, aortic stenosis, regurgitation or pulmonary pathology. Given presumed new onset and symptoms regardless of position or activity, this would be concerning for an obstructive pathology such as a myxoma.

History and physical

Focused history to elicit risk factors for infective endocarditis (recent dental visit), risk factors for acute cardiomyopathy (recent viral illness, peri-partum state, alcohol abuse, history of coronary artery disease, family history of sudden death or cardiomyopathy), or additional history consistent with myxoma such as prior history of myxoma, fever, cachexia, hemoptysis or new tachycardia. Physical examination for signs of left sided involvement or obstruction include peripheral embolic phenomenon (limb, renal, cerebrovascular, ischemic bowel), pulmonary edema, arrhythmia, systolic murmur, diastolic murmur ("tumor plop"), and conjunctival pallor consistent with anemia. Right sided involvement may manifest with pulmonary emboli or tricuspid obstruction and related signs of jugular venous distension, peripheral edema or ascites. Ask about pulmonary pathology as well including asthma or COPD.

Tests

- *CXR*. Chamber obstruction can be seen either as enlarged cardiac silhouette or increased pulmonary vascular markings or pulmonary edema/effusions.

- *EKG*. Non-specific commonly, however may show bundle branch block, complete heart block or arrhythmias.
- *Lab*: anemia common, elevated CRP and ESR common but non-specific.
- *Echocardiogram*: transthoracic or transesophageal (preferred) echocardiogram is often diagnostic for cardiac tumor, particularly myxoma.
  - *Evaluate*: tumor size, extent, mobility, stalk, degree of obstruction, chamber and wall involvement, and proximity to valvular/electrical intracardiac structures to plan therapy.
- *Cardiac catheterization*. Coronary artery evaluation should be considered if procedural embolization risk is minimal. Beneficial in evaluation of ventricular involvement of malignant tumors (blush) or existence of concomitant coronary disease.
- Cardiac CT or MRI is performed to evaluate tumor burden, wall penetration and relation to extracardiac structures. Also of benefit to ascertain consistency of mass (i.e., solid, lipomatous, hemorrhagic).
- Focused imaging important for peripheral emboli for co-morbid risk stratification based on symptoms (neuro, peripheral vascular, pulmonary, GI).

Index scenario (additional information)

"This patient does have significant SOB on high supplemental oxygen, and some necrosis of tip of left fingers. CXR shows increased pulmonary markings and enlarged cardiac silhouette of left heart border. EKG is non specific. TEE shows EF of 50%, 4 cm, mobile, left atrial septal mass, producing intermittent obstruction to mitral valve orifice. Pulmonary artery pressures are half systemic. All head CT scans are negative. How would you like to manage this clinical process?"

Treatment/management

This patient is demonstrating signs of left atrial enlargement, pulmonary hypertension and obstructive heart failure due to the tumor in the left atrium causing diastolic mitral orifice inflow obstruction. Digital necrosis represents distal embolization. Myxoma is the most common cardiac tumor and presents most commonly with signs and symptoms of cardiac chamber obstruction followed by tumor embolization. Some patients present with prodromal symptoms of fatigue, fever, cachexia, anemia, and malaise. Complete surgical excision including a minimum of 5 mm circumferential atrial septal excision with the stalk is the mainstay of the treatment with associated rare recurrences. Preoperative critical assessment of all cardiac chambers is necessary to rule out presence of additional tumor burden, myocardial wall involvement or extracardiac involvement (TEE, Cardiac MRI if available).

Operative steps

Goals – adequate exposure, minimal cardiac manipulation prior to aortic cross clamp, complete excision of mass along with a minimum of 5 mm cuff of normal tissue and reconstruction of cardiac chamber, often using an atrial septal patch.

- *Invasive monitoring*: arterial line and central venous access. Careful consideration of jugular PA and CV catheters should be done in cases of right sided tumors to prevent tumor embolization.
- Intra operative TEE is essential to re-evaluate tumor size, mobility, extent, particular cardiac chamber involvement, degree of obstruction and plan excision and conduct of operation.
- Standard midline sternotomy, marsupialization pericardium and heparinize.
- It is important for minimal to no cardiac manipulation until aortic cross-clamp is applied.
- Standard aortic cannulation.
- *Bicaval venous cannulation.* In the case of right sided tumors, cannulate high on SVC and low on IVC. Snare cavae in preparation for complete cardiopulmonary bypass (CPB). Likely avoid pre-clamp retrograde in case right sided involvement or risk of embolization with intracardiac pre-bypass manipulation.
- Vent the left ventricle through aortic root. Do not use right superior pulmonary vein (RSPV) vent especially in case of left sided tumors as it risks tumor embolization.
- Myocardial protection can be achieved utilizing only antegrade cardioplegia as these patients are often young and do not have coronary artery disease or myocardial hypertrophy.
- Systemic cooling is often not necessary for left atrial myxoma excision.
- Commence CPB, cross-clamp and arrest. Mobilize SVC and IVC.
- Options for exposure for a left atrial myxoma are bi-atrial or right atrial approaches.
  - *Right atrial*: snare cavae and make standard right atriotomy and exposure with retraction sutures. You can often detect the stalk penetrance of the left sided myxoma by the visual thickening of the septum. Incise atrial septum lateral to suspected location with an 11 blade then very carefully extend after directly visualizing tumor to assure avoidance or manipulation of the tumor or stalk. Perform wide local excision of atrial septum by a minimum of 5 mm circumferentially around tumor mass and stalk. Remove involved atrial septum and mass in toto and send to pathology. Aggressively inspect entire left atrium, atrial appendage, mitral valve and even left ventricle for any

438

residual tumor burden, residual tissue or damage to mitral leaflet (that may require repair). Irrigate clean and patch septal defect with patch (Gore-Tex or autologous pericardium).

- Another option for complex tumors is a bi-atrial approach. This can either be done with separate left and right atriotomies to gain exposure or a bi-atrial incision from the RSPV vestibule extended over to right atrium to attain biatrial approach. This approach can be helpful but does carry with it a slight increase risk for postoperative arrhythmias.

- Be wary of tumor fragmentation and utilize outside suction during tumor excision. Following excision, aggressively irrigate and suction the cardiac chamber.

- Following excision check for residual ASD or VSD as appropriate and valvular integrity.

- Avoid primary closure of defect. Close right atrium with 4-0 or 5-0 prolene.

- De-air through root vent, wean CPB. Once off bypass re-evaluation of all cardiac chambers with TEE is important to rule out any ASD or VSD, new mitral or tricuspid insufficiency.

- Heart block is relatively uncommon but placement of atrial and ventricular wires can prevent post operative complications from transient rhythm abnormalities. Reverse heparin, place drainage tubes and proceed with closure.

Potential questions/alternative scenarios
"Patient arrests on induction of anesthesia."
Loss of vasomotor tone can lead to drop in preload to the left atrium leading to tumor potentially obstructing mitral inflow causing low to no cardiac output, lack of coronary perfusion pressure and shock. ACLS protocols to be followed. Once secure airway is confirmed and presuming that arrest/shock does not reverse after catecholamine administration and CPR while prepping, then perform immediate midline sternotomy, heparinize and place on CPB.

Following sternotomy simultaneous with heparinizing, open pericardium and proceed with rapid cannulation of aorta and right atrium (provided known isolated LA myxoma). If there is foreknowledge of bi-atrial involvement, central aortic and isolated SVC partial or peripheral venous drainage can be initially established. Once CPB and full circulation is established then can change to bi-caval cannulation and proceed as above.

"An atrial septal defect is seen after coming off bypass."
Attempt to determine the size and location of the defect by TEE in order to plan management. Only if tiny leak is noted conservative post-protamine approach may be adequate. However this is often an iatrogenic error and will likely require surgical correction. Resume bi-caval CPB, open the right atrial incision, and assess defect size, atrial septal wall and tissue integrity. If the sutures have pulled through (particularly if you tried to close it primarily the first time), use a pericardial patch closure. Small defect due to improper suture technique can be closed by reinforcement sutures provided healthy surrounding atrial tissue.

"Tumor is in right atrium causing obstructive symptoms, ascites, and hepatomegaly."
Pre-operative assessment of tumor location and extent is of critical importance. Along with TEE, CT/MRI or even venography may be helpful to evaluate the extent of caval involvement. During operative set up, it is imperative to use TEE to best guide venous cannulation. For extensive caval involvement, the patient may need right internal jugular (IJ) and femoral venous cannulation. Often the tumor and its atrial base can be readily excised via a right atriotomy. Rarely those with SVC or IVC extension may either have to be managed by extending the atriotomy onto the SVC (laterally to avoid the SA node) or onto the intrapericardial IVC facilitated by peripheral venous cannulation or, very rarely, facilitated by a brief period of hypothermic circulatory arrest to assure full resection. Always assess all chambers, protect the tricuspid valve while excising the tumor, and be careful to avoid the AV node in Triangle of Koch (Boundaries - Tendon of Todaro, Septal leaflet and coronary sinus).

"Tumor is high in SVC and has embolized to PA."
This patient's cannulation and operative conduct strategy is the key point here. Central aortic and peripheral venous cannulation will be best. Femoral venous multi-stage cannula would be most helpful brought up to just before the RA-IVC junction (i.e., biomedicus 21 or 25 Fr multi-stage venous). Upper drainage will depend on the imaged extent of the SVC involvement. Though right IJ cannulation is often preferred and commonly used for minimally invasive surgery (i.e., percutaneous use of a 15 Fr biomedicus arterial cannula), given the nature of the extent in question, this may need to be in the left IJ or subclavian for venous access to assure avoidance of tumor mass. Preoperative central venous access would likely be best in the contralateral subclavian. High SVC mobilization above the azygous will be important and proximal snaring as appropriate. Clamp, antegrade cardioplegic arrest is achieved. Once on total CPB and snared, if no documented left sided involvement, a small RSPV vent will be helpful. These tumors can often be excised via a right

atriotomy with extension laterally on the SVC to avoid the SA node. Be sure to inspect the RV and RV outflow tract from the right atrium to look for tumor. A separate pulmonary arteriotomy can be used to extract the tumor embolus. Rarely, if visualization is difficult or if emboli are diffuse, a brief period of hypothermic arrest may facilitate full removal of tumor burden from the distal PA.

"Ventricular myxoma"
A more rare entity, right or left ventricular involvement is often first related to an intra-atrial myxoma and secondary extension below the AV valve in the ventricular outflow tract. These can be approached via the outflow tract or via the AV valve. For myxoma arising from the base of the papillary muscle or within chordae of the AV valve, the surgical approach will involve repair or replacement of the valve. Full inspection of the ventricular chamber along with the atrial chamber is important but ventriculotomy is often avoided.

"Small pedunculated mobile density attached to the aortic valve is seen during pre-op Echo for coronary artery bypass graft (CABG). Patient has had no fevers, no history of intravenous drug use and no indwelling venous catheters. Patient has had a normal dental exam."
This small density seen on pre op ECHO is most likely Papillary Fibroelastoma. These are benign tumors that are most commonly incidental findings. Due to their embolic potential, they are excised when diagnosed, particularly during a concomitant cardiac operation. This patient should undergo an on-pump CABG along with transverse aortotomy and primary excision. The fibroelastoma often arises from valvular endocardium at the coaptation zone of the leaflet. Resection is often performed with full leaflet and annular preservation as there is usually a small stalk that can be amputated flush with the leaflet without incurring any leaflet damage. The aortotomy is closed in the standard manner and the proximal anastomoses are performed.

Pearls/pitfalls
- Benign tumors comprise 80% of cases and prognosis is good with surgical excision. They include cardiac myxoma as the most common followed by lipoma then fibroelastoma. Papillary fibroelastoma arise from valvular endocardium and have equal distribution among heart valves. Surgical strategies for complete resection of myxomas are important to mitigate recurrence.
- Malignant tumors comprise up to 20% of cases. They are primarily sarcomas and present often below age 50. They include rhabdomyosarcomas, angiosarcomas, fibrosarcomas, myxosarcoma, and liposarcomas. Long term survival is poor.

- Surgical strategies for cardiac tumor requires careful thought on cannulation, prevention of intraoperative tumor embolization by avoiding over manipulation prior to cross clamp, operative exposure often involving more than one chamber, surgical excision and tension free repair. Obstruction of cardiac output, chamber extension/embolization, and heart block are common pitfalls that should be thoughtfully prepared for.

Suggested readings

- Centofanti P, Di Rosa E, Deorsola L, et al. Primary cardiac tumors: early and late results of surgical treatment in 91 patients. Ann Thorac Surg 1999;68:1236-1241.
- Bireta C, Popov AF, Schotola H, et al. Carney-complex: multiple resections of recurrent cardiac myxoma. J Cardiothorac Surg 2011;6:12.
- Benign Cardiac Tumors: A Review. Reardon MJ et al. Methodist Debakey Cardiovasc J 2010 Jul-Sept;6:20-6.
- Blackmon SH and Reardon MJ. Cardiac Neoplasms. Lawrence Cohn (ed). Cardiac Surgery in the Adult 2012.

Notes

57. Operative management of pulmonary embolism

Emily Downs, MD, and Gorav Ailawadi, MD

Concept
- Diagnosis of pulmonary embolism
- Indications for surgical embolectomy
- Surgical technique
- Chronic pulmonary embolus and management

Chief complaint
"You are called to see a 47 yo woman with a recent diagnosis of localized pancreatic cancer who presented to the emergency department with a 1-week history of progressive fatigue and dyspnea on exertion. She appears short of breath, heart rate is 116 beats/min, blood pressure is 100/66, oxygen saturation is 88% on room air. CT chest with pulmonary arteriography shows a large embolus nearly occluding the right pulmonary artery."

Differential
The diagnosis of pulmonary embolism (PE) is established from the history and high index of suspicion. A PE protocol CT with contrast during the pulmonary phase (CTPA) is diagnostic. Extent of pulmonary and hemodynamic compromise is important in determining management.

History and physical
Key points include contributing factors to thrombosis, determining clinical status and extent of hemodynamic instability. Determine patients risk profile for invasive therapeutic options such as surgery or thrombolytic therapy. Thrombosis risks are summarized by Virchow's triad: venous stasis, endothelial injury, and hypercoagulability. History should evaluate:
- *Venous stasis*: recent immobility due to travel, illness, surgery, prolonged bedrest.
- Endothelial injury from surgery, trauma, venous access procedures.
- Hypercoagulable state associated with malignancy, inherited thrombophilia, use of medications (oral contraception) or history of thrombosis.

Hemodynamic stability is evaluated with close attention to signs of shock and right heart strain. Thrombolysis with tissue plasminogen activator (several formulations available) may be considered, but must rule out absolute contraindications. Ask patients about history of stroke, intracranial tumors, or recent trauma or surgery.

Tests

- *EKG*: most common finding is tachycardia; may have T-wave abnormalities, right bundle branch pattern, atrial arrhythmias, S1Q3T3 (S wave in I, Q wave in III, inverted T wave in III—not common but highly specific).
- *Echocardiogram.* Transthoracic study done at bedside can detect signs of PE but cannot image the pulmonary arteries directly: evaluate for right heart strain (dilation, septal flattening), overall function, intra-atrial thrombus. Transesophageal study (TEE) can directly image the pulmonary arteries and atria.
- *Pulmonary angiography*: may be used to further evaluate clot extent and location.
- CTPA is the diagnostic test of choice for pulmonary embolism.

Stratification of early risk of death from PE

- *Low-risk PE.* Embolus identified without presence of shock/hypotension, RV dysfunction, or myocardial injury (positive troponin). Low-molecular weight heparin, unfractionated heparin infusion, or fondaparinux treatment with transition to long term oral anticoagulation.
- *Intermediate-risk PE.* Embolus present with RV dysfunction and/or myocardial injury, but without shock or hypotension. Options include unfractionated heparin infusion, low-molecular weight heparin or fondaparinux treatment, with transition to long term oral anticoagulation.
- *High-risk PE.* Presence of hemodynamic compromise (shock or hypotension) and RV dysfunction. Heparin infusion with thrombolysis or embolectomy. Risk of imminent death is ~10%, 30-day risk is ~30%.

Regardless of the risk stratification of a pulmonary embolism, it is critical to recognize this condition and initiate anticoagulation promptly. In the case of high-risk embolism, aggressive management and intensive observation is warranted. Survival rate decreases sharply if a patient requires cardiopulmonary resuscitation (CPR). In one study, patients who required CPR demonstrated mortality of 57% compared with 12% in patients who never required CPR.

Index scenario (additional information)
"Heparin infusion is initiated immediately. Echocardiogram is obtained and shows moderate dilation of the right ventricle with floating thrombus in the right atrium. The patient's clinical condition deteriorates shortly after the study is obtained: Blood pressure 78/52, heart rate 132/min, increasing dyspnea with oxygen saturations of 84%

on 100% O2 by nonrebreather mask. What are the options for management?"

Treatment/management

Hemodynamic compromise automatically classifies this as a high-risk pulmonary embolism and intervention is indicated. The recommended treatment is heparin infusion plus thrombolysis or embolectomy. Systemic administration of thrombolytic agent reduces the risk of death in patients with acute PE exhibiting signs of shock, but there is a significant risk of bleeding. Absolute contraindications to systemic thrombolysis include:

1) *Stroke*. Any history of hemorrhagic stroke or stroke of unknown origin, ischemic stroke in the past six months.
2) Central nervous system neoplasm.
3) *Past three weeks*: major trauma, surgery, or head injury.

Additionally, approximately 8% of patients who receive thrombolysis fail this treatment and continue to experience hemodynamic instability with persistent clot burden. In hemodynamically compromised patients with absolute contraindications to thrombolysis or a failed attempt at systemic thrombolysis, surgical intervention should be considered. Patients who have already experienced a code event (pulseless electrical activity or other arrhythmia) have higher mortality rates than those who are hemodynamically unstable but have not experienced PEA. This has led some to advocate more aggressive approach to hemodynamically unstable patients with PE, and even consideration of surgical intervention for intermediate-risk patients without hypotension but already with right ventricular dysfunction and significant clot burden if there is a contraindication to early thrombolysis.

Catheter-based embolectomy has been used in place of surgical intervention in unstable patients with contraindication to systemic thrombolysis or failed attempt at systemic thrombolysis. At centers where this technique is available, it may be used as an alternative to open surgical procedure, but some concern remains that catheter based technique may cause fragmentation of proximal clot and showering to more distal arteries. This approach is highly dependent on the skill of the operator.

Another approach in the case of significant hemodynamic compromise and poor oxygenation is to utilize extracorporeal membrane oxygenation (ECMO) via peripheral cannulation. This provides support while heparin therapy takes place, and may be a viable alternative for poor surgical candidates or those whose burden of clot requires more time for resolution. It may be used as a backup for catheter-based embolectomy.

ECMO does not fully unload the RV and thus it will help with systemic perfusion but myocardial injury may persist until the clot burden is relieved.

Surgical embolectomy has been described in the literature with varying success rates, though there is little data comparing this strategy to medical management. A series of 47 patients by Leacche et al describes prompt surgical intervention in patients with large clot burden and contraindications to thrombolysis or failure of medical therapy. Operative mortality was 6% and 1-year survival was 86% for this series.

Operative steps
Goals – remove clot from pulmonary arteries, remove clot in transit in the right atrium, explore smaller segmental arteries to remove more distal clot.

- Large-bore IV access, arterial line, general endotracheal anesthesia, TEE probe in place, foley catheter.
- Evaluate extent of clot with TEE, examine right atrium and ventricle for clot in transit, evaluate for patent foramen ovale (PFO) as clot has been documented extruding through PFO during embolectomy. Some centers also use epicardial echo to locate emboli and determine cannulation sites.
- Median sternotomy, pericardial stay sutures.
- Heparinization, cannulation for cardiopulmonary bypass with attention to locations of emboli visualized on TEE.
- Normothermia as long as the thrombus is known to be in the main trunk of the PA. If more extensive thrombectomy is anticipated, cool patient depending on plan for circulatory arrest. Cardiac arrest is generally not necessary unless repair of PFO or ASD is needed.
- Longitudinal arteriotomy incision of main pulmonary artery (PA), may extend transversely onto right or left PA, some also perform arteriotomy of the right PA between the ascending aorta and the superior vena cava if preop evaluation indicated presence of clot accessible from this location.
- Removal of clot with suction and gallbladder stone forceps. Intermittent reduction in bypass flow aids visualization of emboli. In some cases with extensive clot distally in branch pulmonary arteries, circulatory arrest may be required to create a bloodless field. Prepare for this ahead of time.
- Removal of distal clot—methods vary; may use a choledochoscope to visualize distal clot, also reports of opening pleura and using gentle lung massage to evacuate clot (careful as this may cause pulmonary hemorrhage; not all centers advocate entering the pleura for this purpose).

- IVC filter placement within 24 hours of surgery if not placed intraoperatively. Some centers report using right atrial purse-string cannulation site to place the IVC filter after performing the embolectomy.

Table 57-1. Summary of treatment options for high-risk pulmonary embolism.

	Systemic thrombolysis	Catheter-based technique	Surgical embolectomy
Patient candidates	Poor operative candidates; no contraindications to thrombolysis	Poor operative candidates, proximal clot accessible via catheter, contraindication to systemic thrombolysis	Patients with high-risk emboli, significant proximal clot burden, contraindication to thrombolysis
Mortality rate*	7-30%	10-20%	14-27%
Major risks	Bleeding, failure of treatment in 8% with persistent clot burden	Distal showering of clot, damage to vessels from mechanical thrombectomy	Risks associated with bypass, sequelae of distal clot burden

* Mortality rate for acute massive pulmonary embolism with any management strategy is approximately 30% at one month after diagnosis.

Potential questions/alternative scenarios

"Chronic pulmonary embolism and pulmonary hypertension: A 58 yo man presents to clinic with chief complaint of progressive shortness of breath. Three years ago, he underwent hip surgery complicated by a large pulmonary embolus one month postoperatively and was treated with thrombolysis. He recovered from this event but over the past several months has had increasing dyspnea. Echocardiogram demonstrates pulmonary artery pressure of 64 mmHg. What are the next diagnostic steps?"

The patient presents with symptoms and echocardiogram findings consistent with chronic thromboembolic pulmonary hypertension (CTEPH). Approximately 1-5% of patients who experience acute pulmonary embolism go on to develop this complication, presenting with vague dyspnea and fatigue after initially recovering from the acute embolic event. Further workup includes pulmonary angiography to assess the location of the vasculopathy causing pulmonary hypertension. Right heart catheterization provides helpful hemodynamic information but wedge pressures may be difficult to obtain due to irregular contour of pulmonary arteries. Pulmonary function testing should be used to evaluate coexisting obstructive or restrictive lung disease, which if severe would steer away from surgical intervention.

If a patient is evaluated and felt to be a good candidate for surgery for CTEPH, there are some key differences between the surgical procedure for acute massive pulmonary embolus versus CTEPH. For patients with chronic disease, the intervention is a pulmonary artery endarterectomy with removal of thickened scar-like tissue from the vessel intima, in addition to removal of the gross thrombus which characterizes the procedure for acute PE. Pulmonary endarterectomy is performed under hypothermia with intermittent circulatory arrest to facilitate thorough removal of intraluminal fibrinous material and optimally reduce pulmonary hypertension. This procedure has a mortality rate of 4-7% when performed at high-volume centers.

"TEE performed just prior to pulmonary endarterectomy for CTEPH demonstrates moderate to severe tricuspid regurgitation. How should this be addressed?"
Many patients with CTEPH will exhibit some degree of tricuspid regurgitation. In general, once the pulmonary arterial pressure is reduced and the right ventricle is unloaded, the valvular insufficiency resolves. One option is to wean bypass support and evaluate valve function after the embolic burden is relieved, then repair the valve if regurgitation warrants this. Consider repair for severe
tricuspid regurge with structural damage to the tricuspid valve or annular dilation (> 40 mm).

"72 hours after pulmonary endarterectomy the patient is noted to have a diffuse opacity in the right middle and lower lobes."
Reperfusion syndrome occurs in 8-10 percent of patients after endarterectomy. Treatment is mainly supportive with ventilation and pressors as needed. Patients should be diuresed and FiO_2 should be weaned. Rarely iNO or ECMO are required. The syndrome tends to resolve after 7-10 days.

Pearls/pitfalls
- Diagnosis of PE with hemodynamic instability (shock, signs of RV dysfunction), contraindication to thrombolysis or failure of initial attempt at thrombolysis—consider surgical embolectomy.
- Chronic thromboembolic pulmonary hypertension—thorough endarterectomy can help reduce pulmonary hypertension and symptoms.

- Tricuspid regurgitation with CTEPH—repair usually not needed, regurgitation decreases as right ventricle remodels postoperatively.

Suggested readings

- Leacche M et al. Modern surgical treatment of massive pulmonary embolism: Results in 47 consecutive patients after rapid diagnosis and aggressive surgical approach. *Journal of Thoracic and Cardiovascular Surgery* 2005; 129: 1018-1023.
- Madani MM, Jamieson SW. Pulmonary Endarterectomy for Chronic Thromboembolic Disease. *Operative Techniques in Thoracic and Cardiovascular Surgery.* 2006; 264-274.

Notes

58. Pericardial disease/pericardiectomy

Vakhtang Tchantchaleishvili, MD, and Peter A. Knight, MD

Concept
- Causes of chronic pericardial disease
- Pathophysiology, physical findings and diagnostic workup
- Operative indication
- Critical operative steps
- Alternative scenarios
- Pearls/pitfalls

Chief complaint

"A 67 yo man who was treated for stage II thymoma, including thymectomy done two years ago by you returns with fatigue, dyspnea on exertion, and peripheral edema."

Differential

Radiation-induced chronic pericarditis, congestive heart failure, restrictive cardiomyopathy, recurrence of malignancy

History and physical

Inquire about duration, progression and severity of symptoms. Inquire about dyspnea at rest or orthopnea. Ask about risk factors for constrictive pericarditis such as history of acute pericarditis, infections, renal failure, lupus, rheumatoid arthritis, radiation, prior MI, trauma or cardiac surgery. On physical examination, look for evidence of decreased atrial filling and elevated RV diastolic pressure - jugular venous distention, hepatomegaly, peripheral edema, ascites, decreased breath sounds (effusions) and pericardial knock (early rapid ventricular filling with elevated pressures during diastole - "S3").

Tests

Purpose of these tests are to confirm the diagnosis of constrictive pericardial disease and differentiate it from restrictive myocardial disease. The later is treated by transplantation and not pericardial stripping. The CT scan/MRI/echo showing pathology of the surrounding pericardium often gives the most valuable information for making this distinction. The physiology of constrictive pericarditis becomes evident on cardiac catheterization, echo or physical exam. The primary problem is decreased atrial and ventricular compliance. This "stiffness" results in higher atrial pressures with rapid filling of the ventricle during diastole. The stiff ventricles give off an audible S3 during diastole. On cardiac catheterization the ventricular pressure readings show a classic square root sign (rise in ventricular pressure at end diastole). During inspiration the preferential inflow to the right heart over the left is met with increased RV stiffness leading to the classic bowing of the RV to the LV seen on echo. This discordance shows up on catheter derived pressure tracings.

- *CXR*: pericardial calcification (40%) or signs of compression.
- *CT scan or MRI*: (90% sensitivity) helpful in visualizing thickened and/or calcified pericardium.
- *EKG*: non-specific ST-T changes.
- *Echo*: constrictive physiology = bowing of the interventricular septum to the left with inspiration, thickened pericardium.
- *Cardiac catheterization pressure readings suggestive of constrictive pericarditis*: square root sign, RV end diastolic pressure greater than 1/3 of the RV systolic pressure, equalization of pressures across the atria during diastole, equalization of pressures across the ventricles during end diastole (except during inspiration).
- *Distinguishing features of restrictive disease*: small or normal size heart, reduced LV function, pulmonary and hepatic congestion, prominent x and y descents on atrial pressure readings. If diagnosis is still in doubt, endomyocardial biopsy or ultimately mini-exploratory thoracotomy with inspection of the pericardium. BNP levels are not elevated with constrictive pericardial disease, but may be significantly increased with restrictive cardiomyopathy.

Index scenario (additional information)
"The patient had radiation in addition to thymectomy. His fatigue and dyspnea on exertion has been going on for several months. Recently he developed peripheral edema. Jugular venous distension is noted. On physical exam, there is systolic retraction and a pericardial knock. CXR demonstrates pericardial calcification. There are nonspecific ST-T changes on EKG. Right and left heart catheterization shows a square root sign, elevated RV end diastolic pressures with equalization of right and left atrial pressures during diastole. How do you proceed?"

Treatment/management
The patient has a radiation-induced chronic constrictive pericarditis. The basis of the disease is formation of pericardial scar from a wide range of pathologic processes (infectious, postoperative, therapeutic radiation), which results in compromised filling of the ventricles and leads to venous congestion and low cardiac output. Surgery is curative for constrictive pericarditis, thus the diagnosis in the setting of symptoms is a general indication for pericardial stripping. As mentioned, it is imperative to differentiate constrictive pericardial disease from restrictive cardiomyopathy which, despite similar clinical presentation, is not an indication for pericardial stripping. Notably in some cases like radiation-induced heart disease, there may be a concurrent presence of both

451

conditions. If only minimally symptomatic from constrictive pericardial disease, patients with serious concomitant disease may forgo surgery. Although surgery improves or alleviates symptoms in vast majority of patients, long term survival is diminished in patients with radiation induced constrictive pericarditis.

Operative steps
Goals – excise the pericardium from phrenic nerve to phrenic nerve anteriorly, diaphragm, AV groove and around the entrance of caval/pulmonary veins posteriorly.

- Median sternotomy is used most commonly, however some surgeons prefer a thoracotomy approach.
- You can begin the dissection on the right but cardiopulmonary bypass is often needed for resection of the left sided heart structures.
- After developing a plane on the left side of the heart and freeing up the diaphragm it helps to retract the heart towards the right in order to dissect out the left sided pulmonary veins. Release as much as you can posteriorly along the AV groove but be careful not to injure the esophagus. Check for the TEE probe and stay clear of it.
- The lack of surgical plane can lead to significant blood loss, epicardial coronary vessels and major venous structures are at risk of damage during the dissection (see Chapter 29, Vascular injuries).
- Complete pericardial resection may not always be possible, especially in cases of radiation induced pericardial disease and small islands of pericardium can be left behind especially over the coronaries.

Potential questions/alternative scenarios
"You begin dissecting the right atrium and start getting small tears that you are able to oversew. You've lost nearly 500 mL from the atrial dissection alone and still do not have it well exposed. You experience too much hypotension to perform the left sided dissection safely. What is your cannulation strategy?"

Always have your cannulation strategy in mind prior to starting a pericardiectomy. Bypass is not always necessary and it is hard to predict when it is. In this case, keep manual pressure over the atrial tear while you work on getting aortic access for cannulation. Once the aorta is exposed heparinize, cannulate the aorta and cannulate the atrium through the tear. Once the procedure is complete, switch to bicaval cannulation and repair the tear with a patch if needed. If you cannot expose the aorta and cannot control the tear with manual pressure then heparinize, dissect out the groin and cannulate the femoral vessels. These procedures can be difficult. Have blood available and the groins well marked prior to starting. Having the groin vessels exposed is not an unreasonable approach if you anticipate a particularly hazardous dissection.

"The patient was found to have constrictive pericardial disease. He has some fatigue but minimally decreased exercise tolerance, and no edema. He also has advanced COPD, chronic renal insufficiency, and a history of stroke with residual deficits. How would you proceed?"
Given patient's serious concomitant disease, the operation can be delayed until more significant symptoms develop from his pericardial disease.

"The patient who is status post CABG 6 weeks ago presents to your clinic for postoperative follow-up. He has a significant dyspnea. His exercise tolerance, which initially improved after the surgery, has been worsening again. How do you proceed?"
Perform a physical exam, EKG, chest X-ray, and echo.

"Your workup demonstrated constrictive pericarditis. You take the patient to OR for pericardiectomy, however during the operation you enter one of the bypass grafts. How do you proceed?"
Go on cardiopulmonary bypass, be aware of the territory the graft supplies and its significance. Check the EKG and hemodynamics for changes. Depending on the extent of the injury and hemodynamics you could give partial dose heparin, clamp the graft and do a primary repair. Alternatively you can do an interposition graft with vein or go on CPB, arrest the heart and do a completely new bypass.

"The patient has a remote history of lymphoma. His workup shows constrictive pericardial disease. You take him to the operating room and find large implants on the pericardium which were not visualized on preoperative imaging. How would you proceed?"
Remove a diagnostic sample of the pericardium and send for frozen pathology.

"Frozen pathology results are concerning for malignancy."
Abort the operation and refer the patient to oncologist.

Pearls/pitfalls
- Early clinical symptoms of constrictive pericarditis include dyspnea, fatigue, decreased exercise tolerance. Late symptoms include peripheral edema, hepatic congestion and ascites. May see "square root sign" on cardiac catheterization.
- Physical examination can reveal jugular venous distention, peripheral edema, and pericardial knock.

- With diagnostic tests, look for for constrictive physiology on echocardiography, thickened and/or calcified pericardium on CT/MRI, equal end-diastolic pressures in heart chambers on cardiac catheterization.
- Pericardial stripping is curative and either completely alleviates or significantly reduces the symptoms.
- Median sternotomy is the most commonly used operative approach, however a thoracotomy can be used as well.
- Cardiopulmonary bypass is not necessary, but may be needed. Thus, OR with cardiopulmonary bypass capability is preferred and have cannulation options in mind ahead of time.
- The lack of surgical plane can lead to significant bleeding, epicardial coronary vessels are at risk of damage as are major venous structures (see Chapter 29, Vascular injuries).
- Long term survival is diminished in patients with radiation induced constrictive pericarditis.

Suggested readings

- Cho YH, Schaff HV. Surgery for pericardial disease. Heart Fail Rev. 2012 Aug 15.
- Napolitano G, Pressacco J, Paquet E. Imaging features of constrictive pericarditis: beyond pericardial thickening. Can Assoc Radiol J. 2009 Feb;60(1):40-6.
- Leya FS, Arab D, Joyal D, et al. The efficacy of brain natriuretic peptide levels in differentiating constrictive pericarditis from restrictive cardiomyopathy. J Am Coll Cardiol. 2005 Jun 7;45(11):1900-2.

Notes

III. Congenital Cardiac Surgery

59. Patent ductus arteriosus

Kristopher B. Deatrick, MD, and Richard G. Ohye, MD

Concept
- Presentation of PDA
- Diagnostic methods
- Medical and surgical treatment options
- Indications for surgery
- Conduct of the operation and pitfalls

Chief complaint
"An infant born at 28 1/7 weeks estimated gestational age with a weight of 1100 g is admitted to the neonatal intensive care unit for treatment of respiratory distress syndrome with mechanical ventilation and multiple doses of surfactant. Her ventilator course has been characterized by persistent inability to wean. She is noted to have a continuous murmur."

Differential
Aortopulmonary window, truncus arteriosus, atrial septal defect, ventricular septal defect, Tetralogy of Fallot, Pulmonary stenosis

History and physical
Suspicion of a PDA is based upon the presence of a continuous murmur, the low birth weight and the early gestational age. Hemodynamically significant PDAs may be present in up to 45 percent of infants with a birthweight of less than 1750 g and up to 85 percent of infants with a birthweight of less than 1200g. Respiratory failure, pulmonary edema and inability to wean from mechanical ventilation may also be present. Physical examination should focus on the presence of murmurs, with the classic "machinery-like" holosystolic murmur being most characteristic. Infants presenting with PDA may also have signs of congestive heart failure, tachypnea, recurrent respiratory infections and failure to thrive.

Tests
- *CXR.* Presence of concomitant pulmonary disease, evidence of pulmonary overcirculation (increased pulmonary vascular markings, pulmonary edema).
- *Echocardiogram.* Presence of patent ductus arteriosus (PDA), direction of flow, degree of shunting, size and function of chambers, presence of associated intracardiac defects. Exclusion of other lesions is essential so as not to close a physiologically necessary left-to-right or right-to-left shunt.

- *Cardiac catheterization*: reserved for device closure or in older children with suspected right to left shunting to determine reversibility of pulmonary hypertension.

Index scenario (additional scenario)

"The patient is noted to have a regular rate and rhythm with a normal S1 and S2. She has a grade 2 out of 6 continuous systolic murmur heard best at the left upper sternal border, radiating towards her midclavicular line. A CXR shows bilateral hazy opacities consistent with respiratory distress syndrome. The cardiac silhouette is normal. The echocardiogram shows a large patent ductus arteriosus with left-to-right flow in both systole and diastole, and a mildly dilated left atrium. There is normal left ventricular size and hyperdynamic systolic function. No other intracardiac defects are noted."

Treatment/management

A PDA may be closed medically, via percutaneous transcatheter intervention (infants > 5 kg), or by open or minimally invasive surgical ligation. Closure by any of these methods is indicated in children with a hemodynamically significant PDA (significant shunt [Qp:Qs > 1.2] and/or evidence of pulmonary overcirculation). Ninety percent of PDAs are hemodynamically insignificant and will close by 8 weeks. Approximately 1 in 2000 infants will have persistent ductal flow. Even small, asymptomatic PDAs are at risk of causing endocarditis and should be closed. Medical closure is the first line of treatment in neonates and infants. This usually is accomplished with indomethacin (0.2 mg/kg infused over 20 minutes and repeated at 12 and 24 hours). Indomethicin acts by blocking the action of endogenous prostaglandins. Indomethacin treatment is usually given in combination with diuresis and fluid restriction, if there are symptoms of heart failure and volume overload. Up to 80% of premature infants will have successful closure of the PDA with medical treatment. It is rarely successful in full term infants. Side effects of indomethacin include impaired renal function, impaired platelet aggregation and impaired host defenses. Contraindications to treatment with indomethacin include sepsis, renal failure, and known bleeding disorders.

If medication fails or is contraindicated, surgical or percutaneous closure should be undertaken for all hemodynamically significant PDAs. Percutaneous closure with coils or the Amplatzer Occlude (St. Jude Medical, St. Paul, MN) is commonly used except in patients with PDA > 4 mm in diameter, pulmonary hypertension with right-to-left shunting, and weight < 5 kg (small femoral vessels). Thus, due to size restrictions, percutaneous closure is generally not indicated in neonates. In the present scenario, the failure of respiratory improvement and failure to wean from mechanical ventilation are due to a clinically significant PDA and surgical closure should be undertaken.

Operative steps

PDA ligation in premature infants with left sided arch

- General endotracheal anesthesia through a single lumen endotracheal tube.
- Left posterolateral thoracotomy at third or fourth interspace.
- Retract lung anteriorly.
- Open the mediastinal pleura and reflect it anteriorly and posteriorly.
- Division of the the left superior intercostal vein may aid the exposure.
- Identify the ductus just opposite to the left subclavian artery (LSCA). Knowledge of the location of the left pulmonary artery, descending aorta, aortic arch, LSCA, and recurrent laryngeal nerve is a critical part of the operation since most misadventures result from inadvertent ligation of structures other than the PDA.
- Avoid cautery near the recurrent laryngeal nerve and take great care to ensure that you do not clamp the recurrent laryngeal nerve.
- Avoid unnecessary dissection around the ductus. Life-threatening hemorrhage may result from tearing a friable ductus.
- Ultimately, the duct is divided either with a simple clip (< 10 mm duct), silk ligature or using small vascular clamps with suture ligation (short, wide ducts > 10 mm).
- Prior to dividing the duct, temporarily occlude it with forceps. This should be followed by an augmentation of the diastolic pressure, with continued pulsatility in the aorta. An esophageal stethoscope used by the anesthesiologist may be helpful to identify loss of the murmur.

Potential questions/alternative scenarios

"The patient is noted to have a calcified ductus. How should surgical closure be approached?"

This can be hazardous and is the type of case that may have been best served with transcatheter occlusion. In the operating room, it is safest to approach the PDA via median sternotomy using CPB. After CPB is initiated, ductal flow can be controlled initially by inverting the anterior wall of the main pulmonary artery against the ductus while cooling to 28-32° C. Low-flow CPB can then be instituted and the MPA opened. The opening of the ductus is then patched closed with PTFE. Care must be taken to prevent the entrainment of air into the systemic circulation. A brief period of deep hypothermic circulatory arrest may be necessary.

"The test occlusion is performed and the patient becomes hypotensive, bradycardic, and the SpO2 begins to fall. What is the likely cause and what is your strategy?"

First ensure that you have not clamped the aorta or the left main PA. Release the clamp and resuscitate as needed. Make sure you clearly see the LSCA, ductus, aortic arch, descending aorta and left PA. If you confirm that you have clamped the ductus, then this patient may have a ductal dependent systemic circulation and further diagnosis is required.

"A PDA is identified in a previously asymptomatic adult. Is closure indicated? How will you proceed?"

A PDA in an adult should be closed. There is a risk of endocarditis even in clinically insignificant PDAs. Any PDA that becomes symptomatic should be closed. Transcatheter closure is ideal if feasible.

"An aneurysmal PDA is detected in a patient with a history of endocarditis on preoperative imaging."

Plan for a median sternotomy, CPB, and resection of the aneurysmal ductus. In the absence of dense left pleural adhesions, a left thoracotomy with left heart bypass would be an acceptable alternative.

"As you clamp and divide the PDA through a left thoracotomy a tear develops in the left PA with severe hemorrhage."

This is an uncommon event, but you should anticipate this if the duct is wide and friable. Obtain local hemostasis with direct digital pressure. Heparinize and cannulate the descending aorta and left atrium. Once on CPB the hemorrhage should significantly decrease allowing you to close the defect in the PA.

"Post operatively, you notice an elevated left hemidiaphragm."

This is due to left phrenic nerve damage. Conservative management should be attempted first since these injuries often represent blunt trauma or stunning of the nerve from nearby cautery rather than complete avulsion or transection. An US showing lack of diaphragmatic movement is a poor prognostic sign. If hemidiaphragm paresis is persistent and impairs the patient's ventilatory status, reoperation with diaphragmatic plication is indicated.

"The patient has persistent milky white chest tube output after 5 days of conservative management."

Chylothorax is a risk of PDA ligation due to lymphatic channels near the aortic arch and around the PDA. It is rare for the actual thoracic duct to be ligated or injured. A conservative trial of observation is not unreasonable, as many will stop spontaneously. A low fat diet, a trial of NPO, or octreotide infusion may be attempted.. Some would return to the

OR sooner as the culprit lesions may be easier to identify earlier rather than later in the postoperative period. Most often you will enter the same left thoracotomy site. An alternative would be a right thoracotomy with supradiaphragmatic mass ligation of the thoracic duct (see Chapter 14, Chylothorax).

Pearls/pitfalls

- PDA is common, affecting between 1 in 1200 and 1 in 5000 births.
- Physiologic closure may fail in neonates due to lack of normal O2 tension, decreased sensitivity to signals for closure, and increased sensitivity to vasodilators.
- Medical closure is highly successful and is first-line therapy for most neonates.
- Decision for surgical closure in a neonate is based on symptoms and hemodynamic significance.
- Closure can be accomplished via a limited thoracotomy and often at the bedside in the neonatal intensive care unit.
- Attempted medical closure (Indomethacin, 0.2 mg/kg, 3 doses) is indicated for all *neonatal* PDA unless there is a contraindication.
- Elective closure of even small PDAs should be undertaken due to the late risk of bacterial endocarditis.
- Before attempting any closure, the presence of ductal dependent circulation must be excluded.
- Complications usually result from injury to surrounding structures during dissection including: left recurrent laryngeal nerve, lymphatics, phrenic nerve, transverse aortic arch, descending thoracic aorta, left main pulmonary artery.
- Knowledge of surrounding structures is critical, as the PDA may be larger than the aortic arch in some cases.

Suggested readings

- Khonsari S., Sintek C. Patent Ductus Arteriosus. Khonsari S., Sintek C., (eds).*Cardiac Surgery: Safeguards and Pitfalls in Operative Technique.* 4th ed. Philadelphia, PA: Lippincott Williams and Wilkins, 2008: 201-208.
- Tsang, V.T., Stark, J. Persistent Ductus Arteriosus. Tsang, V.T., Stark, J. (eds.) *Surgery for Congenital Heart Defects.* 3rd ed., West Sussex, England: John Wiley & Sons, Ltd, 2006: 275-284.
- Tsia T., Wu J.J., Ringel R. Patent Ductus Arteriosus. Yuh D.D., Vricella L.A., Baumgartner W.A. (eds). *The Johns Hopkins Manual of Cardiothoracic Surgery.* New York, NY: The McGraw-Hill Companies, Inc.: 2007: 1049-1056.

Notes

461

60. Atrial septal defects

William Stein, MD, and Brian Kogon, MD

Concept

- Indications for surgical repair of ASD
- Preoperative evaluation of patients with ASD
- Surgical management of secundum and sinus venosus ASDs

Chief complaint

"A 7 yo boy with reduced exercise tolerance is referred to you by a pediatric cardiologist for evaluation after an atrial septal defect (ASD) was identified on a transthoracic echo."

Differential

The diagnosis has already been made in this patient. The type and size of defect and the presence of any other associated cardiac malformations should be determined as described below.

History and physical

A focused history and physical should be performed to assist in determining the degree of shunting through the ASD. Symptoms of pulmonary overcirculation such as respiratory infections, dyspnea on exertion, and failure to thrive should be discussed. A past history of arrhythmias or paradoxical emboli should be elicited. The physical exam in these patients is typically non-revealing. However, the presence of a fixed split second heart sound, a soft systolic flow murmur over the pulmonary valve, and a left parasternal lift can be indicative of a larger Qp:Qs.

Tests

- *CXR*. The size of the cardiac silhouette and increased pulmonary vasculature is proportional to the amount of shunting across the ASD. The presence of anomalous pulmonary veins can be seen as extra vascular markings in the right hilar region.
- *Transthoracic echo (TTE)*. Two dimensional TTE is the diagnostic modality of choice for ASDs. Images with microcavitation injection ("bubble study") may be helpful. Detection rates for secundum ASDs is nearly 100%. The detection rate for sinus venosus ASDs is approximately 70%. Transesophageal echo (TEE) has a nearly 100% detection rate for sinus venosus ASDs. Qp:Qs can be estimated by echo as well.
- *EKG*. Although not essential for diagnosis, will typically show evidence of RV hypertrophy.

- *Cardiac catheterization.* Cardiac catheterizations are not typically needed for uncomplicated ASDs. Three situations in which a cardiac catheterization may be necessary are the presence of severe heart failure, concern for pulmonary hypertension, or the failure to adequately define the anatomy by either TTE or TEE.
- *Cardiac MRI or CT.* Not indicated in the management of uncomplicated ASDs, however, may be useful in identifying anomalous venous drainage in sinus venosus ASDs.

Index scenario (additional information)

"The child's history is significant for occasional dyspnea at recess and a chronic cough. He also has an iodine allergy. On physical he is a well appearing child that is in the 45th percentile for height and weight. His physical exam is notable for a fixed split second heart sound. A review of the TTE reveals a 20 mm secundum ASD, a Qp:Qs of 1.7:1, and no evidence of pulmonary hypertension."

Treatment/management

This child meets the criteria for surgical closure of his ASD. The three options for management of secundum ASDs include observation, catheter based closure, and surgical closure. Observation is appropriate for small asymptomatic ASDs (< 8 mm) with a Qp:Qs of less than 1.5:1. Regardless of size, if the shunt is larger than 1.2:1, the child is symptomatic, and/or the ASD fails to close by 3-5 years of age then intervention is warranted to extend survival. Similar recommendations are made for adults with a shunt > 1.5:1 or evidence of prior stroke or embolic events. The decision to undergo surgical closure should be made prior to the development of symptoms and prior to beginning school. Catheter based treatments are acceptable for closure of uncomplicated ASDs. They should not be used for patients with large defects (> 38 mm), those with insufficient rims especially in the subaortic region, primum or sinus venosus ASDs, patients with pulmonary hypertension or those where deployment would potentially interfere with AV valve function or coronary sinus drainage.

Operative steps

- Typically performed through a partial or complete median sternotomy.
- Standard aortic cannulation and bicaval venous cannulation is performed after the administration of heparin. Caval snares are placed around the SVC and IVC.
- A cardioplegia catheter is placed in the ascending aorta. After the cross clamp is applied, a single dose of antegrade cardioplegia is given and the caval snares are tightened.

- An oblique incision is made in the right atrium and the anatomy is examined paying particular
- attention to the relative locations of the coronary sinus, tricuspid and mitral valves (evaluate for cleft if primum ASD), and the pulmonary veins, as well as the presence of a second defect.
- The defect is closed with a piece of autologous pericardium with/ without fixation in 0.6% gluteraldehyde or Gore-Tex® using a running prolene. The left atrium is deaired prior to completing the suture line. The cardioplegia catheter is converted to an aortic vent and the cross clamp is removed.
- The right atrium is closed in two layers and the caval snares are removed.
- After the heart is deaired the patient is weaned from bypass, and the patch is inspected via TEE.

Potential questions/alternative scenarios

"Preoperative TTE reveals that the ASD is located at the superior aspect of the septum near the SVC. How would you proceed?"

This situation is concerning for a sinus venosus ASD and during examination of the ASD in the OR the presence of PAPVR must be determined. Preoperatively, if the TTE is not diagnostic then a TEE would be helpful. Patient with sinus venosus ASD and PAPVR tend to have higher Qp:Qs and are symptomatic at an earlier stage than secundum ASDs. Closure of SV ASDs with PAPVR require the creation of a baffle of autologous pericardium directing pulmonary blood through the ASD into the left atrium. This can be accomplished through a right atrial incision, a superior vena caval incision, or through an incision crossing the RA-SVC junction lateral to the region of the SA node. If the SVC is large, the ASD may be closed primarily with a running suture. To prevent the development of an SVC syndrome due to narrowing of the RA-SVC junction, a second patch of autologous pericardium can be incorporated into the right atrial suture line. Regardless, care should be taken to avoid narrowing of either the systemic or pulmonary venous drainages into their respective atria.

For a SV ASD with anomalous pulmonary veins that drain particularly high onto the SVC, creating this baffle can be challenging. Instead, a Warden procedure can be performed. This entails transecting the SVC above the highest anomalous pulmonary vein. The cardiac end of the SVC is over-sewn and the entire SVC/RA orifice is baffled across the ASD in order to close the defect and correct the PAPVR. The cephalad end of the SVC is then anastomosed the RA appendage to re-establish appropriate systemic venous drainage.

"A 4 yo boy is referred after a TTE revealed a 2 mm patent foramen ovale with left to right shunting. The echo is otherwise normal. He is asymptomatic. How would you proceed?"

The echo is diagnostic of a patent foramen ovale. They occur due to failure of the septum primum and secundum to fuse after birth. In the absence of symptoms there are currently no indications for closure. The presence of a right to left shunt, cryptogenic stroke, or the need for other cardiac surgery are the current scenarios in which closure should be considered.

Pearls/pitfalls

- The preferred diagnostic modality is a 2D transthoracic echo, not catheterization or cardiac CT. The alternative modalities are only necessary if there is inadequate visualization via echo.
- Uncomplicated ASDs should be repaired if they fail to close by 3-5 years old and have a Qp:Qs greater than 1.2:1.
- Sinus venosus ASDs are frequently associated with anomalous pulmonary veins. When repairing these defects pulmonary venous flow must be redirected into the left atrium and the SVC should be augmented as needed to prevent development of a SVC syndrome.

Suggested readings

- Troise D et al. Atrial septal defects and partial anomalous pulmonary venous connections. Yuh D, Vricella LA, and Baumgartner WA (eds). Johns Hopkins Manual of Cardiothoracic Surgery. 2007; 1057-1076.
- Bichell D and Christian K. Atrial septal defect and cor triatrium. Del Nido PJ, and Swanson SJ (eds) Sabiston and Spencer - Surgery of the Chest. 2010; 1797-1816.
- Turbendian H and Chen H. Atrial septal defects. Franco K and Thourani V (eds.) Cardiothoracic Surgery Review. 2011.

Notes

61. Anomalous pulmonary venous return
Eric Griffiths, MD, and James Gangemi, MD

Concept
- Initial management
- Preoperative considerations
- Operative interventions
- Critical steps of repair
- Pitfalls and alternative solutions

Chief complaint
"A 4 day old baby boy with cyanosis, hypoxemia and respiratory distress is found on echocardiogram to have total anomalous pulmonary venous return."

Differential
See differential for cyanotic heart disease (see Chapter 66, Transposition of the great arteries). Although the diagnosis has been established in this case, important information regarding the defect is required.

History and physical
A focused history should aim to identify symptoms of congestive heart failure (failure to thrive, feeding intolerance). Physical exam should focus on vitals, degree of cyanosis and evidence of CHF, or other physical abnormalities.

Tests
Echocardiography (essential information needed)
- *Anatomical diagnosis*: total anomalous pulmonary venous connection (TAPVC) versus partial anomalous pulmonary venous connection (PAPVC).
- TAPVC.
- Location of venous confluence and systemic venous connection.
  - Supracardiac (45%) vs. cardiac (25%) vs. infracardiac (25%).
- Presence and location of shunt(s).
  - Survival is dependent on a right-to-left shunt which is almost always a nonrestrictive PFO.
  - *Evidence of obstruction*: color Doppler demonstrating turbulent flow in venous pathway is indicative of obstruction.
- Evidence of right heart overload.

CXR
- Evidence of pulmonary edema, older babies may have cardiomegaly.

Cardiac angiography
- Rarely performed.

MRI/CT
- May rarely be needed, most information obtained through echo. Though CT may provide better anatomical detail, MRI provides information regarding flow and velocity which can reveal differential lung perfusion and venous stenoses.

Index scenario (additional information)
"The baby has a supracardiac confluence of veins with evidence of obstruction."

Treatment/management
TAPVC
Limited options for preoperative medical management. Patients requiring resuscitation should be intubated, kept on low oxygen settings and high PEEP to decrease pulmonary blood flow and limit pulmonary edema. Inotropes should be used as necessary. Prostaglandins and pulmonary vasodilators should be avoided.
- *TAPVR with obstruction*: surgical emergency
- *TAPVR without obstruction*: may optimize with diuretics and supplemental oxygen, proceed with early elective repair

Operative steps
Goals – identify the anomalous connection and reroute flow to the left atrium (LA). Close the interatrial connection (PFO/ASD).
- Cardiopulmonary bypass often with DHCA.
  - Single arterial and venous cannula (bicaval cannulation optional).
  - Ligate PDA if present.
- *Supra and infracardiac venous confluence*: direct anastomosis to left atrium.
- *Cardiac venous confluence*: unroofing of the coronary sinus. Make an incision that unites the ASD and coronary sinus ostia. Then place a patch over the whole defect so that the sinus drains directly into LA.

- *Sutureless repair*: Anastomotic stricture is a serious concern for TAPVR procedures. Sutureless repair is used for small veins or obstruction at venous confluence.
  - LA is incised as well as the pulmonary veins including areas of obstruction or narrowing.
  - LA sutured to the pericardium adjacent to the pulmonary veins with continuous suture line.
  - Creates a "controlled bleed" into the LA.

Potential questions/alternative scenarios

"Postoperatively, the baby has difficulty weaning from ventilator, CXR shows right pleural effusion and congestion."
This patient likely has an obstruction at the anastomosis of the right veins. Obtain an echo (transthoracic) to evaluate the right sided pulmonary venous return. Consider contrast enhanced MRI, CTA of the heart, or possibly catheterization to look for obstruction. May need surgical revision with sutureless technique (see above).

"A 6 month old baby boy with failure to thrive is found to have drainage of the right upper pulmonary vein into the superior vena cava with an associated atrial septal defect."
This patient has a sinus venosus ASD with partial anomalous venous return (PAPVC). Other forms of PAPVC include PAPVC to SVC without ASD and Scimitar syndrome. Scimitar syndrome consists of right pulmonary veins draining into the IVC, anomalous arterial supply from the abdominal aorta, and often pulmonary sequestration. For these patients, the history and physical should focus on evidence of CHF, arrhythmias, failure to thrive, and paradoxical embolus. Treatment of PAPVC is discussed below.

Treatment/management

PAPVC
Evaluate for evidence of pulmonary hypertension (clinical, radiographic, or echocardiographic). PAPVR with ASD leads to excess volume load on the right heart and pulmonary over circulation which can result in irreversible pulmonary hypertension.
- If no pulmonary hypertension then proceed with repair.
- If pulmonary hypertension is present then proceed with cardiac catheterization to evaluate pulmonary vascular resistance (PVR).
  - *If normal*: proceed with surgical correction.
  - *If increased PVR but responsive to 100% O2 and/or inhaled nitric oxide*: proceed with surgical correction

.

- *If elevated PVR, not responsive (8-12 U/m2)*: may require ASD closure and lung transplant, or possible heart/lung transplant.

Operative steps
PAPVC with sinus venosus defect
- Median sternotomy, bicaval cannulation, caval tapes, superior right atriotomy.
- Intra atrial patch (bovine pericardium or autologous pericardium) used to baffle venous opening into left atrium.
- Second patch often used to close the opening over the superior cavoatrial junction.

Potential questions/alternative scenarios
"The venous confluence is too high on the SVC to baffle to left atrium."
Warden procedure: transect the SVC at the cavoatrial junction and relocate it to right atrial appendage, the pulmonary venous return is then baffled to left atrium through the ASD.

Pearls/pitfalls
- Obstructed TAPVC represents a surgical emergency.
- Limited role for medical management in TAPVC beyond intubation and inotropes. Prostaglandins and pulmonary vasodilators should be avoided.
- *Approach*: bicaval cannulation, DHCA may be used for better intraatrial visualization.
- Repair depends on site of confluence: supracardiac, cardiac, or infracardiac.
- Consider sutureless repair for small veins or obstruction at confluence.
- PAPVR requires evaluation for pulm HTN.
  - If pulmonary hypertension is suspected, proceed to cardiac catheterization to determine PVR (normal or reversible, may proceed with repair).
- Fixed PVR requires ASD closure and lung transplant, or possible heart/lung transplant.

Suggested readings
- Delisle G, Ando M, Calder AL, et al. Total anomalous pulmonary venous connection: report of 93 autopsied cases with emphasis on diagnostic and surgical considerations. *Am Heart J* 1976;91:99-122.

- Kang N and Tsang VT. Total anomalous pulmonary venous connection. Yuh D, Vricella LA, and Baumgartner WA (eds). *Johns Hopkins Manual of Cardiothoracic Surgery* 2007.
- Calderone CA.(2009, Oct 7) "Sutureless" pulmonary vein stenosis repair. Retrieved Dec 28, 2012 from http://www.ctsnet.org/sections/clinicalresources/congenital/expert_t ech-3.html.

Notes

62. Ventricular septal defects

George Dimeling, MD, and Olaf Reinhartz, MD

Concept

- Definition
- Morphology
- Natural history
- Treatment
- Pathophysiology
- Indications for surgery
- Surgical procedure

Chief complaint

"A 4 month old boy presents with poor feeding and growth failure. On physical exam he has a precordial pansystolic murmur. His EKG demonstrates biventricular hypertrophy. Cardiomegaly is evident on CXR."

Differential

VSD of any variety (Perimembranous, Muscular, Doubly Committed Subarterial, Inlet, or Malalignment), VSD associated with any cardiac anomaly (i.e., TOF, TGA), ASD

History and physical

Most VSD are small, restrictive and asymptomatic. Many of these will close spontaneously. Patients with larger and more clinically significant VSD may present with signs and symptoms of pulmonary overcirculation (tachypnea, poor feeding, growth failure, repeated respiratory infections). On exam patients may have a palpable thrill on the lower left sternal border with a loud high-frequency holosystolic murmur. The patient may be small for age and have evidence of pulmonary congestion on exam. Cyanosis in a patient with an isolated VSD can indicate Eisenmenger's physiology.

Tests

- *CXR.* May show increased pulmonary vascular markings with an enlarged heart.
- *Echocardiography.* The diagnostic gold standard for VSDs. Given the curved ventricular septum, multiple echo windows are required to determine the location and size of the defect. Color Doppler greatly enhances the sensitivity. The sensitivity approaches 100% for inlet and outlet defects, 80-90% for perimembranous defects, and 50% for trabecular/muscular lesions. Trabecular/muscular defects can be missed on exam due to differences in contractility,

equalization of ventricular pressure gradient, and there can be multiple defects obscured by the overlying trabecular muscle. The echo should give an estimation of ventricular function and RV systolic pressure. It should identify any associated cardiac anomalies (i.e., ASD, coarctation, PDA, TGA, TOF, etc.).

- *Cardiac catheterization*: indicated when echo and clinical findings suggest advanced pulmonary vascular disease. Catheterization allows calculation of Qp:Qs, PA pressures, PVR, response of high PVR to vasodilators such as inhaled nitric oxide and delineation of unclear anatomy.
- *EKG*: helpful for establishing the baseline rhythm prior to surgery.

Index scenario (additional information)
"Echo reveals a 10 mm perimembranous VSD with normal RV pressures and a left to right shunt."

Treatment/management
Spontaneous closure occurs at a rate inversely proportional to age. Eighty percent of VSDs at 1 month and fifty percent of VSDs at 6 months eventually close. Of the primary VSDs that do not close, eighty percent are perimembranous and border the tricuspid valve and conduction system. Thus, patients with small VSDs that are restrictive and asymptomatic may be followed. All asymptomatic residual VSDs > 3 mm after 2-3 years of age should be closed. If the patient is symptomatic (failure to thrive, symptoms of pulmonary overcirculation) then closure should be planned electively but soon. If the Qp:Qs is greater than 2:1 or the pulmonary vascular resistance is high (4 units/m² or greater) then closure is warranted. If the VSD is associated with aortic valve prolapse (with or without regurgitation), a history of endocarditis, or ventricular dilation, then the lesion should be repaired. All inlet or outlet VSDs should be fixed. In general, all VSDs found during another cardiac procedure should be fixed. Short of symptomatic VSDs, all other VSDs that meet an indication for repair should ideally wait until the child is between six months and one year old. Medical treatment attempts to decrease L-R shunting using diuretics, digitalis, and afterload reducing agents often as a prelude to surgery. If medical therapy is effective at reducing symptoms, it may enable the child to delay surgery until he or she is closer to six months of age.

Operative steps
Right atrial approach
- Supine, standard lines, shoulder roll, TEE.
- Median sternotomy.

- Resect or retract thymus, open pericardium +/- harvest pericardium for fixation and possible patch, suspend pericardium.
- Dissect between aorta and PA, evaluate for patent ductus arteriosus.
- Heparinize, aortic and bicaval cannulation. LV vent.
- Check ACT. Commence CPB. Dissect and ligate PDA if present. Allow temperature drift down.
- Place SVC and IVC occlusion tapes and snare.
- Place antegrade cardioplegia stitch and cannulate. Cross clamp and arrest.
- Oblique right atriotomy parallel to the AV groove.
- Place stay stitches in the atrium and tricuspid valve septal and anterior leaflets.
- Identify and measure the VSD. Trim patch material to desired size (Dacron or PTFE).
- Perform a running or interrupted patch repair. Rewarm.
- De-air prior to closing the defect (LV vent off to allow it to fill). Float tricuspid valve. Support anteroseptal commissure with a stitch if needed.
- Remove cross clamp. LV vent back on. Root vent on.
- Close atriotomy in running fashion.
- Check TEE for residual or other undetected VSDs, aortic insufficiency, tricuspid valve regurgitation, and function.

Potential questions/alternative scenarios

"A 6 mo old child is found to have multiple defects along the muscular septum. The Qp:Qs is > 2:1 and the shunt is left to right. How would you repair this defect?"
An uncommon but extreme example of multiple muscular VSDs is the so called "Swiss Cheese Deformity" which is best approached initially by pulmonary artery banding. Many of these defects will close over time.

"A 6 mo child has a conal (supracristal) defect. How will you approach it for closure?"
A transpulmonary approach is used most often. Exposure is via a longitudinal incision in the main pulmonary artery (MPA), extending nearly to the annulus. Patch closure is recommended to prevent injury to or distortion of the aortic valve. The MPA is closed primarily.

"A 1 yo child has an outlet VSD with AI."
Outlet VSD can cause the right aortic cusp to prolapse into the defect causing aortic insufficiency. In this setting surgery is indicated before permanent damage is sustained to the valve cusp or ventricular function.

"A 2 yo child presents with a large VSD and cyanosis."
Patients with cyanosis or right to left shunting on echo require a catheterization to investigate the degree of pulmonary vascular disease. If PVR is > 8-10 U/m^2 and Qp:Qs is < 1.3 then the child has pulmonary vasoconstriction. Check for reversibility with supplemental oxygen or inhaled nitric oxide (iNO). Reversibility is suggested if the Qp:Qs rises above 1.5:1 and the PVR drops below 8 U/m^2.

"Describe flow patterns across the VSD and how they affect Qp:Qs."
Flow through a VSD occurs during systole. Several factors of fluid dynamics contribute to flow through the defect and whether or not it is restrictive. An non-restrictive VSD is defined by equalization of pressures in the right and left ventricle. The difference between the systemic and pulmonary vascular resistance is the chief factor determining direction of flow through a VSD. In the setting of a non-restrictive VSD, the difference between the pulmonary and systemic vascular resistance will determine the Qp:Qs. In a restrictive VSD, the Qp:Qs will be determined by the sum of the PVR and the gradient across the VSD minus the SVR. The second factor determining flow is the size of the defect relative to the aortic annulus size. As the size of the VSD approaches or exceeds 50% of the aortic annulus size, the defect becomes non-restrictive. Other factors that play a role in flow are viscosity (hematocrit) and velocity (contractility).

"Describe the different types of VSD and their relative incidence."
VSD can be broadly defined as inlet, outlet, perimembranous and muscular. Clinically and conceptually it can be advantageous to classify VSD as those that are tissue deficient and those that are tissue sufficient. Five to ten percent are doubly committed subarterial VSD or "outlet/conotruncal" VSD and are bordered by the semilunar valves. Five percent of VSD are muscular and are further delineated by location relative to the right ventricle (i.e., outlet, trabecular, inlet, apical, or anterior). Less than 5% of VSD fall into the inlet type/AV cushion defects. Tissue deficient lesions include muscular, perimembranous, and endocardial cushion defects. Muscular defects occur in the trabecular muscle and are completely surrounded by muscle. A more common situation is a single muscular VSD that only requires clinical follow up and eventually closes. The other subcategory of VSD has sufficient tissue but is malaligned. In this set of lesions the infundibular septum and the muscular septum fail to grow in the same plane and are in near parallel planes. This occurs during the "looping" phase of development. In anterior malignment VSDs the infundibulum is anterior with respect to the muscular septum causing the LVOT to crowd the RVOT, this is frequently associated with Tetralogy of Fallot. Posterior Malalignment VSD are associated with interrupted aortic arch. Rotational VSD are seen

in the Taussig-Bing Heart where the infundibular septum and the muscular septum are in different non-parallel planes.Tissue deficient VSDs have the potential to close spontaneously, usually occurring between 6 months and 1 year of life. Depending on heart failure symptoms, these lesions can be watched for up to two years before an intervention is needed. Muscular VSDs are the most likely to close spontaneously as the ventricular muscle fills in the defect. Perimembranous VSDs may close spontaneously. Malalignment and rotational VSDs never close without intervention and should be repaired electively with in the first two years of life.

"Describe the relationship of the conduction system to the various types of VSDs."

Conal: remote.
Perimembranous (d-looped ventricles): posterior and inferior to defect. place sutures on RV side only.
Perimembranous (l-looped ventricles): anterior and superior to defect.
Inlet: apex of the triangle of Koch (formed by the TV annulus, the tendon of Todaro, and the orifice of the coronary sinus).
Muscular: remote.

Pearls/pitfalls
- The most common type of VSD encountered at surgery is perimembranous.
- The approach for supracristal VSDs is usually transpulmonary and patch repair is recommended.
- Medical treatment attempts to decrease L-R shunting by using diuretics, digitalis, and afterload reducing agents (typically ACE inhibitors) as a prelude to surgery.
- Knowledge of the expected location of the conduction system is critical.

Suggested readings
- Ventricular Septal Defect. Kouchoukos NT, Blackstone EH, Hanley FL, and Kirklin JK (eds). *Kirklin/Barratt-Boyes Cardiac Surgery, 4th ed.*1274-1325.
- Ventricular Septal Defect. Jonas RA. (ed). *Comprehensive Surgical Management of Congenital Heart Disease*: 242-255.
- Ventricular Septal Defects, Mavroudis C and Becker CL. *Pediatric Cardiac Surgery*. 298-320.

Notes

63. Atrioventricular canal defects

Walter F. DeNino, MD, and Minoo N. Kavarana, MD

Concept
- Classification of atrioventricular (AV) canal defect
- Preoperative considerations
- Methods of repair
- Critical steps in repair
- Pitfalls and alternative scenarios

Chief complaint

"The parents of a 3 month old boy infant present with their son. The baby was born with Down Syndrome and therefore followed by a cardiologist. At about 8 weeks of life, he began to have difficulty with feeding, appeared to be breathing 'quickly and shallowly', would occasionally sweat excessively and has fallen behind on the growth curve."

Differential

Atrial septal defect (ASD) with or without anomalous pulmonary venous drainage, ventricular septal defect (VSD), Tetralogy of Fallot (TOF), AV canal defect, cystic fibrosis

History and physical

Elicit signs and symptoms of congestive heart failure (including difficulty feeding, excessive sweating, failure to thrive, tachypnea, cyanosis) and/or pulmonary vascular disease. Pansystolic murmurs of variable grades may be found. 50% of children with Down syndrome have an AV canal defect and 75% of patients with complete AV canal have Down syndrome.

Tests

- *Echocardiogram*: presence and size of ASD and/or VSD. Degree of AV Valve (AVV) regurgitation as well as balance of the canal (right vs. left ventricle), morphology of the left AVV with respect to size of left lateral leaflet, number and spacing of papillary muscles, right ventricular outflow tract and pulmonary valve morphology. If AVV regurgitation is present, the degree and location should be noted. Presence of any other associated anomalies should also be noted.
- *CXR*: increased pulmonary markings, possible left atrial enlargement (see elevation of left mainstem bronchus).
- *EKG*: counterclockwise axis shift as Bundle of His displaced inferiorly (as opposed to clockwise axis shift in secundum ASD).

- *Right heart catheterization*: usually not indicated unless there is a concern regarding irreversible pulmonary hypertension.

"The ECHO demonstrates a complete AV canal defect."
Classification system
Partial (PAVC), transitional (TAVC) or complete AV canal (CAVC) [Rastelli A, B, C].
PAVC = primum ASD with complete cleft of the anterior leaflet of mitral valve.

Transitional = pressure restrictive inlet VSD. VSD ranges in size from point of continuity of septal leaflets of mitral and tricuspid valve to a larger VSD with dense chordal attachments from crest of ventricular septum to undersurface of superior and inferior common leaflets. In this type it is possible to see two separate AV valve orifices. Loss of ventricular component of AV septum displaces the hinge plane of the mitral and tricuspid valves apically, thus increasing the length of the LVOT. This lengthening is otherwise referred to as a "gooseneck deformity."

Complete AV canal (CAVC) is defined as an AV canal defect with a primum ASD, inlet VSD and a single AV valve orifice. They are classified according to the Rastelli classification which is based on the morphology of the superior bridging leaflet, the degree of bridging and the nature and position of chordal attachments. The three types are:

- *Rastelli A*: most common (75%) based on complete division of superior bridging leaflet over the crest of septum with chordal attachments from crest of septum to left and right septal components of the superior bridging leaflet. Division of the inferior leaflet over crest of septum is rare. VSD under inferior leaflet usually small due to dense, short chords as opposed to superior leaflet with larger VSD component secondary to longer, less dense chordal attachments.
- *Rastelli B*: rare, exceedingly so in balanced ventricles. Straddling chords from contralateral component.
- *Rastelli C*: second most common (25%). Undivided (or "free-floating") superior bridging leaflet. Most commonly associated with TOF complex.

Associated anomalies include TOF, double outlet right ventricle, left ventricular outflow tract obstruction (LVOTO), double orifice mitral valve, single papillary muscle.
Pathophysiology
Left to right shunt exists in all classifications therefore increasing

pulmonary blood flow. In CAVC, the VSD is unrestrictive so pulmonary hypertension will result if left untreated. Additionally, all four chambers of the heart dilate, impeding valve leaflet coaptation and resulting in AVV regurgitation. Pulmonary vascular disease appears to be accelerated in patients with Down Syndrome.

Treatment/management
Diuretics, vasodilators and digoxin are the standard medical treatment. Feeding tubes may be necessary to supplement nutritional intake.

Timing of surgery
Partial and transitional AV Canal
Pulmonary vasculature is relatively protected in this setting so it is acceptable to wait until the child is of preschool age to undertake repair unless the patient is symptomatic or has worsening AVV regurgitation.

CAVC
Early surgical intervention is necessary to avoid accelerated pulmonary vascular disease. Surgery is scheduled electively at 3-6 months of age even in asymptomatic patients. Surgery would be scheduled earlier in life if the baby experiences failure to thrive and worsening pulmonary over-circulation from the large left to right shunt or worsening left AVV regurgitation.

Operative steps
Partial AV canal
- Median sternotomy.
- Ascending aorta cannulation.
- Two right angle venous cannulae.
- +/- left atrial vent.
- Cool to 28° C.
- Antegrade cardioplegic arrest.
- Right atrial incision.
- Inspection and testing of valve and sub-valvar anatomy.
- Closure of cleft with direct suture (continuous 6/0 polypropylene or 5/0 for larger children) vs. horizontal mattress (6/0 with pledgets) up to free edge.
- Commisuroplasty if annulus dilated (prefer lateral commisure to avoid conduction). Caution: circumflex artery. 5/0 doubly pledgeted horizontal mattress.
- Close the ASD with bovine/autologous pericardium or PTFE. A row of 7-10 interrupted 5/0 or 6/0 prolene horizontal mattress sutures are first placed through the division point of the AV valves. These sutures are then placed through the base of the ASD patch. The two corner sutures are preserved and used to close the ASD in a

479

continuous running fashion. Care is taken at the inferior aspect by suturing first wide of the coronary sinus and then inside the mouth of the coronary sinus to avoid the inferiorly displaced AV node. Care is taken at the superior aspect where the aortic valve is anticipated.

- Leave suture line untied at highest point to de-air.
- Fill left heart with blood, vent via cardioplegia site in ascending aorta, valsalva. Tie suture line. Release cross clamp. Close atriotomy.
- Left atrial monitoring line via right superior pulmonary vein (RSPV) if needed.
- Bipolar temporary A and V pacing wires.
- Transesophageal ECHO to confirm absence of intracardiac air, assess valve competence and degree of stenosis if present, ventricular function and presence of residual ASD or VSD.

Transitional AV canal
- Setup same as for PAVC above.
- Modified single patch "Australian" technique: Transitional AV canals most often have small VSDs which are amenable to this repair. Single non-pledgeted or pledgeted interrupted horizontal mattress sutures are placed into the right ventricular (RV) side of the crest of the ventricular septum, 5 mm away from the margin and subsequently through the line of division of the left and right AV valves and then into the base of the ASD patch to close VSD over the ventricular septum. The ASD is then closed using a continuous running technique taking care to avoid injury to the AV node (inferiorly) and the aortic valve (superiorly).
- Two patch technique: If the VSD is large a separate crescent shaped patch of either PTFE, bovine or autologous pericardium is sutured to the crest of the ventricular septum using a continuous or interrupted technique. Interrupted sutures are then placed through the superior free edge of the VSD patch and then into the line of division of the left and right AV valves. The same sutures are then placed into the base of a separate ASD patch. The ASD is then closed in a continuous running fashion.

CAVC: two-patch technique (our preferred technique)
- Cool to 28° C.
- Two right angle venous cannulae.
- Control branch PAs to effect a bloodless field for repair of VSD.
- LV vent via RSPV.
- Inspect/test valve with ice cold cardioplegia or saline.
- Approximate superior and inferior common leaflet over the

ventricular crest with singe 6/0 prolene untied to predict and predetermine the AV valve division points and cleft closure.

- Continuous running 6/0 prolene sutures through crest of septum and through a crescent shaped bovine or autologous pericardial patch or PTFE. Sutures are brought out through the atrial side of the AVV. Interrupted 6/0 sutures are placed through the crest of the VSD patch and through the middle of the AVV leaflets for Type A defects and a predetermined division point in the superior bridging leaflet for Type C defects. These sutures are placed into the base of a separate ASD patch. Sutures are tied down while preserving the needles on the two corner stitches.
- Close cleft in bridging leaflet with interrupted horizontal mattress sutures.
- Close ASD as above with preserved corner stitches of 6 or 5/0 prolene.
- De-air as above.
- Intracardiac RA line.
- A and V wires.

Single patch technique
- Setup same as for above.
- Division of superior and inferior bridging leaflets (err slightly to the right of the middle of crest of ventricular septum when in doubt of precise division point).
- Patch is sutured to crest of ventricular septum with continuous sutures of 5/0 prolene.
- AVV leaflets are then re-suspended to the patch with interrupted 6/0 prolene. The suture is passed from right side of bridging leaflet, through the patch, then through the left side of the bridging leaflet.
- Inspect and test competence of mitral valve.
- Close cleft as above.
- Close ASD using the same patch as above with same de-airing technique prior to completion of suture line.

Potential questions/alternative scenarios
"After weaning from bypass you notice complete heart block."
It is hard to tell whether this will be temporary or not. The most likely culprit are the sutures near the coronary sinus. It would be challenging to take down the entire patch and reconstruct. More than likely the block is due to edema and may subside with time. Thus, place reliable but temporary pacing wires prior to closure.

"The patient has PA pressures that are double from baseline and decreased MAPs."

Pulmonary hypertensive crisis can develop following correction of AVC defect. Prompt recognition and treatment is lifesaving. Keep the patient intubated, use a PA pressure monitoring line, avoid acidosis, ventilate to keep the CO_2 low, paralyze, vasopressors and use iNO as needed to weather the crisis. The patient should improve within the first 24-26 hours.

"Residual shunt is discovered on intra-op TEE."

This can be confirmed with PA and SVC saturations and calculating the shunt fraction (Qp:Qs). If Qp:Qs > 1.5 this may potentially warrant repair/revision.

Pearls/pitfalls

- Caution! Damage to Bundle of His on crest of ventricular septum during VSD closure and AV node (which is displaced inferiorly) during ASD closure.

- During VSD repair sutures should be placed on the RV side of the ventricular septum and 5 mm away from the margin on the posterior-inferior aspect of the VSD to avoid conduction tissue.

- During the ASD repair, interrupted sutures at the inferior end of the division point of the AV valves should only be taken through leaflet tissue until suturing well past the area of the nodal triangle. Extend the inferior suture line first wide of and then into the mouth of coronary sinus to avoid conduction (alternatively can proceed inferior and around the coronary sinus redirecting drainage into the LA (cannot use this technique if the patient has a left SVC).

- Unnecessarily deep suture bites in the superior aspect of the annulus can damage the aortic valve.

- Excessively wide bites when performing a commissurotomy can damage or kink the circumflex coronary artery.

- A short or small left lateral leaflet can result in varying degrees of mitral valve stenosis if the cleft is closed completely. In this circumstance the cleft may be partially closed or not closed at all. Intraoperative measurement of valve orifices with Hegar dilators to predetermined diameters based on body surface area (BSA) based z-scores can be helpful. Other mitral valve abnormalities i.e., double orifice valve, single papillary muscle with parachute valve, very closely spaced papillary muscles etc may modify the ability to close the cleft.

- Pulmonary hypertension in the immediate post-op period is a known predictor of mortality though much less frequently encountered when repair is undertaken at an earlier age.

482

Suggested readings

- Jonas RA. Complete Atrioventricular Canal. Comprehensive Surgical Management of Congenital Heart Disease: 386-401.
- Atrioventricular canal defects. Mavroudis C and Becker CL (eds). Pediatric Cardiac Surgery:321-338.

Notes

64. Aortic coarctation

Bryan Barrus, MD, and George Alfieris, MD

Concept

- Indications for repair of coarctation of the aorta
- Preoperative considerations
- Steps of coarctation repair
- Pitfalls and alternative solutions

Chief complaint

"A 4 day old girl with a normal birth history is referred to you by her pediatric cardiologist with a 1 day history of poor feeding, tachypnea, and prominent brachial pulses with diminished femoral pulses. Echocardiography shows coarctation of the aorta."

Differential

The diagnosis has been established. It is important to confirm the diagnosis as detailed below and rule out concomitant pathology.

History and physical

Symptoms may occur abruptly with closure of the ductus arteriosus but may be more gradual in older children as collaterals develop. Evaluate vitals, focus on pulse exam of all 4 extremities, heart, and lung exam. Classic physical exam findings include brachiofemoral pulse delay, diminished or absent femoral pulses, and blood pressure gradient between upper and lower extremities. Diminished pulses in all extremities may signify heart failure. Listen for murmurs along left sternal border radiating to the back and an ejection click (bicuspid aortic valve). Look for differential cyanosis.

Tests

- *Labs.* Arterial blood gas, serum lactate, BUN, creatinine, electrolytes, septic workup in patients presenting in shock (blood, urine, CSF cultures).
- *CXR.* Normal unless heart failure present (cardiac enlargement, pulmonary congestion); > 5 years old look for rib notching by intercostal vessels.
- *Echocardiography*: diagnostic. Obtain Z-score of transverse arch, isthmus, and descending aorta. Score ≤ -2 indicates severe stenosis and must be addressed during surgery. Associated VSD (11%), bicuspid aortic valve (27-46%), distal arch narrowing (50-65%), other valvular anomalies, and ventricular hypoplasia must be ruled out. Measure doppler gradient across coarctation.

- *EKG*: normal; may have left ventricular hypertrophy (LVH) in late presentations.
- *Catheter angiography*: warranted in older children and adults with disparate clinical findings and echocardiography. May be warranted in neonates and infants if the anatomy is not clear.
- *CTA*: helpful in older patients and adults.

Index scenario (additional information)

"The patient is tachypneic, tachycardic, and has absent femoral pulses with weak brachial pulses. The lower half of the body is cyanotic. The blood pressure in the right brachial artery is 50/30 and undetectable in the legs. In addition to coarctation of the aorta, echocardiography shows a left aortic arch with a mildly hypoplastic transverse component, closed ductus arteriosus, and no associated intracardiac defects. The pH is 7.2 and the lactate is 5. How would you proceed?"

Treatment/management

The patient is in cardiogenic shock with a metabolic acidosis and must be resuscitated prior to surgery. Infuse prostaglandin E1 to open the ductus arteriosus and improve antegrade blood flow through the aorta. Support heart failure with mechanical ventilation, inotropes, and diuretics. Correct acidosis with bicarbonate. Monitor ventricular dysfunction and ductus arteriosus patency with serial echos. Monitor liver and renal function.

Operative steps

Goals – relieve obstruction, minimize risk of spinal cord injury, decrease rate of recurrence.
- *Positioning/monitoring*. Right lateral decubitus position with axillary roll, rectal and nasopharyngeal temperature probe, BP cuff and pulse oximetry on legs, right radial artery catheter, foley. Allow proximal hypertension during aortic cross-clamp. For older patients or adults a femoral arterial line may be considered to monitor distal perfusion during cross clamp.
- Allow patient to passively cool to ~34-35° C by dropping the ambient temperature and using cooling blankets as needed.
- Left posterolateral thoracotomy via 4th intercostal space. Retract the lung medially. Incise mediastinal pleura overlying descending thoracic aorta and left subclavian artery (SCA).
- Aggressively mobilize descending aorta, transverse arch, branch vessels and ductus arteriosus.
- Identify phrenic, vagus, and recurrent laryngeal nerves to avoid injury.

- Mobilize intercostal vessels to allow caudal mobility of the arch. Divide as few intercostals as possible.
- Give heparin 100 units per Kg.
- Ligate the ductus arteriosus with silk suture.
- Place vascular clamp proximally as high as possible across the transverse arch. The clamp is positioned in such a way as to occlude the LSCA, LCCA and the arch just distal to the innominate artery. The distal clamp is placed on the mid descending thoracic aorta.
- Divide the aorta just distal to the left SCA and just distal to coarctation segment. Divide the ductus, thereby removing the whole coarct segment and ductus en bloc.
- Incise undersurface of transverse arch proximally to allow for the largest anastomosis possible. Bevel the distal aortic segment accordingly.
- Begin the anastomosis on backwall with 7-0 polypropylene. Use small bites without a lot of tension to avoid stricture or purse string effects. Complete the anastomosis. Prior to closing the anastomosis, irrigate with heparinized saline solution. Make sure the anastomosis is tension free. Try to limit the anastomotic time to less than 20-30 minutes.
- Remove the distal clamp first then the proximal clamp. Thrombin soaked gel foam may be used to help with hemostasis.
- Check for pedal pulse at the end of the procedure. Assure hemostasis prior to closure. Close pleura over the aorta.
- Place a single chest tube and close the chest.

Potential questions/alternative scenarios

"Same patient as above but now with a severely hypoplastic aortic arch. How will you proceed?"
- Median sternotomy, ligate the ductus arteriosus prior to or just after initiating cardiopulmonary bypass (CPB).
- Cross clamp the aorta, give cardioplegia, and cool for deep hypothermic circulatory arrest (DHCA).
- Extensively mobilize the arch, arch vessels, and descending thoracic aorta.
- Begin DHCA at 18° C.
- Frequently, for better mobilization the left SCA will need to be sacrificed; divide the aorta just distal to the left carotid artery and just distal to the coarctation.
- Incise the undersurface of the proximal aortic arch to level of the innominate.
- Complete extended end-to-end anastomosis with 7-0 polypropylene suture versus Norwood-style patch augmentation with homograft depending on the degree of arch hypoplasia.

- Reinstitute CPB, remove the aortic cross clamp, rewarm.
- Wean off CPB, drain the mediastinum and left pleural space if necessary.
- Close.

"On echo, the patient is noted to have a large perimembranous ventricular septal defect (VSD) in the muscular septum in addition to the coarctation. How will you proceed?"

- Restrictive VSDs in the muscular septum are likely to close spontaneously and can be monitored alone. Unrestrictive VSDs can be repaired in either a one-stage or two-stage approach. The one-stage approach is preferred in cases where the VSD is unlikely to close spontaneously (perimembranous, large, inlet, outlet, malaligned). In a single incision approach, perform a median sternotomy. Repair the arch as described above. During rewarming, repair the VSD through a right atriotomy.

- A two-stage approach in which the coarctation is repaired first +/- pulmonary artery banding followed by VSD closure in 2-3 months can also be employed. If preoperative congestive heart failure (CHF) does not resolve, a second operation is required to close the VSD or if the VSD does spontaneously close a debanding procedure is performed. This approach is falling out of favor.

handwritten note: Swiss cheese defect

"The patient has a bicuspid aortic valve in addition to the coarctation of the aorta."

Usually does not need to be addressed at time of coarctation surgery.

"A 14 yo boy presents to his pediatrician with headaches and dyspnea on exertion. His blood pressure is 140/75 in his right arm but 100/70 in his right leg. His femoral pulses are diminished with a delayed upstroke. Rib notching is noted on a chest X-ray. How would you repair this anomaly?"

Obtain an echo and CT angiography to determine anatomy. Large collaterals may impede mobilization of the aorta. Perform a left thoracotomy. The initial dissection is the same as the end-to-end anastomosis described in the initial scenario.

"A 10 yo female presents with headaches, epistaxis and is found by her primary care physician to have a right brachial blood pressure of 160/90. Her mother reports she had repair of coarctation of the aorta as an infant. Echo shows a recoarctation. How would you approach treatment?"

Balloon angioplasty +/- stent placement is 90% successful. Mortality rate is 2.5%. The risk of recurrent coarctation following surgery is 5-10%.

Angioplasty +/- stenting for native coarctation has recurrence rate of 11-15%.

"A 20 yo immigrant with discrete coarctation not previously diagnosed presents to your office. What is the treatment of choice?"
Balloon dilatation and stenting is a reasonable first approach for discrete coarctation of the descending aorta although recurrence is likely to be higher when compared with open surgery.

"After arrival to the intensive care unit, an infant's blood pressure is noted to be severely elevated. Why does this occur? If left untreated, what may occur?"
Early phase (first 24 hours) caused by increased sensitivity of the aortic and carotid baroreceptors. Late phase (48-72 hours) increased levels of renin and angiotensin. Untreated hypertension following surgery is associated with mesenteric arteritis which may require laparotomy.

"You notice a white, milky substance coming out of the chest tube when the child begins to feed. What is your management strategy for the finding?"
Most often chyle leaks are injuries to tributaries of the thoracic duct, not the duct itself. An initial attempt at conservative measures include NPO, somatostatin, and hyperalimentation. If the patient fails to improve, take the patient back to the operating room for exploration.

"How can you limit the chances of paraplegia during repair of coarctation of the aorta?"
Paraplegia occurs 0.5% of the time. This can be prevented by limiting cross clamp time, passive cooling, and avoid hypotension during the clamp period.

Pearls/pitfalls
- Echocardiography is the mainstay of diagnosis.
- Open the ductus arteriosus with a prostaglandin E1 infusion in infants with heart failure.
- Extended end-to-end anastomosis shows the lowest rates of recurrence.
- Angioplasty is the preferred treatment for recurrent coarctation.
- Extensive mobilization of the entire aorta and its branches is required to avoid tension.

Suggested readings
- Backer CL, et al. Repair of coarctation with resection and extended end-to-end anastomosis. *Ann Thor Surg.* 1998;66:1365-1370.

- Fiore AC, et al. Comparison of angioplasty and surgery for neonatal aortic coarctation. *Ann Thor Surg.* 2005;80(5):1659-1665.
- Husain SA, Mokadam NA, Permut LC, and Rodefeld MD, Coarctation of the aorta and interrupted aortic arch. Yuh D, Vricella LA, and Baumgartner WA (eds). *Johns Hopkins Manual of Cardiothoracic Surgery.* 2007.

Notes

65. Tetralogy of Fallot

Asad A. Shah, MD, and Andrew J. Lodge, MD

Concept
- Understand the diagnosis and management of Tetralogy of Fallot (TOF) in infants
- Operative techniques and pitfalls
- Timing of operation
- Long-term post-operative complications

Chief complaint
"A 6 month old infant is referred to you with recurrent cyanotic episodes."

Differential
Tetralogy of Fallot, transposition of the great vessels, tricuspid atresia, total anomalous pulmonary venous return, truncus arteriosus. Other considerations include Ebstein's anomaly of the tricuspid valve and pulmonary atresia. However, the recurrent pattern of this presentation is characteristic of TOF.

History and physical
The history should include the prenatal and birth history, any other illnesses or co-morbid conditions, a feeding history, and events associated with cyanosis such as agitation or crying. The physical exam should include visible evidence of cyanosis (mucous membranes), cardiac and lung exam and peripheral pulses. A typical scenario: Born at term, 30th percentile for height and and 50th for weight, one previous episode of cyanosis while he had a cold, mid-systolic ejection murmur loudest in left 2nd and 3rd intercostal space; clear lungs.

Tests
- *CXR*: boot shaped heart, right sided arch in 25%, clear lungs.
- *EKG*: right ventricular hypertrophy (RVH).
- *Echocardiography*: ventricular septal defect (VSD) anterior malalignment of the conal septum, aortic override, right ventricular outflow tract (RVOT) obstruction, RVH.
- *Cardiac catheterization*: if concern over pulmonary artery anatomy, accessory sources of pulmonary blood flow such as aorto-pulmonary collaterals or coronary artery anatomy. Typically not needed.
- *Magnetic resonance imaging and CT angiography*: may provide information about unusual pulmonary artery anatomy but is

infrequently used due to the need for sedation/anesthesia.

"The patient is diagnosed with Tetralogy of Fallot. His cyanotic spell resolves and his room air oxygen saturation is 75%. What are your options in regards to timing of treatment?"

Treatment/management
Management of hypercyanotic episodes (TET spells)
- Oxygen.
- IV fluids.
- Sedation.
- Place patients' knees to chest to increase systemic vascular resistance and increase pulmonary blood flow.
- Alpha agonists such as phenylephrine.
- Beta blocker (generally not used in acute setting, but may be used in patients felt to be at increased/increasing risk of spells).
- These episodes and/or need for pharmacologic management are generally grounds for surgical repair.

Timing of surgery
- If child can maintain oxygen saturation of 80% or above with normal growth and development, elective surgical repair is preferred.
- Hypoxemic spells are an indication for operation.
- In patients without symptoms, repair should be performed by one year of age. At most institutions, complete, early repair by 3-6 months of age is performed. Late repair has been shown to be a risk factor for late poor outcomes.
- Pre-operative hydration is paramount, as dehydration can trigger cyanotic episodes.
- Some surgeons perform a two-stage procedure in patients less than 6 months old. In this case, a systemic to pulmonary artery shunt is performed first. Other indications for shunting include pulmonary atresia, significant hypoplasia of the branch pulmonary arteries, contraindications to cardiopulmonary bypass (CPB), and other severe congenital anomalies.

Operative steps
Goals – close intracardiac shunts, provide unobstructed pulmonary blood flow, maintain normal function of the right ventricle and tricuspid valve +/- pulmonary valve, and maintain normal sinus rhythm.
- Median sternotomy, bicaval cannulation, aortic cannulation, CPB w/moderate hypothermia.

- Inspect anterior surface of right ventricle for major coronary artery branches crossing the right ventricular outflow tract.
- Divide systemic to pulmonary shunts (if present), ligate patent ductus arteriosus.
- Left ventricular decompression via the pulmonary vein, left atrium or patent foramen ovale (PFO).
- Oblique right atriotomy and place stay sutures on the anterior and septal tricuspid leaflets.
- Transect obstructing muscle bundles in the right ventricular outflow tract including the parietal extension of the septal band. Avoid damage to the tricuspid papillary muscle.
- Close VSD with PTFE or Dacron patch. Use superficial suturing at posterior-inferior margin of defect to avoid conduction system.
- Close co-existing ASD if present. A PFO may be left patent in neonatal cases if large transannular patch is required, or if there is concern for post op RV dysfunction (allows some R to L shunting to preserve cardiac output).
- Probe pulmonary valve with graded dilators.
    - If valve is too small for age, make longitudinal incision in PA and make full commissurotomies if possible, then reassess valve size.
    - If valve still remains too small, place transannular patch by extending the pulmonary arteriotomy across the valve annulus onto the ventricular muscle. Make the ventriculotomy as small as possible to relieve the obstruction adequately; transannular patch may be constructed of PTFE, or autologous (glutaraldehyde fixed) pericardium. Note that leaving some residual RVOT obstruction (up to 50-75% systemic RV pressure) is preferable to too large of a transannular incision.

Potential questions/alternative scenarios

"After dividing obstructive fibers in the RVOT and making your longitudinal pulmonary arteriotomy you feel that the annulus is inadequate for the patients age and size. You decide to make a transannular incision but are impeded by an anomalous LAD originating from the RCA. How would you proceed?"

Anterior descending coronary artery arising from right coronary artery and crossing the RVOT is found in 3-5% of patients. Some patients may have a large conal branch of the right coronary artery that also limits the transannular incision. These anomalies should be detected preoperatively by CT, MRI, and/or echo and then be confirmed by visual inspection early in the operation. If there is an anomalous anterior descending coronary artery that precludes transannular patch, an RV-PA conduit (homograft) may be used to relieve RV outflow tract obstruction. The ventriculotomy is made on the RV free wall below the anomalous artery. The conduit is anastomosed distally to the main pulmonary artery or pulmonary artery bifurcation.

"What is the operative and late survival after repair of TOF?"
Operative survival ≥ 95%; late survival approximately 90%.

"What are some perioperative complications?"
Right ventricular dysfunction - treat with inotropic support and avoidance of pulmonary hypertension. Arrhythmia [heart block, junctional ectopic tachycardia (JET)] - for heart block the best treatment is prevention with careful suturing of the posterior margin of the VSD. Ensure properly functioning pacing wires prior to closure. JET is classically treated with cooling to 35° C, electrolyte correction, reducing exogenous catecholamines, and more recently amiodarone.

"A 22 yo man with a history of Tetralogy of Fallot repair with transannular patch presents with decreasing ability to exercise. What are the potential causes of this and what are some long term risks of transannular patch repair of TOF?"
- Chronic pulmonary insufficiency (PI) resulting in right ventricular dilation.
- Pulmonary valve replacement (PVR) when there is severe PI and RV enlargement (EDVI > 160 mL/m², ESVI > 80 mL/m², RV dysfunction, worsening tricuspid regurgitation, decreased exercise tolerance, or QRS duration of ≥ 180 ms.
  - Homograft or bioprosthetic valve (mechanical valves generally not used due to higher risk of thrombosis). Percutaneous PVR may be appropriate for some patients.
  - Other long term sequelae of transannular patch repair for TOF include atrial and ventricular arrhythmias and sudden death.

"A 2-week old boy presents with cyanosis and is diagnosed with Tetralogy of Fallot. Additional comorbidities include liver dysfunction due to biliary atresia. What is the management of this patient?"
- Staged procedure is ideal for any patient who cannot tolerate full CPB, or patients with pulmonary atresia, significant hypoplasia of the branch pulmonary arteries, or other major comorbidities. The first stage involves placement of a shunt.
- Classic or modified Blalock-Taussig shunt.
  - Median sternotomy preferred; may be performed through thoracotomy.
  - Performed on side opposite the aortic arch.

- For a modified BT shunt, 3.5 or 4 mm PTFE tube graft is used for an infant weighing approximately 3-4 kg.

"You are called to the delivery of a newborn with a prenatal diagnosis of TOF and absent pulmonary valve. The child demonstrates respiratory distress with a respiratory acidosis on arterial blood gas. Two-dimensional echo shows enormous dilation of the main, right, and left PAs. The child is intubated and stabilizes with positive pressure ventilation. A CT shows severe main pulmonary artery dilation with tracheal and bronchial compression. What is your surgical plan?"

Although with this diagnosis there is a wide spectrum of severity based on the degree of tracheal/bronchial involvement, this case represents a surgical emergency. In a sick infant who is difficult to ventilate, the decision to pursue CT prior to proceeding to the OR should be deferred. The diagnosis of TOF/absent pulmonary valve alone is an indication for surgery as there are no good medical alternatives for management. In an infant presenting with wheezing or recurrent respiratory infections, repair should take place soon after the diagnosis. In an asymptomatic child, surgery should be scheduled in the first months of life or shortly after diagnosis. In the case presented, CPB should be established using aortic and single venous cannulation as bicaval cannulation can be very difficult in the setting of severe mediastinal crowding. Moderate systemic cooling is initiated (if low-flow CPB is needed for visualization during the case, further cooling may be required). After aortic cross clamping, the MPA is transected at the level of the pulmonary annulus. The right and left PAs are transected leaving a cuff of tissue. A bifurcated pulmonary homograft is chosen and thawed. The VSD is closed followed by division of obstructing RV muscle bundles. The valved homograft is anastomosed to the native annulus and the pulmonary arteries. The PFO is generally left open. Persistent tracheobronchomalacia may be a persistent problem and delayed sternal closure is common. Reduction pulmonary arterioplasty can be used instead of a homograft in cases with less severe PA dilation.

"You come off bypass and TEE shows a residual VSD."

Typically residual patch leaks are due to aneurysmal tricuspid valve tissue or chordae obscuring the true margins of the VSD during patch placement. TEE is helpful in localizing the defect and determining its approximate size. The TEE should be used to differentiate a peripatch leak from a muscular VSD. Muscular VSDs that were not seen previously or appeared small may be more visible once RV pressure is subsystemic following repair. Residual VSDs are poorly tolerated in TOF due to an increased RV volume load in the setting of diastolic dysfunction. This scenario can lead to a low cardiac output state. One general rule of thumb is residual defects > 2.5 mm should be repaired as long as the child can tolerate it. Ideally a simple pledgeted suture at the most likely site will resolve the leak. Muscular VSDs requiring a transventricular approach should be managed on a case-by-case basis to evaluate the risk of ventriculotomy versus the potential benefit of closing the residual left to right shunt.

"You come off bypass and TEE shows severe TR."
Use TEE to help determine the etiology of the valve dysfunction. May be due to the nearby patch causing distortion of the TV at the anteroseptal commissure by "splaying" the leaflets apart, or may be due to trapped chordae. A leak at the commissure can usually be treated with one or two mattress stitches at the commissure to support this area. A more serious potential complication is damage to the anterior papillary muscle during division of obstructing fibers in the RVOT. Repair should be attempted.

Pearls/pitfalls
- Tetralogy of Fallot is the most common cyanotic congenital heart defect.
- Recurrent cyanotic spells and room air oxygen saturation of less than 80% are indications for immediate operation. Otherwise, "complete repair" is electively performed between 3-6 months of age, and certainly before the age of one.
- The key steps of repair include closure of the VSD, division of muscle bundles to relieve the RVOT obstruction, and pulmonary valvotomy or transannular patch.
- Indications for a staged, palliative approach (shunt) include extreme instability or systemic illness, significant noncardiac comorbidities, diminutive pulmonary arteries, and contraindications to CPB.
- Pulmonary regurgitation resulting in RV dilation is a late complication, particularly after transannular patch, and is treated with PVR.

Suggested readings
- Duncan BW. Tetralogy of Fallot with Pulmonary Stenosis. Selke FW, del Nido PJ, Swanson SJ (Eds). Sabiston & Spencer - Surgery of the Chest, 8th Edition. 2010. pp 1877-1896.
- Hirsch JC, Bove EL. Tetralogy of Fallot. Mavroudis C, Becker CL (Eds). Pediatric Cardiac Surgery, 3rd Edition. 2003. pp 383-397.
- Jaquiss RDB. Tetralogy of Fallot. Kaiser LR, Kron IL, Spray TL (Eds). Mastery of Cardiothoracic Surgery, 2nd Edition, 2007. pp 907-15.

Notes

66. Transposition of the great arteries
Muhammad Aftab, MD, Elizabeth Pocock, MD, and Charles D. Fraser, Jr., MD

Concept
- Presentation
- Differential for TGA
- Diagnostic evaluation
- Surgical repair
- Pitfalls

Chief complaint
"A one day-old, full term and 3.2 kg boy is transferred to your center for the management of complex cyanotic heart condition. Patient's mother is a 17 yo primigravida with the history of bipolar disorder who has received no prenatal care. At birth the infant was found to be severely cyanotic. PGE 1 has been initiated and because of the lack of advanced cardiac intervention capability, the patient is transferred to your center for the further care. What is your differential of cyanotic heart disease and how would you proceed?"

Differential
The differential diagnosis of cyanotic congenital heart condition at birth includes:
1) Transposition of great arteries (TGA)
2) Tetralogy of Fallot (ToF)
3) Truncus arteriosus (TA)
4) Tricuspid atresia
5) Total anomalous pulmonary venous return (TAPVR)
Other cyanotic congenital heart conditions include:
6) Single ventricle anomalies
7) Hypoplastic left heart syndrome (HLHS)
8) Pulmonary atresia or pulmonary stenosis (PA/PS)
9) Double outlet right ventricle (DORV)
10) Ebstein's anomaly
11) Single atrium

History and physical
TGA is a common cause of cyanosis in infants accounting for 7-8% of all congenital cardiac defects. The degree of cyanosis is affected by the extent of intracardiac shunting. Neonates with TGA and intact ventricular septum (IVS) have the most severe cyanosis which is immediately discernible. TGA and non-restrictive VSD may present with very mild cyanosis which can be clinically unappreciated.

The patients with TGA/VSD may present with the signs and symptoms of CHF secondary to pulmonary overcirculation after the physiological fall in pulmonary vascular resistance in neonatal period.

Systolic murmurs may be audible in almost 50% of patients.

Tests

- *Transthoracic echocardiography (TTE)*: the mainstay of diagnosis. The classic echocardiographic findings are: great vessels seen parallel to each other instead of classic wrapping pattern (on the long axis view), two semilunar valves (mitral-pulmonary contiguity) visible within the same slice (on the short axis view) and an early branching pattern of the great artery associated with the left ventricle (pulmonary artery). The echocardiogram should also be able to define the relative position and size of great vessels, the relative size of aortic and pulmonary valves and the location of coronary ostia.
- *CXR*. Classically demonstrates the "egg on a string" sign suggestive of a narrow superior mediastinum. The initial CXR in the patients with TGA/IVS as well as TGA/VSD typically may not show the pulmonary plethora. However later on, with the fall in pulmonary vascular resistance, the pulmonary vascular markings and cardiomegaly becomes more prominent in patients with TGA/VSD compared to TGA/IVS. In contrast, patients with TGA/PS may have oligemic lung fields.
- *EKG*. Usually normal for age in the beginning. In neonates with TGA/IVS, it may later demonstrate RV hypertrophy with the right axis deviation. In patients with TGA/VSD, it usually shows biventricular hypertrophy with a normal axis.
- *Cardiac catheterization*. Not usually indicated preoperatively. Therapeutic cardiac catheterization to perform balloon atrial septostomy may be warranted in TGA/IVS patients with an absent or restrictive atrial septum.

Index scenario (additional information)

"Two dimensional echocardiogram showed the two great vessels parallel to each other, with a patent ductus arteriosus (PDA), a small restrictive atrial septal defect (ASD) and an intact ventricular septum (IVS)."

Treatment/management

Medical management

The goal of medical management of a neonate with TGA is stabilization of the patient and correction of metabolic derangements caused by impaired perfusion and cyanosis. PGE1 is immediately initiated to increase pulmonary blood flow. Balloon atrial septostomy should be performed within hours of diagnosis of TGA in the absence of sufficient shunting at the atrial (ASD), ventricular (VSD), and/or arterial (PDA) level. If a prenatal diagnosis has already been established, the child should be delivered in a center where balloon atrial septostomy can be performed expeditiously.

Typically, the neonate is stabilized and resuscitated in the ICU for a day or two prior to surgery.

Surgical management
The diagnosis of TGA in a neonate is an indication for surgery.

TGA/IVS. An arterial switch operation (ASO) is indicated in patients with simple TGA early in the neonatal period. In infants with simple TGA who present beyond 4-6 weeks after birth, LV deconditioning is a matter of concern. In these patients if the LV muscle mass is adequate and the LV posterior wall thickness is normal for the age, a single stage ASO can be performed. For patients with an unprepared or marginal LV a two stage approach is used. This consists of LV retraining by placement of pulmonary artery band (PAB) with or without modified Blalock-Taussig shunt (BTS) followed by an ASO.

TGA/VSD. An arterial switch operation with VSD closure is indicated for TGA/VSD diagnosed at any age, provided that there is a non-restrictive VSD and a patient has not developed the fixed pulmonary vascular obstructive disease (PVOD). A non-restrictive VSD or a PDA of sufficient size to maintain LV pressure > 2/3 of the RV (systemic) pressure will prevent the deconditioning and keep the LV prepared for one-stage ASO.

TGA/VSD/PS (LVOTO). The surgical options for patients with TGA/VSD/PS include ASO, Bex-Nikaidoh, Réparation à l'Etage Ventriculaire (REV) and the Rastelli operation.The choice of operative procedure varies based on the size of pulmonary valve annulus, degree and etiology of pulmonary stenosis and the resectability of LVOT. For patients with an isolated pulmonary valve abnormality (i.e., focal area of pulmonary stenosis), it is possible to resect the obstruction and perform a primary ASO.

For the subset of patients having TGA/VSD/PS (LVOTO) with moderate pulmonary valve hypoplasia and septal malalignment, an anatomical repair can be performed using the Bex-Nikaidoh operation. These patients usually have a VSD non-committed to the great arteries (inlet or trabecular type), so construction of a LV to aorta tunnel is not possible.

Patients with TGA/VSD/PS (LVOTO) having pulmonary atresia, significant valvular pulmonary stenosis or hypoplasia can undergo anatomic repair using the REV procedure or Rastelli operation. These procedures can be performed safely only after the neonatal period, so it is crucial to carefully monitor these patients for any worsening cyanosis. A palliative modified BTS may be necessary for these patients before the definitive repair.

TGA/VSD/aortic arch obstruction. For patients with TGA/VSD/aortic arch obstruction secondary to IAA/ arch hypoplasia or coarctation, a single stage arch repair should be included in the definitive operative procedure.

Operative steps
Arterial switch operation (ASO)
- Place TEE probe.
- Median sternotomy is performed and partial thymectomy is carried out.
- Pericardium is opened and portion of pericardium is harvested for the later reconstruction of the defects created by excision of coronary buttons from the native aortic root (neopulmonary artery).
- Cardiopulmonary bypass is established using bicaval cannulation and the arterial cannula is placed in the ascending aorta.
- Cooling for moderate hypothermia is initiated. The repair of TGA/IVS and TGA/VSD usually do not require deep hypothermic circulatory arrest.
- The PDA is dissected out, doubly ligated and divided.
- A left atrial vent is placed either via the right superior pulmonary vein or via right atriotomy into the left atrium.
- Extensive mobilization of pulmonary arterial branches is performed.
- The ascending aorta is cross clamped and the heart is arrested with antegrade cardioplegia. Interval doses of cardioplegia are then given every 15-20 minutes in either retrograde fashion or directly into the coronary ostia.
- Both the aorta and the main PA are divided above the semilunar valves.
- The Lecompte maneuver is performed by translocation of the pulmonary artery confluence in front of the aorta after repositioning of the aortic cross clamp.
- Coronary buttons are excised from the native aortic root and reimplanted into the native pulmonary root (neoaortic root) taking great care to avoid twisting, kinking, and excess tension. (Coronary

reimplantation may also be accomplished after anastomosis of the neoaortic root. A "closed technique" uses marking stitches on the outside of the neoaortic root to identify the commissures so that a safe location for button reimplantation can be found after the anastomosis is complete when the root is temporarily filled).

- Aortic continuity is established by anastomosing the native pulmonary root (neoaortic root) to the ascending aorta.
- The defects of coronary buttons in the native aortic root (neopulmonary root) are patched using autologous pericardium. Pulmonary arterial continuity is then reestablished by anastomosing the neopulmonary root to the pulmonary artery bifurcation.
- A VSD, if present, is usually repaired through the right atriotomy via the tricuspid valve using autologous pericardium or Gore-Tex®. The ASD is usually closed primarily or by patch closure.
- Rewarming is started, the aortic cross clamp is removed and deairing is accomplished under TEE guidance.
- The patient is separated from the cardiopulmonary bypass, protamine is administered to reverse the heparin and the heart is decannulated.
- Hemostasis is secured. Chest tube(s) are placed. Some groups also place a peritoneal dialysis catheter at this point.
- The sternum is closed in the standard fashion.

Potential questions/alternative scenarios
"What is the morphology of TGA and what are the clinical subtypes and most common coronary patterns?"

Morphology of TGA
Morphologically, TGA is characterized by isolated ventriculo-arterial discordance. The aorta arises from the right ventricle and the pulmonary artery from left the ventricle. The looping of ventricles is normal i.e., d-looping; right atrium is related to the right ventricle and left atrium to left ventricle. TGA is further classified into:

- *Simple TGA* (75%). These patients have an Intact Ventricular Septum (IVS) and no other cardiac anomaly except a patent ductus arteriosus (PDA) and patent foramen ovale (PFO).
- *Complex TGA with ventricular septal defect-VSD* (20%). VSD are more commonly conoventricular (perimembranous) or outlet morphology. Approximately 25% of the patients with TGA and VSD have pulmonary stenosis resulting in LVOTO. TGA with anterior malalignment VSD is also frequently associated with Interrupted Aortic Arch (IAA) or marked hypoplasia of aortic arch with coarctation.

Although the coronary anatomy is variable among patients with TGA, the most common (60%) distribution consists of the left main coronary artery originating from the leftward and posterior facing sinus and right coronary artery arising from the rightward and posterior facing sinus. In almost 1/3 of the patients with TGA, the coronary arteries are found looping either anterior or posterior to the great arteries. Other coronary variations include all arteries arising from a single sinus and intramural coronary arteries. The coronary branching pattern is usually variable and is related to the technical complexity of the treatment.

Clinical variations of TGA and physiologic implicaitons
1) Transposition of Great Arteries with Intact Ventricular Septum TGA/IVS.
2) Transposition of Great Arteries with Ventricular Septal Defect (TGA/VSD).
3) Transposition of Great Arteries with Ventricular Septal defect and Left Ventricular Outflow flow tract obstruction (TGA/VSD/LVOTO).
4) Transposition of Great Arteries with Ventricular Septal Defect (TGA/VSD) and Aortic Arch Obstruction (IAA/Arch Hypoplasia or Coarctation).

The circulation in patients with TGA consists of two parallel circuits. The first circuit consists of the deoxygenated blood returning from the Venae cavae to RA, then going to the RV, then into the aorta. In the second circuit oxygenated blood cycles from the lungs to LA, then to the LV and through the PA and returns to lungs. The survival of the neonate depends upon the communication between these two circuits at the level of the ASD, VSD, and/or PDA.

In patients with TGA/IVS, the PDA must be maintained by a PGE1 infusion to allow survival, as closure of the PDA and loss of mixing may result in significant cyanosis and hemodynamic compromise. Balloon atrial septostomy should be performed early if warranted. Occasionally patients with TGA/IVS may survive undiagnosed due to adequate atrial level shunting. In these neonates, with the fall of pulmonary vascular resistance, the LV becomes deconditioned and loses its ability to support the systemic circulation. These patients will need LV reconditioning by pulmonary artery banding (PAB) prior to ASO.
Patients with TGA/VSD (nonrestrictive) typically have more effective mixing between both pulmonary and systemic circuits resulting in pulmonary overcirculation. Moreover because of the equalization of pressure between both ventricles, the LV maintains its ability to support the systemic circulation. These patients are at significant risk of early onset pulmonary vascular obstructive disease (PVOD) from pulmonary

overcirculation.

Neonates with TGA/VSD and PS have a physiology similar to Tetralogy of Fallot. Mild PS protects the lungs from the development of pulmonary vascular obstructive disease. Usually these patients have adequate intracardiac mixing. Moreover, the LV pressure load from PS and the VSD prevents deconditioning of the LV. Patients with significant pulmonary stenosis may require a PGE1 infusion to provide adequate pulmonary blood flow by maintaining the PDA.

Patients with TGA/VSD and aortic arch obstruction (i.e., IAA, arch hypoplasia or coarctation) have blood flow to lower body dependent upon the PDA. The lower body is supplied with fully saturated blood from the left ventricle through the PDA while the upper body is desaturated resulting in characteristic *blue fingers and pink toes*; diagnostic for TGA with arch obstruction, also known as reverse differential cyanosis.

"What is the REV procedure and how does it compare with the Rastelli operation?"

A Rastelli is the classic corrective operation for the patients with TGA/VSD/PS. In this procedure the left ventricular blood flow is diverted by an intraventricular baffle across the VSD to the aorta. The right ventricle to pulmonary artery continuity is then established using an extracardiac valved conduit. The reported mortality from this procedure ranges from 10-29% with the acceptable long-term results. Long-term survival is usually affected by LV dysfunction and conduit stenosis/subaortic stenosis requiring multiple reoperations.

The Réparation à l'Etage Ventriculaire (REV procedure), which consists of reconstructing the RVOT without the prosthetic conduit, was introduced by Lecompte to decrease the number of reoperations from conduit replacement. This procedure consists of:

1) Extensive resection of the conal septum for the VSD enlargement, even if the VSD is non-restrictive, thus creating a short and straight LV to aortic tunnel without reducing the size of RV cavity.
2) Creation of an intraventricular baffle to divert the LV flow to the aorta.
3) Aortic transection to perform the Lecompte maneuver.
4) Pulmonary artery is directly reimplanted into the RV. RVOT reconstruction is completed using an anterior patch.

The operative mortality of the REV procedure is less than 5%. The advantage of the REV procedure over the Rastelli operation is that the LV function remains preserved among most of the survivors with a very low risk of subaortic stenosis.

"What is the Bex-Nikaidoh operation?"

This procedure consists of harvesting the aortic root, as in the Ross procedure, and reconstructing the LVOT by the translocated the aortic root. LVOT obstruction is relieved by dividing the outlet septum and or enlarging the outflow tract with a patch if necessary. Coronary arteries are individually reimplanated after translocation or transferred enbloc with the root. The RVOT is then reconstructed by anterior translocation of the pulmonary artery (or using pulmonary homograft) and direct anastomosis to the right ventricle.

The advantage of the Nikaidoh procedure is that it is an anatomic repair in which both the LVOT and RVOT are normally aligned compared to the right angle turns constructed in the Rastelli repair.

"What are the outcomes of an Arterial Switch Operation and how would you follow your patient after ASO?"

The reported 30 day mortality rate following an ASO is 1.6%. The expected long term survival is > 95% with a normal life style and LV function.

Close long-term follow-up is necessary because some of the patients may develop complications requiring reoperation such as: 1) proximal coronary artery stenosis - especially in patients with complex coronary ostial origins, 2) supravalvar pulmonary stenosis and, 3) dilatation of neoaortic root resulting in aortic insufficiency.

"What is the relevance of left ventricular outflow tract obstruction in TGA?"

Isolated LVOTO sometimes occurs in patients with TGA and IVS. This is a functional obstruction, usually caused by the leftward bulging of the septum due to higher RV (systemic) pressure compared to the lower pressure LVOT. The functional LVOTO usually resolves with anatomic correction resulting in a rightward shift of the septum. However sometimes this can progress into fixed organic LVOTO.

Hemodynamically significant organic valvular and sub-valvular stenosis causing LVOTO is more common in patients with TGA/VSD. Organic LVOTO results in reduced pulmonary blood flow which, in combination with TGA physiology, causes a profound cyanosis. This may also affect surgical decision making.

"After coming off pump following an ASO, significant ST changes are noted on EKG with hemodynamic instability. LV function is severely depressed on TEE. What would you like to do?"

The scenario describes myocardial ischemia due to coronary insufficiency. Poor myocardial preservation or an intraoperative complication of coronary transfer must be considered. Assuming myocardial protection was adequate, coronary insufficiency may be due to proximal occlusion, stenosis, or dissection. Proximal occlusion or stenosis can be caused by twisting of the artery during coronary artery button rotation prior to implantation, stretching of or tension on the coronary artery, or by other distortion. Coronary artery dissection is possible during manipulation of the artery before, during, and after harvesting the buttons, or may be due to a retraction injury. The most important treatment is prevention of these conditions! Reimplantation of a coronary button with repositioning and patching can be attempted, but is very difficult and usually requires taking down the pulmonary anastomosis and re-arresting the heart. Most common management strategies include proximal patch (autologous pericardium) coronary arterioplasty, coronary artery bypass grafting (usually with the internal thoracic artery), or both techniques combined. Stenting has been successfully used to treat coronary artery dissection following a Ross procedure, and may be an option in bigger patients after ASO. Management decisions should be based on patient characteristics, surgeon comfort level and institutional practice, as well as the availability of a catheterization lab and a skilled interventionalist.

Pearls/pitfalls
- Classic echo finding is two great vessels running parallel to each other in the long-axis view, or the "double-barrel" appearance of the great vessels in the short-axis view. Classic CXR description is "egg on a string."
- After birth, PGE should be initiated to maintain ductal patency. Balloon atrial septostomy should be performed urgently if there is insufficient shunting at the atrial (ASD), ventricular (VSD), and/or arterial (PDA) level. Usually at least two levels of shunting are needed for adequate mixing.
- The diagnosis of TGA in a neonate is an indication for surgery.
- In infants with simple TGA who present beyond 4-6 weeks after birth, LV deconditioning is a matter of concern. For patients with an unprepared or marginal LV, a two stage approach consisting of LV retraining by placement of pulmonary artery band (PAB) with or without modified Blalock-Taussig shunt (BTS) followed by an ASO is undertaken.
- The surgical options for patients with TGA/VSD/PS include ASO, Bex-Nikaidoh, Réparation à l'Etage Ventriculaire (REV) and the Rastelli operation.
- Avoiding coronary complications is critical, as surgical correction can be very difficult.

Suggested readings

- Coronary artery anomalies. Mavroudis C. and Backer CL (eds). *Pediatric Cardiac Surgery*, 3e Philadelphia, PA: Mosby; 2003.
- Transposition of the Great Arteries. Jonas R. (ed). *Comprehensive Surgical Management of Congenital Heart Disease.* Hodder Arnold Publication. 2004.
- Khonsari S, Sintek CF. *Cardiac Surgery: Safeguards and Pitfalls in Operative Technique.* 4th ed.Philadelphia, PA: Lippincott Williams & Wilkins; 2008.
- Franco KL, Thorani VH (editors). *Cardiothoracic Surgery Review.* 1st ed. Philadelphia, PA: Lippincott Williams & Wilkins; 2012: 315-327.

Notes

67. Ebstein's anomaly

Damien J. LaPar, MD, MSc, and Pedro J. del Nido, MD

Concept
- Indications for surgical repair of Ebstein's anomaly
- Critical steps of tricuspid valve repair (cone procedure)
- Alternative surgical techniques
- Pitfalls and alternative solutions

Chief complaint
"A 9 yo boy with a known history of Ebstein's anomaly presents with worsening cyanosis, new onset palpitations and fainting episodes."

Differential
The diagnosis has been established in the patients medical record and the patient was observed throughout the neonatal period. It is likely that the degree of malformation and regurge at birth was not sufficient enough to warrant repair. The new symptoms are most likely related to a progression of his Ebstein's. If cyanosis is present in the neonatal period one should consider other causes of cyanotic congenital heart disease including: Tetralogy of Fallot, total anomalous pulmonary venous return, hypoplastic left heart syndrome, d-transposition of the great arteries, truncus arteriosus (persistent), tricuspid atresia, pulmonary atresia, and critical pulmonary stenosis.

History and physical
Focused history for presence of cyanosis, palpitations, fatigability, reduced exercise tolerance, dyspnea on exertion, or other manifestations of reduced cardiac functional status. Most patients with Ebstein's anomaly have an atrial shunt (PFO or secundum ASD) which accounts for the cyanosis. The presence of cyanosis suggests a malformation severe enough to warrant surgery. A focused physical exam should clarify the presence of cyanosis, a systolic murmur of tricuspid regurgitation (TR), a prominent jugular venous "v" wave, as well as evidence of irregular cardiac rhythm and tachyarrhythmia.

Tests
- *Laboratory analysis*: may reveal polycythemia.
- *EKG*. Right bundle branch block with right axis deviation, atrial arrhythmia, tachyarrhythmia (Wolff-Parkinson-White (WPW) syndrome).

- *Imaging*
  - – *CXR*: cardiomegaly (enlarged right atrium (RA) and atrialized right ventricle (RV), decreased pulmonary vascular markings.
  - – *Echocardiography*: diagnostic test of choice.
    - o LV function, right atrial and RV size and function.
    - o Doppler - estimate severity of TR and RV outflow obstruction.
    - o Atrial shunt type and direction (ASD, PFO).
    - o Degree of tricuspid valve (TV) leaflet malformation, apical displacement of the septal leaflet, restriction of the anterior leaflet, degree of tethering, extent of RV atrialization.
    - o Carpentier classification of Ebstein's anomaly (helps determine severity of malformation and depicts important components of the echo and gross inspection):
      - ▪ *Type A*
        - ◊ small atrialized RV (adequate-sized functional RV)
        - ◊ moderate displacement of septal/posterior leaflets
        - ◊ normal anterior leaflet
      - ▪ *Type B*
        - ◊ large atrialized RV (small functional RV)
        - ◊ marked displacement of septal/posterior leaflets
        - ◊ hypoplastic adherent septal leaflet
        - ◊ normal anterior leaflet
      - ▪ *Type C*
        - ◊ large atrialized RV (very small functional RV)
        - ◊ marked displacement of septal/posterior leaflets
        - ◊ hypoplastic, adherent septal and posterior leaflet
        - ◊ restricted anterior leaflet (may cause obstruction)
      - ▪ *Type D*
        - ◊ almost completely noncontractile atrialized RV
        - ◊ marked displacement of septal/posterior leaflets

◊ hypoplastic, adherent septal and posterior leaflet
◊ adherent anterior leaflet
○ *Great Ormond Street (GOS) score*: ratio of combined RA area and atrialized RV to the combined areas of the functional RV and left heart chambers in diastole on 4 chamber view (Score 1-4).
▪ Score 1: ratio < 0.50
▪ Score 2: ratio 0.50-0.99
▪ Score 3: ratio 1.00-1.49
▪ Score 4: ratio > 1.50
▪ Studies demonstrating Scores 3-4 (ratio > 1.00) predict high mortality (44-100%).
- *Cardiac catheterization*: rarely necessary. May precipitate arrhythmias. Only useful if ruling out severe pulmonary vascular resistance.
- *MRI*. May help to measure chamber size.
- *Associated anomalies*: rare, bicuspid AV, mitral valve prolapse, and ASD are the most common considerations.

Index scenario (additional information)

"EKG demonstrates WPW syndrome, CXR with cardiomegaly (cardiothoracic ratio 0.66), and echocardiography demonstrates severe TR, Ebstein's malformation and the presence of an ASD."

Treatment/management

Treatment is dictated by age of presentation, constellation of clinical features, and anatomy. Indications for surgical management include the presence of the following: 1) symptomatic NYHA functional class III or IV; 2) NYHA functional class I or II in the presence of cardiomegaly (cardiothoracic ratio ≥ 0.65) or severe tricuspid regurgitation; 3) cyanosis; 4) paradoxical embolism; or 5) tachycardia and accessory AV bundle. Early surgical intervention encouraged prior to deterioration of right and/or left ventricular function. Mortality for late-stage operations increases significantly.

Operative steps

Biventricular TV repair-cone reconstruction

Goals – there are fundamental goals to most techniques for correction of Ebstein's malformation.
• Preoperative electrophysiologic mapping of accessory conduction pathways in patients with ventricular preexcitation
• If present, closure of ASD (+/- fenestration)

- Ligation of prior shunts and correction of associated cardiac anomalies
- Performance of any indicated antiarrhythmia procedure (such as cryoablation of AV nodal reentrant tachycardia, right MAZE, etc).
- Tricuspid valve repair (versus replacement with bioprosthetic) whenever a good to excellent result can be expected
- Possible plication of the atrialized right ventricle
- Reduction (right) atrioplasty
- Avoiding the major pitfalls - injury to the coronary sinus, right coronary artery or conduction.
- Place TEE probe
- Access via median sternotomy
- Aortic and bicaval venous cannulation and initiation of cardiopulmonary bypass (CPB)
- Moderate hypothermia (28-34° C), aorta cross clamped with antegrade cardioplegia, snare IVC and SVC
- Oblique right atriotomy parallel with AV groove
- Left heart vent (often placed through PFO/ASD if present)
- Investigate presence of ASD
- Inspection of TV leaflets and annulus; assessment of size and extent of atrialized RV (see Carpentier's classification above)
- Incise anterior leaflet at 12:00 (surgeon's view), a few millimeters from the true annulus and extend in a rightward/clockwise fashion using scissors. Detach ("delaminate") the anterior and posterior leaflets from the underlying RV myocardium, leaving all attachments and chordae to the leading edge intact.
- Mobilize the septal leaflet off of the true annulus and underlying myocardium in a similar fashion if sufficient tissue is present. Leave all apical attachments intact. The septal leaflet is typically diminutive and displaced toward the apex more so than the other leaflets.
- Rotate the free edge of the anterior/posterior leaflet complex clockwise and suture its septal edge (interrupted 5-0 or 6-0 monofilament) to the septal leaflet, thus increasing the height of the septal leaflet. If too little septal leaflet tissue, suture free edge of posterior leaflet to the septal edge of the anterior leaflet.
- Annuloplasty (usually partial/posterior +/- prosthetic ring)
- Suture the 360° cone-shaped valve to true tricuspid annulus.
  - Superficial bites near AV node to avoid heart block.
- Test valve while occluding PA
- Closure of ASD (may leave fenestration)
- +/- ablation or right MAZE
- Right reduction atrioplasty. Close RA, remove cross clamp

- Patient rewarmed and weaned from CPB
- PRN inotropic support and RV afterload reduction (dopamine, milrinone, iNO)

"Describe the approach to medical management in neonatal period."
Approach to treatment is dictated by clinical presentation. Aggressive medical management is required in neonatal period in preparation for surgery or until native pulmonary vascular resistance (PVR) falls to reduce right-to-left shunting. Tenants in the medical management include intubation and mechanical ventilation, efforts to decrease PVR (hyperventilation, alkalosis, nitric oxide), eliminate ductal patency (discontinue prostaglandin E_1), and aggressive management of congestive heart failure with inotropic ventricular support (dopamine, dobutamine, milrinone, etc.). If medical management alone is not satisfactory, significant cyanosis persists, or there is evidence of ventricular deterioration, the patient should proceed to surgical repair. Even if patients are weaned from this form of medical support, elective surgical repair should be undertaken if any of the surgical indications mentioned above are met (see treatment/management).

"If initial TV repair proves inadequate, what other surgical options are available?"
Re-repair of residual anatomic defect is preferred. If repair is not possible, TV replacement (TVR) is an option. In order to avoid damage to the conduction system, the coronary sinus may be left to drain into the RV if there is not enough room between it and the AV node during valve implantation. Also, to protect the RCA, the valve suture line may need to deviate above (cephalad to) the tricuspid annulus posterolaterally where tissues are typically thin. Choices for TVR include both tissue and mechanical valve prostheses. Mechanical valves require lifetime anticoagulation; however mechanical valves on the right side of the heart are also more prone to thromboembolism despite systemic warfarin therapy. In general, tissue valves are preferred due to decreased thromboembolic risk, although in a young patient there will be a high incidence of degeneration requiring reoperation. Valve replacement in a young patient will likely require future upsizing of valve prosthesis due to annular growth. Endovascular therapies may be an option in the future.

"Describe alternative options for patients that are not candidates for bi-ventricular repair alone."
For most patients, a biventricular repair alone is possible and the cone procedure has become the procedure of choice. Some patients, however, benefit from a 1.5-ventricle repair (addition of a bidirectional cavopulmonary shunt to either TV repair or replacement) to reduce TV

volume and hemodynamic stress if significant RV dilation or dysfunction exists or if TV repair leaves a small effective orifice. For patients who are not candidates for biventricular repair, surgical options include a single ventricle repair that usually involves TV bovine patch exclusion of the RV (typically with fenestration to allow RV decompression from thebesian drainage) with enlarging of an intra-atrial connection and placement of a systemic-to-pulmonary artery shunt (Starnes procedure), palliative shunt alone (systemic or cavopulmonary shunt or Fontan operation), or cardiac transplantation (opportunities may be limited due to donor shortage for this patient population).

Pearls/pitfalls
- *Common clinical presentation includes*: cyanosis, palpitations, arrhythmia.
- *Classic CXR finding*: cardiomegaly (cardiothoracic ratio > 0.65).
- Wolff-Parkinson-White syndrome may be associated with Ebstein's anomaly and may predispose to tachyarrhythmia presenting as fainting spells (syncope). Use preoperative EP mapping for localization/ablation of accessory conduction pathways. Consider right MAZE.
- Aggressive medical management required in early neonatal period to support RV dysfunction until reduction of PVR.
- Cone reconstruction is the preferred biventricular TV repair technique.
- Post-operative atrial arrhythmias are common following repair.
- Bioprosthetic prosthesis preferred for TV replacement if repair not possible.
- Early surgical repair encouraged to avoid ventricular deterioration (associated with increased mortality).

Suggested readings
- Dearani JA, Bacha E, and da Silva JP. Cone Reconstruction of the Tricuspid Valve for Ebstein's Anomaly: Anatomic Repair. Oper Tech Thorac Cardiovasc Surg 2008;13(2):109-125.
- da Silva JP and da Silva Lda F. Ebstein's Anomaly of the Tricuspid Valve: The Cone Repair. Semin Thorac Cardiovasc Surg Pediatr Card Surg Annu. 2012;15(1):38-45.
- da Silva JP et al, Baumgratz JF, Fonseca L, et al. The cone reconstruction of the tricuspid valve in Ebstein's anomaly. The operation: early and midterm results. J Thorac Cardiovasc Surg; 133: 215-23.
- http://www.ctsnet.org/sections/videosection/videos/vg2012_Caputo M_coneReconstruct. html

Notes

68. Congenital aortic stenosis

Ashok Muralidaran, MD, and Katsuhide Maeda, MD, PhD

Concept
- Clinical presentation in infancy and childhood
- Diagnostic modalities
- Indications for balloon valvuloplasty
- Surgical considerations
- Steps of the Ross-Konno procedure

Chief complaint
"A one month old acyanotic boy is referred to you by his primary pediatrician with congestive heart failure symptoms and a systolic murmur. A transthoracic echo suggests aortic stenosis."

Differential
Differential for CHF symptoms and a systolic murmur can be extensive. A few considerations include: Left ventricular outflow tract obstruction (LVOTO) with either valvular, subvalvular or supravalvar obstruction. Others include: Ventricular septal defect (VSD), Atrial Septal Defect (ASD), AV canal defect, Coarctation of aorta, Ebstein's anomaly, Anomalous origin of the left coronary artery from the pulmonary artery (ALCAPA). In this case, the diagnosis has been suggested by echo as being related to the LVOT.

History and physical
Clinical findings depend on the severity of AS and the ability of the left ventricle to handle a full cardiac output, especially after ductal closure. The typical findings of a prominent apical impulse, precordial and suprasternal notch thrill and an ejection systolic murmur are found in most instances with moderate to severe AS. With critical AS and a failing left ventricle (LV), these findings are overshadowed by signs of circulatory collapse. The neonate is pale, hypoperfused with poor peripheral pulses, tachycardic with a prominent RV impulse and has hepatomegaly. In less severe cases as in the scenario mentioned above, the infant may display signs of poor feeding, tachypnea and failure to thrive.

Tests
- *EKG.* Looking for signs of LV hypertrophy and a strain pattern.
- *CXR*: pulmonary congestion.

514

- *Echocardiography.* 2D-transthoracic echo. Assess the LVOT and determine the level of obstruction (valvular, subvalvular, supravalvular). Assess aortic valve morphology - tricuspid, bicuspid or unicuspid; assess the leaflet mobility and degree of thickening. Measure peak Doppler gradient. Check the size of the annulus, sinus, STJ, and subvalvar area. Assess for presence and severity of left ventricular hypertrophy. Check LV size and function, ductal patency and direction of flow. Check all other valves and rule out other associated anomalies such as AV canal defect, double-outlet right ventricle, and functionally single ventricle mitral valve. Evaluate for coarctation of the aorta. Note: valve areas are indexed to the body surface area in children, with normal being above $2 \text{ cm}^2/\text{m}^2$ and severe being $< 0.5 \text{ cm}^2/\text{m}^2$.
- *Cardiac catheterization.* Provides peak-to-peak gradient measurement between LV and the aorta. Currently utilized predominantly for therapeutic balloon valvuloplasty.

Index scenario (additional information)
"The baby was diagnosed with severe valvar stenosis without any additional anomalies. His EF was 45% and he had evidence of moderate LVH. He underwent a cardiac catheterization and balloon valvuloplasty that resulted in severe AI. How would you proceed?"

Treatment/management
Balloon valvotomy is the preferred primary procedure for critical neonatal aortic valve stenosis. Beyond the neonatal period, a catheter measured peak-to-peak gradient > 20-30 mmHg or a peak Doppler-derived gradient > 30-40 mmHg is an indication for balloon valvuloplasty. With adequate aortic annulus size, there is almost never an indication for primary surgical valvuloplasty in children. Surgical backup should be available in case of acute severe regurgitation which is described in the scenario.

The Ross procedure combined with the Konno root enlargement is the preferred surgical approach for neonates and older children who fail balloon valvotomy. An alternative for older children and young adults is aortic valve replacement with annular enlargement maneuvers like the Nicks or the Manouguian procedure as needed.

Operative steps
Ross-Konno procedure
- Median sternotomy, bicaval cannulation and hypothermia to 25° C.
- After aortic cross clamping, a transverse aortotomy is performed, aortic leaflets are excised and coronary buttons mobilized.

515

- Branch pulmonary arteries are snared and the pulmonary artery (PA) is transected proximal to the bifurcation.
- The pulmonary autograft is harvested with a cuff of infundibular muscle.
- An anterior aortic root enlargement incision (Konno) is now performed. The incision is made just to the left of the right coronary artery (RCA) ostium site, extending on to the ventricular septum thus enlarging the subaortic area.
- If significant LV endocardial fibroelastosis (EFE) is observed, it is stripped.
- The pulmonary autograft is now implanted into the aortic annulus and the ventricular septal incision.
- The left coronary button is reimplanted followed by the right button.
- The distal autograft to ascending aortic anastomosis is now performed.
- The crossclamp is removed after deairing maneuvers.
- A pulmonary homograft is now obtained and the distal anastomosis to the PA bifurcation is performed.
- The proximal pulmonary homograft is then anastomosed to the infundibulum taking care at the leftward aspect to not compromise the left anterior descending coronary artery.
- The patient is fully rewarmed, ventilated and weaned off cardiopulmonary bypass.
- Monitoring lines including a left atrial line are placed and the heart function assessed with transesophageal or epicardial echocardiography.

Potential questions/alternative scenarios

"What other preoperative echocardiographic findings are important before a Ross-Konno procedure?"

It is important to assess the pulmonary valve morphology and rule out stenosis or incompetence. Also, the distal ascending aorta and the arch are assessed for potential augmentation during surgery.

"What intra-operative echocardiographic features are assessed post-repair?"

It is important to evaluate biventricular function, look for any residual VSD, and assess coronary flow. As in the arterial switch operation (ASO), complications of coronary transfer are possible and best prevented. See Chapter 66, Transposition of the great arteries for discussion of management.

"A 10 day old neonate is diagnosed with critical aortic stenosis. He has pulmonary congestion, dyspnea, cold and clammy extremities. The NICU has asked for your opinion and evaluation."
This is a surgical emergency. Initial medical stabilization with intubation, mechanical ventilation, and inotropic support is required. Prostaglandin infusion helps to maintain a PDA and improve systemic perfusion. Percutaneous transcatheter balloon aortic valvotomy is the procedure of choice. Nearly 50% of patients will require a repeat procedure within 5 years.

"A 14 yo girl presents with severe symptomatic aortic stenosis. She is 8 years s/p balloon valvuloplasty. What are her surgical options?"
The management of these adolescents can be challenging and essentially requires a discussion of the risks and benefits of a Ross procedure versus mechanical/bioprosthetic AVR (see Chapter 34, Aortic stenosis).

"The echo on a 6 yo child with chest pain and syncope is consistent with subaortic stenosis. How would you proceed?"
Most often this presents with a discrete fibrous membrane or diffuse fibromuscular tissue leading to LVOTO. You need to inspect the mitral valvular apparatus carefully on echo as there may be papillary muscle abnormalities or abnormal insertion of the leaflets. The treatment depends on whether the stenosis is due to a discrete fibrous membrane or diffuse fibromuscular disease. Surgical indications vary between institutions but generally include symptomatic obstructions or a peak Doppler gradient > 40-50 mmHg in asymptomatic patients. The onset of new AI is also an indication for surgery. A transverse aortotomy extended into the non-coronary sinus and the aortic leaflets are retracted gently. The membrane is completely excised often with a small amount of septal tissue. AI may progress in a quarter of patients at 10 year followup and recurrent obstruction requiring reoperation is seen in up to 15% of patients at 5 years.

For diffuse fibromuscular subaortic stenosis a similar procedure is performed with the addition of a modified Konno procedure.

Pearls/pitfalls
- The primary intervention for critical neonatal aortic stenosis is balloon valvuloplasty with surgical backup available.
- Depending on the type of LVOTO and the institution, indications for surgery vary. Generally accepted indications for surgery are:
  - *Discrete subaortic membrane*: symptoms, peak Doppler gradient 40-50 mmHg, or new onset AI.

- *Diffuse subAS*: generally a slightly higher peak Doppler gradient (50-60 mmHg) used as a guideline for surgery due to complexity of procedure, or symptoms.
- *Hypertrophic obstructive cardiomyopathy*: symptoms rather than gradient typically dictate need for surgical intervention. Surgery for HOCM in children is rare.

- In the Ross-Konno procedure, the autograft harvest should include a generous anterior free-wall lip to fill the ventricular septal incision.
- Any septal perforator injury should be repaired immediately to prevent coronary steal.
- The Konno incision on the ventricular septum should be made leftward and not directed toward the LV apex, to avoid the conduction system.
- The pulmonary autograft to ventricular septal anastomosis should be adequately reinforced to prevent any residual septal defects.
- *Posterior root enlargement maneuvers* (see Chapter 34, Aortic stenosis for more details).
    - *Nicks*. The aortotomy is extended down the middle of the non-coronary cusp just across the aortic annulus. A Dacron patch is sewn from the apex of the incision. Interrupted valve sutures are placed from the outside-in along the width of the patch.
    - *Manouguian*. The aortotomy is initiated as in the Nicks maneuver but extended beyond the aortic annulus onto the anterior mitral leaflet. The left atrium is hence incised and should be closed along with a patch repair of the Mitral leaflet onto the aortic annulus.

Suggested readings
- Douglas J. Schneider, John W. Moore. Aortic Stenosis. Allen, Hugh D.; Driscoll, David J.; Shaddy, Robert E.; Feltes, Timothy F.(eds). *Moss and Adams' Heart Disease in Infants, Children and Adolescents: Including the Fetus and Young Adults*. 2008;968-986.
- Richard A. Jonas. Left Ventricular outflow tract obstruction: aortic valve stenosis, subaortic stenosis, supravalvar aortic stenosis. Richard A. Jonas (ed). *Comprehensive surgical management of congenital heart disease*. 2004;320-340.
- Katsuhide Maeda, Rachel E. Rizal, Michael Lavrsen, et al. Midterm results of the Modified Ross/Konno procedure in neonates and infants. *Ann Thor Surg* 2012;94:156-63.

Notes

69. Anomalous origin of the left coronary artery from the pulmonary artery

Michael C. Monge, MD, and Hyde M. Russell, MD

Concept
- Presentation
- Differential for ALCAPA
- Diagnostic Evaluation
- Surgical Repair
- Mechanical assistance
- Pitfalls

Chief complaint
"A two month-old infant presents with diaphoresis, tachypnea, and failure to thrive."

Differential
Dilated cardiomyopathy, myocarditis, Kawasaki disease, Ebstein's anomaly, large ventricular septal defect, ostium primum atrial septal defect, coarctation of the aorta, patent ductus arteriosus, atrioventricular canal, congenital aortic stenosis, left ventricular outflow tract obstruction, aortic or mitral regurgitation.

Anomalous Origin of the Left Coronary Artery from the Pulmonary Artery (ALCAPA) must be excluded with a thorough diagnostic work-up.

History and physical
Although symptoms of ALCAPA may begin to develop shortly after birth, these are rarely severe enough to prompt medical attention when other abnormalities are absent. After ductal closure, and as the pulmonary vascular resistance drops, there is increasing coronary artery steal with gradual myocardial ischemia. Feeding, the most strenuous activity in which an infant engages, may be poor due to angina, resulting in failure to thrive. Worsening ischemia leads to heart failure by 2 to 12 months of age, heralded by diaphoresis, tachypnea, and tachycardia. As with cardiomyopathy, a precordial lift from cardiomegaly is frequently appreciated. In addition, a systolic murmur from mitral regurgitation may be auscultated at the apex, in association with a gallop rhythm. Lung auscultation will reveal rales due to interstitial pulmonary edema and hepatomegaly can be palpated.

Tests

- *CXR*: severe cardiomegaly, pulmonary edema.
- *EKG*. Q-waves and ST segment elevation from anterolateral ischemia are frequently present. Evidence of left ventricular hypertrophy may be apparent.
- *Labs*. Biomarkers may suggest myocardial ischemia (elevated troponin) and heart failure.
- *Echocardiography*. Dilated left ventricle with markedly reduced function. Dilated right coronary artery (RCA) may be evident. Color Doppler echocardiography can detect retrograde flow from the anomalous coronary artery into the pulmonary artery. Mitral regurgitation is often present. The hyperechogenicity of endocardial fibroelastosis may be observed.

Although echocardiography can establish ALCAPA, it is not adequate to rule-out the diagnosis. Only cardiac catheterization can rule-out ALCAPA in patients presenting with classic symptoms.

- *Cardiac catheterization*. Single right coronary artery arising from the aorta. Characteristic blush in the pulmonary artery from retrograde filling of the left coronary artery. Prominent collaterals are observed in adult-type ALCAPA. An oxygen step-up in the pulmonary artery will be present from left-to-right shunting through the anomalous coronary artery and collateral vessels. Care should be taken in the already compromised patients undergoing invasive diagnostic testing.
- *Magnetic resonance angiography (MRA)*: similar sensitivity and specificity to coronary angiography in diagnosis of ALCAPA.
- *Computed tomographic angiography (CTA)*: assessment of coronary anatomy may be difficult because of tachycardia.

Index scenario (additional information)

"An apical pansystolic murmur was auscultated. Left-axis deviation was noted on EKG with Q-waves and ST elevation in I, aVL, and V4-V6. CXR demonstrated cardiomegaly. A dilated left ventricle with markedly reduced function is evident with echocardiography. Severe mitral valve regurgitation with calcification of the papillary muscles is observed. The coronary arteries are not well-visualized. What additional studies, if any, would you like to perform?"

Treatment/management

Although an anomalous coronary artery from the pulmonary artery was not seen on echocardiography, further diagnostic testing is mandatory to rule-out ALCAPA. Cardiac catheterization, demonstrating retrograde flow through from the coronary artery into the pulmonary artery should be performed. Alternatively, CTA may be used, although the quality may

521

be limited by tachycardia. Identification of ALCAPA is an indication for surgical intervention, which should be performed within days of the diagnosis to promote rapid left ventricular recovery. Several surgical strategies were previously used to treat ALCAPA, including ligation, creation of an aortopulmonary fistula, subclavian artery anastomosis, and ligation with coronary artery bypass grafting. More recently, creation of an intrapulmonary tunnel from the aorta to the anomalous coronary artery ostium was described by Takeuchi and colleagues. This approach may be useful in selected patients in whom the coronary os arises far from the aorta. However, the experience with coronary artery transfer gained from the arterial switch operation has made aortic implantation, with the creation of a two-coronary system, the preferred technique.

Operative steps

Aortic implantation of ALCAPA

Goals – intraoperative myocardial preservation with adequate delivery of cardioplegia, restoration of two-coronary system, myocardial support with mechanical assistance as needed.

- *Place transesophageal echocardiography (TEE) probe*: used to assess postoperative patency of re-implanted coronary artery, assess postoperative ventricular function, assess degree of mitral valve regurgitation.
- Prep and drape right neck into field in case postoperative extracorporeal membrane oxygenation (ECMO) is needed.
- Median sternotomy.
- Harvest pericardial patch.
- Ischemic myocardium with poor ventricular function is prone to ventricular fibrillation. Myocardial contact should be minimized prior to initiation of cardiopulmonary bypass.
- *Cannulation*. Cannulate ascending aorta near innominate artery to provide sufficient length for aortic implantation of anomalous coronary artery. Bicaval cannulation is utilized to protect myocardium from warm blood entering heart. Cardioplegia is delivered via an angiocatheter in aortic root. A left ventricular vent is placed via the right superior pulmonary vein to decompress the left ventricle.
- Bilateral pulmonary arteries should be mobilized and the ligamentum arteriosum divided. The branch pulmonary arteries are encircled with Rumel tourniquets, which are snared once bypass is initiated to increase pressure in the left coronary artery system by preventing run-off.

- Ligation and division of collateral vessels prior to or at the time of commencing cardiopulmonary bypass will minimize the risk of uncontrolled bleeding, requiring the re-institution of cardiopulmonary bypass, following the repair. Cauterization of these vessels may result in troublesome bleeding.
- The aorta is cross-clamped and cardioplegia is delivered into the aortic root.
- The main pulmonary artery is transected after fully mobilizing the branch pulmonary arteries.
- A large coronary artery ostial button is developed. The left main coronary artery is mobilized off the epicardium.
- An atraumatic vascular clip is used to occlude the orifice of the left coronary artery while a second dose of cardioplegia is administered.
- With care taken to prevent injury to the aortic valve, an opening is created in the left posterolateral wall of the ascending aorta, approximately 30-40% smaller than the coronary button. By excising a large ostial button, the pulmonary wall can be used to extend the coronary artery to create a tension-free repair. A flap of aortic wall can be created to augment the anastomosis as needed to prevent tension at the coronary button anastomosis.
- The left coronary artery-to-aorta anastomosis is performed with 7-0 prolene suture.
- After completion of the anastomosis, the aortic root is de-aired via the angiocatheter. The aortic cross-clamp is removed.
- The sinus of the pulmonary artery, in which the ostial button was harvested, is reconstructed with a fresh autologous pericardial patch using 6-0 prolene suture.
- The pulmonary artery is re-anastomosed at the site of transection with 6-0 prolene suture.
- Inotropic support with epinephrine and milrinone is initiated as the patient is warmed.
- Left atrial pressure is monitored with a catheter placed through the vent site in the right superior pulmonary vein.
- The patient is weaned from cardiopulmonary bypass by allowing venous return to fill the left side of the heart.
- TEE will demonstrate poor ventricular function unimproved from the preoperative study; and therefore, careful monitoring of blood pressure and left atrial pressure is required.
- If the left atrial pressure is consistently above 20 mmHg, the patient is unlikely to be able to be weaned from cardiopulmonary bypass, and consideration should be given to initiating mechanical assistance (i.e., ECMO or left ventricular assist device (LVAD)).

- Modified ultrafiltration should be used as it improves myocardial contractility, decreases central venous pressure, and reduces myocardial edema.
- Delayed sternal closure after placement of a silastic skin patch should be considered if significant myocardial or pulmonary edema is present.

Potential questions/alternative scenarios

"The preoperative echocardiogram demonstrates severe mitral regurgitation with severely reduced left ventricular dysfunction."

The majority of patients present with some degree of mitral regurgitation related to annular dilatation from left ventricular enlargement or to ischemic papillary muscle dysfunction. Although the severity of mitral regurgitation has been proposed as a risk factor for operative mortality, this has not been supported unanimously. However, the severity of left ventricular dysfunction has been shown to be the main risk factor for mortality in several studies. Left ventricular function has been shown to recover to normal or near-normal levels within one to two years following repair. With the improvement in left ventricular function, the mitral regurgitation improves in the majority of patients, and secondary mitral valve operations are rarely necessary. The increased cross-clamp time required to repair the mitral valve can be detrimental to the already compromised myocardium.

In older children, usually with well-developed collaterals, severe mitral regurgitation may be present despite preserved left ventricular function. Intervention on the mitral valve may be considered at the initial operation if the regurgitation is predominantly due to ischemic changes of the papillary muscle as opposed to annular dilatation.

"Upon weaning from cardiopulmonary bypass, the patient is hypotensive with an elevated atrial pressure."

The left ventricular function may remain markedly depressed in the early postoperative period. Because significant improvement in function is expected, an aggressive approach to supporting the damaged myocardium with mechanical assistance should be used. If significant hypotension or supraventricular or ventricular arrhythmias persist, total cardiopulmonary support with ECMO should be instituted. In the absence of arrhythmias, a left ventricular assist device is another option. The surgical team should select the mechanical assist system with which they are most comfortable. Most patients demonstrate myocardial recovery in 48 to 72 hours.

"After routine closure of a ventricular septal defect, a patient develops myocardial ischemia with severe left ventricular dysfunction."

Patients with patent ductus arteriosus (PDA) or ventricular septal defects (VSDs), with unrecognized ALCAPA, may be protected from myocardial ischemia due to the elevated pulmonary artery pressure and oxygen saturation. Upon ligation of the PDA or closure of the VSD, with the subsequent drop in pulmonary artery pressure and oxygen saturation, coronary steal with myocardial ischemia develops. Cardiopulmonary bypass should be promptly resumed and the anomalous coronary reimplanted into the aorta.

"Three years after successful repair of ALCAPA, a patient is noted to have worsening mitral regurgitation with persistent left ventricular dysfunction."

Although rare, stenosis of the re-implanted coronary artery must be assessed in the setting of persistent or worsening mitral regurgitation or ventricular dysfunction.

"Upon transection of the pulmonary artery, the origin of the anomalous coronary artery is observed to be from the non-facing sinus."

The majority of anomalous coronary arteries originate from the posterior facing sinus of the pulmonary artery. Even anomalous coronary arteries that arise from the non-facing sinus of the pulmonary artery can be successfully re-implanted. A large segment of the pulmonary artery wall is excised and fashioned into a tube, lengthening the proximal end of the coronary artery. Alternatively, an intrapulmonary aortocoronary tunnel can be performed, although this approach has been associated with supravalvar pulmonary artery stenosis and baffle leaks.

"A 30 yo asymptomatic woman is incidentally found to have an anomalous origin of the left coronary artery from the pulmonary artery on CT imaging."

A small subset of patients, often with pronounced right coronary dominance and/or a restrictive ostium of the anomalous coronary, survive to adulthood. Significant intercoronary collateral vessels develop. These patients may be asymptomatic or present with exertional angina, dyspnea, pre-syncope, or syncope. Mitral regurgitation from ischemic papillary muscle dysfunction can exist, despite left ventricular function being relatively well preserved. Because of the risk of sudden death, these patients should undergo operation on an elective basis.

- In patients presenting with classic symptoms, in whom echocardiography has not confirmed ALCAPA, a cardiac catheterization must be performed to rule-out the diagnosis.
- Mild-to-moderate or greater mitral valve insufficiency is often present preoperatively. The mitral insufficiency improves over time in most patients. Mitral valve repair/replacement is rarely indicated at the initial operation.
- Rapid initiation of mechanical assistance with ECMO or LVAD support should be performed if the patient is unable to be weaned from cardiopulmonary bypass.
- Delayed sternal closure after 48-72 hours to allow for resolution of myocardial and/or pulmonary edema may be of benefit in some patients.

Suggested readings

- Dodge-Khatami A, Mavroudis C, Backer CL. Anomalous origin of the left coronary artery from the pulmonary artery: collective review of surgical therapy. Ann Thorac Surg 2002; 74:946-955.
- Ben Ali W, Metton O, Roubertie F et al. Anomalous origin of the left coronary artery from the pulmonary artery: late results with special attention to the mitral valve. Eur J Cardiothorac Surg. 2009; 36(2):244-8, discussion 248-9.
- Schwartz ML, Jonas RA, Colan SD. Anomalous origin of the left coronary artery from pulmonary artery: Recovery of the left ventricular function after dual coronary repair. J Am Coll Cardiol. 1997; 30:547-553.
- Turley K, Szarnicki RJ, Flachsbart KD et al. Aortic implantation is possible in all cases of anomalous origin of the left coronary artery from the pulmonary artery. Ann Thorac Surg. 1995. 60:84-89.

Notes

70. Pulmonary artery sling

Robroy MacIver, MD, MPH, and Igor E. Konstantinov, MD, PhD, FRACS

Concept
- Differential for vascular anomalies that can cause respiratory issues
- Embryological and anatomical reason for sling
- Diagnostic options prior to surgical therapy if needed
- Conduct of operation and pitfalls

Chief complaint
"A five month-old boy is referred to your clinic from his primary provider with question of tracheal stenosis. The child has had respiratory issues since birth and was intubated for 48 hours two months ago secondary to pneumonia at an outside hospital while the family was on vacation."

Differential
Congenital or acquired tracheal stenosis, vascular ring, pulmonary arterial (PA) sling, tumor, foreign body.

History and physical
The focus should be to elucidate symptoms. PA sling will typically have airway symptoms only. Vascular rings will have both respiratory and feeding symptoms. Timing of symptom development also should be raised. Determining foreign body ingestion in children can be difficult, but a history of choking or new onset of chronic cough can be a clue. Physical exam should identify any murmurs suggestive of coexisting cardiac malformations. History and physical exam should also encompass comorbid conditions such as imperforate anus, genitourinary abnormalities, biliary atresia and Hirschsprung's disease.

Tests
- *CXR*. It is important to review prior CXRs. Either lung may appear hyperinflated secondary to varying location of tracheal stenosis. On a lateral film the left pulmonary artery on end will appear as a mass anterior to the esophagus and posterior to the trachea.
- *Echocardiography*. There is up to a 50% incidence of congenital heart defects with PA sling. These include atrial septal defects, left superior vena cava, ventricular septal defect and patent ductus arteriosus. The anomalous take-off of the left pulmonary artery can usually be diagnosed by echocardiography.

- *Barium swallow.* In PA sling, unlike other vascular rings, the indentation on the esophagus will occur on the anterior margin rather than the posterior aspect. The esophagus will appear deviated slightly to the right.
- *Computed tomography/magnetic resonance imaging (CT/MRI).* Useful to delineate both airway and vascular anatomy. Some groups have begun using MRI to avoid bronchoscopy in planning possible airway surgery. Many groups favor a CT scan over barium swallow.
- *Bronchoscopy.* Important as there is an approximately 50% incidence of complete tracheal rings. The treatment plan is much different when tracheal stenosis is present. Usually the bronchoscopy is performed in the same setting as repair.

Index scenario (additional information)
"The patient's history and physical exam reveal symptoms of respiratory compromise only. The child has no problems with either liquid or solid feeds. He has no other co-morbidities. A CT scan reveals a left pulmonary artery originating from the posterior aspect of the right pulmonary artery and coursing behind the trachea contributing to tracheal compression."

Treatment/management
Originally the operation for PA sling was performed through a left thoracotomy focusing on re-implantation of the left pulmonary artery into the main pulmonary artery. The operation evolved recognizing the need to also divide the ligamentum arteriosum. Today most groups approach the operation through a median sternotomy with the aid of cardiopulmonary bypass and a beating heart. A more extensive dissection of the pulmonary arteries can be performed with the use of bypass. In addition, during the reconstruction of the trachea the endotracheal tube can be withdrawn to aid in creating the anastomosis. The focus of the operation is alleviating external compression on the left pulmonary artery and bronchus or trachea with tracheal reconstruction as needed.

Embryology
Jue et al. described a hypothesis of the embryology of the formation of the pulmonary artery sling. The distal pulmonary arteries develop from the primitive lung buds. These then join with the sixth aortic arch. The anomalous connection of the left pulmonary artery in pulmonary artery sling is felt to be caused by a failure of connection of the lung bud with the sixth aortic arch. Instead of joining with the left sixth arch, the lung bud passes dorsal to the trachea and connects with the right sixth aortic arch.

Operative steps

Reimplantation of left pulmonary artery via median sternotomy.

- If associated tracheal repair is anticipated a low collar neck incision can be added for dissection of the trachea in the neck. Other groups feel the trachea is well viewed from an extended median sternotomy.
- Bronchoscopy should be performed to better determine the extent of the airway stenosis.
- Resect thymus if needed for visualization.
- Dissect out aorta and pulmonary artery. The ductus arteriosus is ligated and divided.
- The trachea is dissected out in the plane between the aorta and the superior vena cava.
  - Care should be taken to avoid the lateral tracheal blood supply.
  - Care should be taken to avoid injury to the recurrent laryngeal nerve that passes in the tracheoesophageal groove.
- Dissect out the left pulmonary artery to the level of the hilar branches.
- CPB with moderate hypothermia is begun through the ascending aorta and a two stage venous catheter or bicaval cannulation can be used. The left ventricle is vented through the right superior pulmonary vein. CPB allows for more aggressive dissection and the option of removing the endotracheal tube during the procedure.
- Any associated cardiac lesion is repaired prior to repair of pulmonary sling.
- At this point the pulmonary artery is brought forward to the carina by either resecting the LPA at its origin or transecting the trachea if a tracheal resection is planned.
- If needed the trachea is reconstructed.
  - If the segment of the tracheal stenosis is short it can be resected with end-to-end anastomosis, however, a slide tracheoplasty is the method of choice if greater than 5 tracheal rings are involved.
  - There are multiple methods of tracheal anastomosis. A polyglyconate suture should be used. A continuous layer through the membranous portion with interrupted sutures on the cartilaginous sections is performed. Alternatively some groups use a continuous circumferential layer.
- Bronchoscopy should be performed to inspect the anastomosis.

- A pedicled pericardial flap can be harvested to separate the tracheal anastomosis from the mediastinum. More specifically, this helps to prevent erosion of the reconstructed trachea into the vessels and also to ensure that the tracheal anastomosis is well sealed.
- The anastomosis is then tested with a peak airway pressure of 35 cm H_2O.
- If not already done, the left pulmonary is transected and the defect in the right pulmonary artery is repaired.
- The left pulmonary artery is inspected to determine the optimal location of insertion on the main pulmonary artery that would avoid kinking and ensure a natural course to the left lung.
- Most often it is best to place the left pulmonary artery slightly posterior on the proximal main pulmonary artery just above the pulmonary valve. Some groups use the origin of the ligamentum arteriosum as a reference point.

Potential questions/alternative scenarios

"After inspection of the trachea by bronchoscopy in the operating room, you realize the child has complete tracheal rings of 3 mm diameter. Do you resect? Perform a tracheoplasty?"

Complete tracheal rings do not necessarily need resection or tracheoplasty. The normal size of the trachea for an infant is 5-6 mm, so a 3 mm sized trachea is approximately 50% of normal lumen size. Good results have been obtained with pulmonary artery reimplantation alone. Many groups feel that the presence of complete tracheal rings with diameter < 50% of expected size warrants operation. The decision to perform a slide tracheoplasty versus resection depends on the length of the stenosis.

"Itraoperative bronchoscopy reveals tracheal rings with tracheal stenosis over 7 tracheal rings. Should you perform a resection or slide tracheoplasty?"

Most groups will perform a resection with five tracheal rings or more. Slide tracheoplasty has become the main treatment method replacing patch tracheoplasty in most series. The method described by Grillo is most common and involves dividing the stenosis at midpoint, incising the proximal and distal narrowed segments vertically on opposite anterior and posterior surfaces and sliding these together.

"After the operation the patient develops dense granulation tissue at the anastomosis causing airway compromise. What are the treatment options?"

Stenting is the most commonly used method, but not the first choice. Balloon dilatations with rigid bronchoscopy must be tried first followed by stenting if needed. Laser therapy can be used if available. Aggressive nebulizer treatments with humidified air and mucolytic therapy must be used while the stent is in place. The majority of patient deaths in series of PA sling with tracheal stenosis center on repeated airway collapse and inability to clear secretions leading to infectious complications.

"The child is 14 yo and presents after a CT scan performed for blunt trauma incidentally shows a PA sling. The child is asymptomatic."
Although most pulmonary artery slings are symptomatic when found, the natural history is unknown. Surgery should be performed only in symptomatic patients. An echocardiogram should be performed as well to rule out coexisting cardiac malformations.

Pearls/pitfalls
- Use caution during the dissection of the pulmonary artery and posterior trachea/bronchus (CPB is helpful for this).
- Always look for coexistent cardiac malformations.
- The left pulmonary artery should be implanted slightly posteriorly on the proximal main pulmonary artery.
- Some groups use the ligated ductus as a guide for re-implantation.
- Extensive tracheoplasty can cause carinal collapse requiring tracheal stenting.

Suggested readings
- Backer CL, Russell HM, Kaushal K, et al. Pulmonary artery sling: Current results with cardiopulmonary bypass. *Journal of Thoracic and Cardiovascular Surgery* 2012;143:144–151.
- Huang SC, Chen YS, Chang CI, et al. Surgical management of pulmonary artery sling: Trachea diameter and outcomes with or without tracheoplasty. *Pediatric Pulmonology* 2012;47:903-908.
- Yong MS, d'Udekem Y, Brizard CP, et al. Surgical management of pulmonary artery sling in children. *The Journal of Thoracic and Cardiovascular Surgery* 2012. Epub June 12.

Notes

71. Congenital tracheoesophageal fistulae

Muhammad A.K. Nuri, MD, and Peter F. Ehrlich MD, MHS

Concept
- Pre-operative evaluation and management of patients
- Risk stratification and decision making
- Congenital cardiac disease and disease management
- Management of long gap atresia
- Conduct of the operation and potential pitfalls

Chief complaint

"A 2.5 kg newborn with an antenatal diagnosis of Tetralogy of Fallot was born via C- section. Maternal history was significant for polyhydramnios during pregnancy. Initial echocardiogram confirmed the diagnosis of Tetralogy of Fallot with no significant gradient across the right ventricle outflow tract and an oxygen saturation of 95%. Upon feeding the child, significant choking, coughing and cyanosis developed. The cyanosis improved with supplemental oxygen. Placement of a nasogastric tube was attempted. Despite multiple attempts, the nasogastric tube could not be passed beyond 10 cm from the alveolar ridge. An X-ray of the chest and abdomen was obtained that revealed coiling of the nasogastric tube in the esophagus with right upper lobe opacification."

Differential

The differential diagnosis of respiratory distress in a newborn is extensive. The common causes of respiratory distress include pneumonia, meconium aspiration, and transient tachypnea of the newborn or structural cardiac conditions. However, the classic triad of choking, coughing and cyanosis or feeding with inability to completely pass a nasogastric tube beyond 10 cm from the incisors is pathognomonic of esophageal atresia with or without a fistula. If there is a scaphoid abdomen and the X-ray shows an abdomen devoid of gas, a diagnosis of pure atresia is more likely.

The most common variety is esophageal atresia with a distal fistula arising from the trachea which is present in 85% of cases (Type C; i.e., *C = most Common*). The second most common presentation is esophageal atresia without a distal fistula (Type A in 8%). The other rare presentations include isolated fistula (Type E), esophageal atresia with proximal fistula (Type B) and esophageal atresia with proximal and distal fistula (Type D).

Associated congenital abnormalities will be found in 50% of patients with TEF. Cardiac abnormalities are the most common and are present in 20-30% of patients. Of those, ventricular septal defect and Tetralogy of Fallot are the most common. In addition, TEF is part of the VACTERL association (Vertebral, Anorectal, Tracheoesophageal, Renal or Radial, Cardiac and Limb abnormalities).

Tests

- *X-ray of the chest and abdomen with a nasogastric tube*: most important diagnostic test. The presence of a nasogastric tube coiled in the superior mediastinum is diagnostic of TEF. The absence of abdominal gas may indicate complete atresia without associated fistula or it may show a double bubble sign indicative of duodenal atresia. Additional rib and vertebral abnormalities may be noted on the chest X-ray as part of the VACTERL syndromes.
- *Contrast study (dilute barium) of the upper esophagus*: to confirm the diagnosis and possibly detect a proximal fistula.
- *Rigid bronchoscopy* is also used at the time of surgery to confirm the diagnosis and for localization of the the fistula.
- *Cardiac echocardiography*: should be obtained in all cases to rule out the presence of structural heart disease. In addition, cardiac imaging is helpful to determine the sidedness of the aortic arch which affects surgical approach.
- *Renal ultrasound*: should be obtained to rule out the presence of renal agenesis.
- *Karyotyping* : should be done to rule out the presence of chromosomal abnormalities; if life threatening chromosomal abnormalities are detected (trisomy 13, 18) further surgical intervention may not be recommended.
- If imperforate anus is present, a spinal ultrasound and a VCUG are also needed to rule out spinal cord anomalies and vesiculo-ureteric reflux.

Index scenario (additional information)

"A 1.2 kg 30 week preterm infant with TEF and respiratory distress syndrome develops progressive respiratory insufficiency requiring high frequency oscillation ventilation. The chest X-ray shows ground glass appearance of the lungs and a very distended stomach. How would you proceed?"

Treatment/management

Pre-operative management

- The neonate should be placed upright at 30-45° C with frequent suctioning to prevent aspiration.

- Prophylactic antibiotics and acid suppression should be administered.
- A nasogastric tube on low intermittent suction should be placed in the pouch to prevent aspiration.
- Vascular access should be established and parenteral nutrition initiated.
- If endotracheal intubation is required, ventilation and oxygenation can be challenging. Gastric distension and poor ventilation can occur if the fistula is large.

Risk stratification and timing of repair

The decision to proceed with definite repair or delayed repair is dependent upon the risk profile of the patient. High risk patients (i.e., low birth weight, ventilated, pneumonia, cardiac anomalies) have traditionally undergone palliation with a gastrostomy followed by delayed repair. The advantage of gastrostomy is in the simplicity of the procedure; however, in some cases it can worsen respiratory status due to escape of ventilatory gases through the gastrostomy. Transpleural ligation of the fistula is being employed with increasing frequency due to these concerns.

In 1962 Waterston proposed a risk classification system for patients with TEF undergoing surgery.

Waterston classification
- *Group A*: Birth weight greater than 2,500 g and well.
- *Group B*: Birth weight between 1,800-2500 g, or any weight with moderate pneumonia and anomalies.
- *Group C*: Birth weight less than 1,800 g, or any weight with severe pneumonia and anomalies.

Significant improvement in diagnosis, neonatal care, anesthetic care and management of associated comorbidities has evolved since the risk classification was initially proposed. It became apparent the risk could not be reliably assessed based upon the Waterston criteria. Sptiz et al from the same institution proposed an additional classification based upon weight and presence of cardiac abnormality.

Sptiz classification
- *Criteria I*: Birth weight > 1500 g without major cardiac disease.
- *Criteria II*: Birth weight < 1500 g or major cardiac disease.
- *Criteria III*: Birth weight < 1500 g and major cardiac disease.

Peonaru et al. (Montreal Classification) recommended that birth weight was not a risk factor; rather pre-operative ventilator dependence and major congenital abnormalities were the major risk factors. Currently, individualized decisions are made and operative approach and timing are dictated by physiologic and clinical status. Premature babies, babies less than 1.2 kg and poor physiologic status are often treated with a staged approach with either fistula ligation or gastrostomy.

Operative steps
Open TEF repair
TEF may be managed with an open or thoracoscopic approach. The operative conduct of a typical open approach is described.

- Left lateral decubitus position.
- A right posterolateral thoracotomy incision is made below the tip of the scapula and extended along the inframammary crease. The chest is entered through the fourth intercostal space and an extra pleural plane of dissection is developed.
- Using blunt dissection, the plane is progressively developed until the azygous vein is encountered. The azygous vein is then ligated or clipped and divided.
- The mediastinal pleura is pushed anteriorly to identify the trachea and esophagus.
- The opening of the esophageal fistula into the trachea is identified and a silastic loop is placed around the distal esophagus for traction. Care should be taken here to confirm that the esophagus has been identified and not the right bronchus. Ligation and division of the right bronchus is an important reported complication.
- The fistula is initially partially divided, ensuring that a small cuff of esophageal tissue is left on the tracheal end to prevent tracheal narrowing. As the fistula is progressively divided, interrupted absorbable 5-0 sutures are used to close the fistulous opening at the tracheal end. The oxygen saturations will often drop during the ligation of the fistula. Communication between the surgeon and the anesthesiologist is important. After ligation of the fistula, water is placed into the thoracic cavity and the inspiratory pressure sustained at 30 cm of water to ensure that there are no leaks.
- The proximal esophagus pouch is identified by gently pushing down with a dilator passed orally by the anesthesiologist. The proximal esophageal pouch is mobilized into the thoracic inlet avoiding injury to the recurrent laryngeal nerve. The distal esophagus is minimally mobilized to preserve its blood supply. If the esophageal ends cannot be brought together after adequate mobilization, a diagnosis of long gap atresia is made (> 3 vertebral bodies - see below under alternative scenarios). The proximal pouch is then opened and the anastomosis between the esophageal ends is

completed using single layer, interrupted non absorbable suture.

- Prior to completion of the anastomosis, a fine nasogastric tube is passed through the anastomosis into the stomach.
- A Jackson-Pratt drain, Blake drain, or chest tube is then anchored to the posterior chest wall, ensuring that it is not adjacent to the suture line.
- The chest is closed with gentle reapproximation of the ribs to prevent overlapping.

Potential questions/alternative scenarios

"You are consulted on a term 3.2 kg neonate with TEF and pulmonary atresia with ductal dependent pulmonary circulation. The patient is maintained on prostaglandins and oxygen saturations are in the low 90s. His hemodynamic status is stable. How would you proceed with timing and sequence of shunt and TEF surgery?"

Patients with cardiac lesions that predispose them to high pulmonary blood flow can safely proceed to esophageal repair in the immediate neonatal period. Since the pulmonary resistance is high, the consequences of high pulmonary blood flow are mitigated. As the pulmonary resistance falls and pulmonary overcirculation develops, appropriate palliative or reparative procedures can be performed. In patients with ductal dependent circulation, the clinical status of the patient dictates timing of esophageal repair. If the clinical condition is good and the duct is patent, prostaglandin infusion is maintained and esophageal repair can be carried out before cardiac surgery. If there is evidence of systemic or pulmonary hypoperfusion with hypoxemia, then a prostaglandin infusion should be initiated and appropriate resuscitation carried out. Once clinically stable, then the patient may undergo esophageal repair. If clinical stability cannot be achieved then the definitive or palliative cardiac procedure should be carried out first. Transpleural ligation of the fistula or emergency gastrostomy can then be subsequently or concurrently performed if there is respiratory embarrassment. It is rare that cardiac surgery precedes palliative or definitive TEF repair.

"You are attempting a thoracoscopic repair and notice a right aortic arch."

The position of the aortic arch should be determined by echocardiography prior to surgery. If a right sided arch is established, a left thoracotomy approach should be undertaken. Although, open repair can be done through the right chest, the aortic arch can be an impediment and limits exposure. In the present scenario, further attempts through a right thoracoscopic approach should be abandoned and a left thoracic approach undertaken.

"After division of fistula, you notice there is a significant gap between the esophageal ends."
Long gap atresia has traditionally been defined as greater than 3 cm or three vertebral bodies. It is a somewhat subjective term which literally means that the gap cannot be bridged together and differs from surgeon to surgeon. It is classically associated with esophageal atresia without fistula. Management of these patients is very difficult and there is no best technique. Esophageal stretching first proposed by Foker et al uses traction sutures on the esophagus that are brought out through the skin. The ends of the esophagus are marked by radio opaque metallic clips. Progressive traction is applied over the course of the next few days and as the esophageal ends overlap, definitive surgery is carried out. The results of this procedure have been controversial. These patients have classically been managed with gastrostomy and bouginage until overlap is seen with serial fluoroscopy and then staged repair is completed. Other methods used to lengthen the esophagus include circular myotomies (achieve 1 cm lengthening with each myotomy), proximal esophageal flap and tubularization and limited mobilization of the distal esophagus. Postoperatively, impaired esophageal function and strictures develop after these procedures that require progressive dilatation. In addition, this anastomosis is under tension and the patient is kept sedated, paralyzed and managed with the neck in flexion for up to five-seven days. If the gap cannot be bridged in patients with long gap atresia even after bouginage, then esophageal replacement options are offered. These include gastric, colonic, or jejunal interposition to bridge the gap.

"You obtain an esophagram after a routine TEF repair on day five and note extravasation of contrast at the anastomosis."
Minor leaks occur in 15-20% of patients after repair; most of these can be managed conservatively with drainage, antibiotics and parenteral or enteral jejunal nutrition. Significant disruptions are rare and present with pneumothorax and signs of sepsis. Most of these disruptions warrant emergency surgery, mediastinal drainage, gastrostomy, and takedown of the anastomosis with possible diverting esophagostomy. Minor leaks are associated with a significant rate of esophageal stricture and should be closely followed with esophagoscopy and dilatation. Aggressive acid suppression with proton pump inhibitors should be initiated.

"You are seeing a patient six months after a TEF repair; parents report poor feeding and regurgitation."
The long term complications of TEF repair include esophageal stricture, esophageal dysmotility, gastroesophageal reflux, tracheomalacia, and scoliosis. In rare cases a missed laryngopharyngeal cleft is diagnosed. Reflux and esophageal strictures predominate due to universal distal esophageal dysmotility. There is approximately a 30% incidence of

stricture formation and about 40% of patients have significant gastroesophageal reflux.

Aggressive screening for stricture with esophagram is recommended and any stricture should be dilated. pH probe monitoring and manometry should be carried out. Failure of acid suppression presents a second set of challenges. Nissen fundoplication has a high early failure rate in patients with TEF. Inherent esophageal dysmotility in children with TEF and the foreshortened esophagus make the wrap difficult. One strategy is to use nasal or gastro-jejunal feeding until the child grows and then reassess the need for an antireflux procedure. Although prokinetic agents are recommended for the esophageal dysmotility, their efficacy and treatment results have been disappointing.

Pearls/pitfalls
- A diagnosis of TEF mandates an aggressive evaluation of concomitant congenital abnormalities.
- Extreme prematurity and unstable ductal dependent neonates are best managed by staged repair.
- Establishing arch sidedness is essential for adopting appropriate surgical approach.
- A small cuff of esophageal tissue should be retained to prevent tracheal narrowing.
- Limited mobilization of the distal esophagus should be undertaken to prevent esophageal necrosis.
- Long gap atresia encountered during surgery is best managed by a staged approach.
- Feeding difficulty is common after surgery due to esophageal strictures, dysmotility and reflux; an aggressive approach to counter these is necessary.

Suggested readings
- Sptiz L. Oesophageal atresia. *Orphanet J Rare Dis* 2007 May 11;2:24.
- Poenaru D et al. A new prognostic classification for esophageal atresia. *Surgery* 1993, 113(4):426-432.
- Foker JE et al. Development of a true primary repair for the full spectrum of esophageal atresia. *Ann Surg* 1997, 226(4):533-41.

Notes

72. Congenital cystic adenomatoid malformation

Immanuel Turner, MD, Jennifer C. Nelson, MD, and
Jennifer C. Hirsch-Romano, MD

Concept

- Indications for resection of congenital cystic adenomatoid malformation
- Preoperative considerations (imaging, classification)
- Method of resection
- Critical steps of resection
- Pitfalls and alternative solutions

Chief complaint

"A 5 day-old 2.2 kg boy presents with respiratory distress and labored breathing. NICU diagnoses him with a CCAM based on the appearance of the prenatal ultrasound as well as the CXR after birth which had multiple gas filled shadows."

Differential

CCAM diagnosis is suspected. Other congenital thoracic lesions to consider include pulmonary bronchogenic cysts, congenital lobar emphysema, pulmonary sequestration, cystic bronchiectasis, pneumatocele formation, foregut malformations, and congenital diaphragmatic hernia. Associated anomalies include cardiac anomalies, intestinal atresia, renal agenesis, congenital diaphragmatic hernias and pectus excavatum.

History and physical

The history and physical exam aids in establishing the diagnosis, and in clarifying the impact that the CCAM had on the pregnancy and on the newborns current state of health. The greater the impact, the earlier and more aggressive the interventions need to be. Elicit whether or not hydrops fetalis or polyhydramnios were present prenatally. After birth, symptoms may include tachypnea, labored breathing, hypoxemia, hypercarbia, poor feeding, and overt respiratory failure requiring invasive or noninvasive ventilatory support. The presence of other associated cardiac, gastrointestinal or renal anomalies should be noted. The physical exam should include general assessment, abdominal exam, and evaluation of heart, lung and periphery.

Prenatal ultrasound: gestational age at diagnosis ranges from 26-28 weeks. Cysts may be unilateral, bilateral, macrocystic or microcystic. There may be associated polyhydramnios, hydrops fetalis, pulmonary hypoplasia, mediastinal shift or ascites. All of these conditions suggest a poor prognosis and are often encountered when the cyst occupies > 50% of the thoracic cavity. CCAM-volume-ratio (CVR) is obtained by dividing the CCAM volume in milliliters by the head circumference in centimeters. This is used to determine the frequency of surveillance. It is based on prenatal ultrasound to correct for gestational age. CVR < 1.2 (weekly surveillance), 1.2-1.6 (twice weekly surveillance), > 1.6 (2-3 times a week).

Postnatal ultrasound: often the only study needed in the newborn.

- *CXR*: multiple air fluid levels or ill-defined shadow within a single lobe. Presence of the nasogastric tube in the chest suggests a congenital diaphragmatic hernia.
- *CT scan*: used to solidify diagnosis, more helpful for older children; multiple cystic or solid lesion with aberrant blood supply. Best test for differentiating CCAM from other congenital lesions.
- *MRI*: helpful in determining the difference between CCAM and congenital diaphragmatic hernia (not routinely used).

Stocker classification is ultimately confirmed by histology but can be predicted preoperatively. This may be helpful for prognosis.

- *Type I*. Macrocystic disease - large cysts (> 2 cm). In rare cases, it is associated with congenital diaphragmatic hernia and can cause pulmonary hypoplasia and pulmonary hypertension secondary to mass effect. Type I has a very good prognosis and is rarely associated with hydrops. It is made up of a layer of respiratory epithelium overlying fibroelastic tissue.
- *Type II*. Mixed CCAM - multiple small cysts (< 1 cm in diameter) develop as a result of airway obstruction during development. These lesions produce distal regional replacement of lung parenchyma. Solid lung is filled with distended bronchioles and alveolar material. This group has a poor prognosis due to association with other cardiac anomalies and prematurity.
- *Type III*. Microcystic CCAM - Solid firm lesions (cysts < 0.5 cm) often with diffuse lung involvement (poor prognosis).

Index scenario (additional information)
"This patient was full term and had no evidence of hydrops fetalis, polyhydramnios, or mediastinal shift on prenatal ultrasound. CXR showed multiple air fluid levels in the right lower lobe. CT scan confirmed multi-cystic lesion with no aberrant pulmonary vasculature.

Tachypnea, increased work of breathing, and poor feeding, were present after birth. No other renal or cardiac anomalies were diagnosed. What are his options and how would you proceed?"

Treatment/management

Presence of a CCAM is an indication for resection. The options are fetal intervention (thoracotomy), termination of pregnancy, preterm delivery with aggressive cardiorespiratory support, or early but elective resection for stable newborns. This patient meets criteria for the later - early but elective resection of the CCAM. Note that management of an asymptomatic CCAM is somewhat more controversial. However, given the risk of malignancy and/or infection that complicates further intervention, the general consensus is to resect.

Operative steps

Goals – completely resect abnormal lung parenchyma to relieve symptoms and prevent infection and malignancy.

- Single lung ventilation (by selective mainstem intubation in neonates).
- Thoracotomy and entrance into the chest cavity through the 5th or 6th inner space or thoracoscopy for smaller lesions amenable to wedge resection.
- Lobectomy is the standard for most CCAM resections although pneumonectomy may be required for Type III lesions that involve the majority of the lung. A parenchymal sparing wedge resection may be appropriate for smaller lesions.

Potential questions/alternative scenarios

"A fetus is noted to have hydrops fetalis at 22 weeks gestational age."

If hydrops fetalis develops secondary to CCAM location and growth, there is a high risk for fetal or early neonatal death. This is usually seen with a CVR > 1.6. Fetal interventional management may be helpful in palliating these patients in attempt to reach full term gestation. This includes administration of steroids and transamniotic drainage of dominant cysts. Sometimes the CCAM will involute. Assessment of overall prognosis and other congenital anomalies is critical before proceeding with operative management given poor outcomes in this population. Termination of the pregnancy may be needed for hyperdynamic maternal states, placentomegaly, and lethal cardiac anomalies. Fetal thoracotomy is an emerging option for young fetuses (< 32 weeks) with hydrops fetalis. If the fetus is > 32 weeks and has hydrops fetalis, then proceed with preterm delivery, cardiorespiratory support, and early resection. Cardiorespiratory support includes intubation, prenatal steroids to enhance lung maturity, inotropes and diuresis for patients with congestive heart failure (cardiac anomalies), and extracorporeal membrane oxygenation (ECMO) for severe cases in patients > 2 kg without contraindications to heparin.

"The patient is born at 32 weeks with a large CCAM causing severe respiratory distress and cardiopulmonary collapse. How would you proceed?"
Intubate, resuscitate and place on ECMO if refractory to medical management. Early surgical resection even on ECMO is warranted.

"The patient is asymptomatic at birth."
Regression may occur in 40-60%. CXR sensitivity is not very good. Ultrasound is the best measure and should be repeated postnatal in patients diagnosed in utero. If the CCAM is still present on CT scan, wait until 6 months of age to minimize risk of operation. In addition, late symptomatic presentation may include those patients with recurrent infection that is an indication for operative management once the infection is cleared. The risk of malignant transformation is not clear for asymptomatic CCAMs. Surveillance imaging and observation has been advocated.

"The patient has both right middle and lower lobe involvement and is asymptomatic."
Traditional approach is for lobectomy leaving only normal lung tissue behind. In this presentation a pneumonectomy could be considered if there is involvement of the upper lobe. A recent study showed no difference in length of stay, early morbidity, and recurrent symptoms from a residual CCAM after parenchymal sparing resection in appropriate candidates. These resections would include lobectomy plus wedge resection and or segmentectomy depending on the anatomy.

"A 3 yo boy presents with recurrent cough and pneumonia. A CXR shows evidence of left lower lobe consolidation. An ultrasound shows an aberrant infra-diaphragmatic blood vessel supplying the left lower lobe. A CT scan is obtained that shows a left lower lobe lung mass with an infra-diaphragmatic aortic blood supply."
This patient has a pulmonary sequestration, which presents differently than a CCAM in that patients tend to be older with more subtle respiratory symptoms. The treatment is resection. In the setting of active infection, resection should be delayed for 3-4 weeks to adequately treat and clear the infection. All sequestrations have aberrant systemic blood supply from the abdominal aorta, thoracic aorta or even subclavian or coronary vessels. They are not generally supplied by the pulmonary arteries. Intralobar sequestrations are more often located in the lower lobes as in this scenario. Intralobar sequestrations are not often associated

with cardiac or gastrointestinal anomalies (unlike extralobar). Intralobar sequestrations drain to the inferior pulmonary veins although right sided lesions may drain into the vena cava. The arterial supply typically emerges within the inferior pulmonary ligament. Extralobar sequestrations drain to the azygous system. Early in the operation the arterial blood supply should be carefully controlled and divided. Note that extralobar sequestrations may connect to the gastrointestinal tract (i.e., esophagus).

Pearls/pitfalls

- If symptomatic, early resection is indicated,and lobectomy is standard of care.
- Hydrops fetalis presenting prenatally is associated with a poor prognosis and fetal intervention may be indicated.
- Controversy still exists regarding the malignant potential for an unresected asymptomatic CCAM.
- If asymptomatic, elective resection after 6 months of age should be considered to minimize risk of recurrent infections and malignant transformation.

Suggested readings

- DiPrima et al. Antenatally diagnosed congenital cystic adenomatoid malformations (CCAM): Research review. J Pren Med. 2012; 6 (2): 22-30.
- Hung-Wen et al. Management of Congenital Cystic Adenomatoid Malformation and Bronchopulmonary sequestration in Newborns. Ped Neonatol. 2010; 51 (3):172-177.
- Kim et al Treatment of Congenital Cystic Adenomatoid Malformation: Should lobectomy always be performed? Ann Thorac Surg. 2008; 86:249-53.
- Laberg JM et al. Asymptomatic congenital lung malformations. Sem Ped Surg. 2005; 14:16-133.
- Nagata et al. Outcome and treatment in an anenatally diagnosed congenital cystic adenomatoid malformation of the lung. Ped Surg Int. 2009; 25:753-757.

Notes

31181983R10325

Made in the USA
Charleston, SC
09 July 2014